Lung Cancer

Translational Medicine Series

Lung Cancer

Translational and Emerging Therapies

Edited by

Kishan J. Pandya
University of Rochester, Rochester, New York, USA

Julie R. Brahmer
Johns Hopkins University School of Medicine, Baltimore, Maryland, USA

Manuel Hidalgo
Johns Hopkins University School of Medicine, Baltimore, Maryland, USA

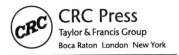

CRC Press
Taylor & Francis Group
Boca Raton London New York

CRC Press is an imprint of the
Taylor & Francis Group, an **informa** business

First published 2007 by Informa Healthcare, Inc.

Published 2019 by CRC Press
Taylor & Francis Group
6000 Broken Sound Parkway NW, Suite 300
Boca Raton, FL 33487-2742

© 2007 by Taylor & Francis Group, LLC
CRC Press is an imprint of Taylor & Francis Group, an Informa business

First issued in paperback 2019

No claim to original U.S. Government works

ISBN 13: 978-0-367-45309-1 (pbk)
ISBN 13: 978-0-8493-9021-0 (hbk)

Visit the Taylor & Francis Web site at
http://www.taylorandfrancis.com

and the CRC Press Web site at
http://www.crcpress.com

Library of Congress Cataloging-in-Publication Data

Lung cancer: translational and emerging therapies / [edited by] Kishan J. Pandya,
   Julie R. Brahmer, Manuel Hidalgo.
       p. ; cm. -- (Translational medicine series ; 3)
   Includes bibliographical references.
   ISBN-13: 978-0-8493-9021-0 (hb : alk. paper)
   ISBN-10: 0-8493-9021-4 (hb : alk. paper)   1. Lung--Cancer--Chemotherapy.
       2. Lungs--Cancer--Treatment--Technological innovations. 3. Lungs--Cancer--
       Molecular aspects.   I. Pandya, Kishan J.   II. Brahmer, Julie R.   III. Hidalgo,
       Manuel, MD.   IV. Series.
   [DNLM: 1. Lung Neoplasms--drug therapy. 2. Antineoplastic Agents--therapeutic
       use.   WF 658 L9637 2007]

RC280.L8L827 2007
616.99'42406--dc22
                                                                    2007007228

Preface

Lung cancer is the most common cancer worldwide, affecting over a million people every year, and it is the leading cause of death. Despite modest improvements in therapy, the five-year survival of this disease is less than 15%. The mainstay of treatment is surgery and adjuvant chemotherapy for early stage disease, concurrent chemoradiotherapy for locally advanced disease, and chemotherapy for metastatic disease. Molecularly targeted treatments are now coming to the fore, and epidermal growth factor receptor tyrosine kinase inhibitors such as erlotinib (Tarceva®) are now approved for use as second-line or third-line treatment of metastatic disease. Although not yet established as standard therapy, there are an ever increasing number of novel and targeted therapies being assessed in the treatment of lung cancer. These therapies are in varied stages of development and include antiangiogenesis inhibitors, epidermal growth factor receptor inhibitors, tumor vaccines, monoclonal antibodies, and endothelial receptor antagonists, to name just a few. Also in development are combination therapies of established treatments with targeted therapies. These emerging therapies reflect our expanding understanding of mechanisms of tumorogenesis and cell growth. This book provides the state-of-the-art information on evolving translational therapies in lung cancer. Currently, there is no text on this topic that assembles, reviews, and synthesizes this material in one volume.

It is appropriate that Drs. Gandara and Gummerlock and their colleagues set the stage and describe the molecular biology of lung cancer as the basis for targeted therapy in their chapter. Dr. Janet Dancey describes some of the more challenging aspects of clinical trial design issues related to clinical evaluation of these novel agents.

Some agents that have shown promise include angiogenesis inhibitors, antibody to vascular endothelial growth factor receptor, small molecule tyrosine kinase, and other multi-targeted agents. Drs. Ramnath and Adjei describe the basis of antiangiogenic therapy as well as provide a comprehensive review of small molecule inhibitors of angiogenesis, followed by a chapter on inhibition of angiogenesis using monoclonal antibodies by Drs. Dubey and Salgia. Drs. Jimeno and Hidalgo discuss the targeting of the epidermal growth factor receptor in the treatment of lung cancer, and Dr. Fred Hirsch and his colleagues discuss the markers of sensitivity and response to treatment with these agents. Drs. Papadopoulos and Tolcher complete the discussion with their chapter on other novel targeted therapies, including such targets as Bcl, tumor necrosis factor–related apoptosis-inducing ligand receptors, inhibitor of apoptosis proteins family, and proteosome.

Vaccine therapy remains a promising area of research, and Dr. Davies and her colleagues update us on cancer immunology and the exciting data on several novel vaccine approaches and other new methods to modify the immune response.

Technological advances in the delivery of radiation as well as newer chemotherapeutic agents have produced improvements in combining these modalities for the treatment of locally advanced disease, as discussed by Drs. Milano and Chen, and also in the treatment of brain metastases, as discussed by Drs. Siker and Mehta. Technological advances in radiological imaging is making it possible to delineate the size and the location of tumors more precisely, as well as detect the presence of metastatic disease, allowing for more accurate staging of the disease as reviewed by Drs. Bhatt and Dogra.

Compared to a decade ago, we have made significant progress in understanding the molecular biology of lung cancer and the potential therapeutic targets in this disease, none of which would be possible without the untiring efforts of researchers and cooperation of the patients and their families.

Kishan J. Pandya
Julie R. Brahmer
Manuel Hidalgo

Contents

Contributors

Alex A. Adjei   Roswell Park Cancer Institute, Buffalo, New York, U.S.A.

Shweta Bhatt   Department of Imaging Sciences, University of Rochester School of Medicine and Dentistry, Rochester, New York, U.S.A.

Yuhchyau Chen   Department of Radiation Oncology, University of Rochester School of Medicine and Dentistry, Rochester, New York, U.S.A.

Janet E. Dancey   Division of Cancer Treatment and Diagnosis, National Cancer Institute, Rockville, Maryland, U.S.A.

Angela M. Davies   University of California Davis Cancer Center, Sacramento, California, U.S.A.

Vikram S. Dogra   Department of Imaging Sciences, University of Rochester School of Medicine and Dentistry, Rochester, New York, U.S.A.

Sarita Dubey   Division of Hematology/Oncology, University of California–San Francisco, San Francisco, California, U.S.A.

Rafal Dziadziuszko   Division of Medical Oncology, Department of Medicine, University of Colorado Health Sciences and Cancer Center, Aurora, Colorado, U.S.A., and Department of Oncology and Radiotherapy, Medical University of Gdańsk, Gdańsk, Poland

David R. Gandara   University of California Davis Cancer Center, Sacramento, California, U.S.A.

Oliver Gautschi   University of California Davis Cancer Center, Sacramento, California, U.S.A.

Paul H. Gumerlock   University of California Davis Cancer Center, Sacramento, California, U.S.A.

Jim Heighway   Cancer Communications, Northwich, U.K.

Manuel Hidalgo   Sidney Kimmel Comprehensive Cancer Center at Johns Hopkins University School of Medicine, Baltimore, Maryland, U.S.A.

Fred R. Hirsch   Division of Medical Oncology, Department of Medicine, University of Colorado Health Sciences and Cancer Center, Aurora, Colorado, U.S.A.

Cheryl Ho   Division of Medical Oncology, British Columbia Cancer Agency, Vancouver, British Columbia, Canada

Antonio Jimeno   Sidney Kimmel Comprehensive Cancer Center at Johns Hopkins University School of Medicine, Baltimore, Maryland, U.S.A.

Primo N. Lara   University of California Davis Cancer Center, Sacramento, California, U.S.A.

Philip C. Mack   University of California Davis Cancer Center, Sacramento, California, U.S.A.

Minesh P. Mehta   Department of Human Oncology, University of Wisconsin School of Medicine and Public Health, Madison, Wisconsin, U.S.A.

Michael T. Milano   Department of Radiation Oncology, University of Rochester School of Medicine and Dentistry, Rochester, New York, U.S.A.

Kyriakos P. Papadopoulos   South Texas Accelerated Research Therapeutics, Division of Medical Oncology, University of Texas Health Science Center at San Antonio, San Antonio, Texas, U.S.A.

Nithya Ramnath   Roswell Park Cancer Institute, Buffalo, New York, U.S.A.

Ravi Salgia   Section of Hematology/Oncology, Department of Medicine, University of Chicago, Chicago, Illinois, U.S.A.

Malika L. Siker   Department of Human Oncology, University of Wisconsin School of Medicine and Public Health, Madison, Wisconsin, U.S.A.

Kristopher M. Skwarski   Department of Respiratory Medicine, Royal Infirmary of Edinburgh, Edinburgh, Scotland, U.K.

Barbara Szostakiewicz   Department of Oncology and Radiotherapy, Medical University of Gdańsk, Gdańsk, Poland

Anthony W. Tolcher   South Texas Accelerated Research Therapeutics, Division of Medical Oncology, University of Texas Health Science Center at San Antonio, San Antonio, Texas, U.S.A.

1

Molecular Biology of Lung Cancer as the Basis for Targeted Therapy

Oliver Gautschi and Philip C. Mack

University of California Davis Cancer Center, Sacramento, California, U.S.A.

Jim Heighway

Cancer Communications, Northwich, U.K.

Paul H. Gumerlock and David R. Gandara

University of California Davis Cancer Center, Sacramento, California, U.S.A.

INTRODUCTION

Here we present recent advances in the molecular biology of lung cancer. This knowledge contributes to our understanding of the mechanisms of carcinogenesis, cancer progression, and metastasis and is essential for the subsequent development of new therapies targeted against disease-relevant genetic pathways. These findings thus provide the background for the following chapters on specific therapeutic approaches. The current state of knowledge regarding the molecular biology of lung cancer at the level of DNA, chromatin, RNA, and protein is summarized, along with the implications of large-scale analysis, biomarker development, and histopathology. Tumor immunology and angiogenesis are discussed in other chapters in this book.

GENETIC ALTERATIONS IN LUNG CANCER

In the beginning of the 20th century, Hansemann and Boveri hypothesized that cancer is the result of genetic lesions (1). Today, we know that the epidemiology of lung cancer is strongly associated with environmental genotoxins, but our understanding of the biological implications of critical genetic alterations is still incomplete. Exposure to cigarette smoke is associated with approximately 90% of lung cancers (2). Cigarette smoke contains more than 50 different carcinogens that induce alterations in a large number of genes controlling the homeostasis of normal alveolar and bronchial cells (3). With the use of cytogenetics, comparative genomic hybridization, and allelotyping, a wide array of genetic changes have been discovered in cancer. As discussed here and as for other cancers, alterations of proto-oncogenes, tumor suppressor genes (TSGs), and chromosome telomeres are particularly important in the etiology and progression of lung cancer.

Proto-oncogenes are genes that contribute to malignant transformation when mutationally activated or overexpressed. In 1917, Rous reported that sarcoma in chickens could be caused by a transmissible agent. This observation led to the discovery of the Rous sarcoma virus and the subsequent isolation of *v-Src*, the transforming component of the viral genome and the first known oncogene. A human gene with homology to *v-Src* (*SRC*) was subsequently identified, and in 1980 Hunter and Sefton found that *v-Src* encodes a mutant kinase, which is constitutively active, thereby transforming cells (4). These and other studies demonstrated that a range of viral oncogenes had related normal counterparts in mammalian genomes. In view of the potential for such sequences to cause malignancy when misregulated, they were termed proto-oncogenes. The human homologue *SRC* was initially thought to be a relatively weak proto-oncogene, but recent data indicate that SRC kinase is an important regulator of migration, proliferation, survival, angiogenesis, and inflammation in normal and cancer cells (5). Potential clinical implications of these findings in lung cancer are now being explored in clinical trials with small molecule inhibitors of SRC kinase (6).

Proto-oncogenes that have been associated with lung cancer include *MYC*, *KRAS*, epidermal growth factor receptor (*EGFR*), *HER2*, and cyclin D1 (*CCND1*) (Table 1) (7). The *MYC* oncogene was isolated in the early 1980s from a retrovirus causing myelocytomatosis and carcinoma in chickens. Human *MYC* family genes were subsequently found to be activated in Burkitt lymphoma (*MYC*, translocation), neuroblastoma (*MYCN*, amplification), and lung cancer (*MYCL*, amplification). Amplification of *MYC* family proto-oncogenes is found in almost all small-cell lung cancers (SCLC) and is reported to confer an aggressive, resistant phenotype (9). *MYC* genes encode transcription factors, which dimerize with the cofactor Max and induce transcription of genes involved in cell cycle progression. MYC/Max dimers can also repress the transcription of genes that lead to cell cycle arrest following DNA damage such as cyclin-dependent kinase (CDK) inhibitor 2A (*CDKN2A*). Several strategies are being pursued to target MYC in

Table 1 Activated Proto-oncogenes in Lung Cancer

Gene	Chromosome	Mode of activation	Frequency in SCLC (%)	Frequency in NSCLC (%)
MYC	8q24	Amplification	90	25
MYCN	2p24	Amplification	25	
MYCL	1p34	Amplification	25	
KRAS	12p12	Mutation	<1	20–40
HRAS	11p15	Mutation		<10
NRAS	1p13	Mutation		<10
ERBB2	17q12	Amplification	<1	10–30
EGFR	7p11.2	Mutation/amplification		5–10 (mutation)

Note: Frequently activated proto-oncogenes and the mechanisms of activation in small-cell lung cancer and non–small-cell lung cancer.
Abbreviations: NSCLC, non–small-cell lung cancer; SCLC, small-cell lung cancer.
Source: From Ref. 8.

cancer. Small molecule inhibitors of MYC/Max dimerization have been shown to repress *MYC*-induced transformation in vivo and serve as lead compounds for cancer drug development (10).

The rat sarcoma viral oncogene homolog (*RAS*) family of proto-oncogenes (*KRAS, NRAS,* and *HRAS*) encodes membrane-bound GTPases, which link signaling from growth factor receptors to the mitogen-activated protein (MAP) kinase proliferation pathway (11). The *RAS* oncogene was first isolated from a virus causing rat sarcoma and its human homologue was identified by Weinberg's group in 1980. *KRAS* is activated by point mutations in up to 35% of lung adenocarcinomas and *KRAS* mutations are associated with smoking (12). Oncogenic mutations of *KRAS*, commonly located in codon 12, 13, and 61, lead to increased GTP binding and constitutive activation of *KRAS* and the MAP kinase pathway. Oncogenic *KRAS* is sufficient to expand murine bronchioalveolar stem cells in culture and in vivo (13). The mutational and stem cell model-derived data indicate that KRAS is a strong oncoprotein in the lung. The function of *KRAS* is reliant on membrane-anchoring of the protein, which in turn is facilitated by several posttranslational modifications, including farnesylation, geranylation, methylation, and palmitoylation. Small molecule farnesyl-transferase inhibitors (FTIs) have demonstrated preclinical activity against lung cancer cell lines and one of these agents, lonafarnib, has shown clinical activity in combination with paclitaxel in non–small cell lung cancer (NSCLC) (14). However, many FTIs have failed to demonstrate single-agent activity in clinical trials. This has been attributed to their lack of selectivity for mutant KRAS and the normal function of wild-type KRAS as a regulator of the MAP kinase pathway. New therapeutic strategies in this field include peptides, which selectively bind and inhibit mutant KRAS protein (15).

The human epidermal growth factor (*EGF*) receptor (*HER*) gene family encodes proto-oncogenes, which belong to the class of receptor tyrosine kinases (16).

This family is also named *ERBB* after the viral erythroblastosis B oncogene and includes the *EGF* receptor (*EGFR/HER1*), *HER2*, *HER3*, and *HER4*. These receptors bind ligands such as EGF and neuregulin 1. Binding of ligand induces receptor homo- or heterodimerization, activation of the intrinsic receptor tyrosine kinase, and activation of intracellular signal transduction pathways that simulate proliferation and survival. The EGFR-HER2 heterodimer has been shown to initiate the strongest and most long-lived signaling in NSCLC models (17). Strong *EGFR* expression is present in 40% to 80% of NSCLC tumor specimens (17). High-level expression of *EGFR* is also present in premalignant bronchial epithelium, suggesting a role for *EGFR* in carcinogenesis (17,18). A common mechanism of *EGFR* overexpression in lung cancer is amplification of the gene copy number (19). Oncogenic mutations of *EGFR* and *HER2*, located in the kinase domain and leading to constitutive activation of the kinase, have been reported in up to 35% and 4% of NSCLC specimens, respectively (20). *EGFR* mutations are mostly found in adenocarcinoma, nonsmokers, and Asian patients. Similar mutations have been detected in the normal respiratory epithelium of up to 43% of patients with *EGFR* mutant adenocarcinomas and are identical to those seen in tumor specimens from the same patient, suggesting that these mutations may be an early event in carcinogenesis, particularly in never-smokers (21). Mutant *EGFR* transforms both NIH-3T3 fibroblasts and lung epithelial cells in the absence of EGF, leading to anchorage-independent growth, decreased contact inhibition, and increased tumor formation in immunocompromised mice (22). Mutant cancer cells are strongly dependent on the signal induced by the aberrant EGFR receptor tyrosine kinase (so-called "oncogene addiction") and undergo apoptosis upon inhibition of the aberrant kinase (23). Taken together, these findings have greatly improved understanding of the critical role that *EGFR* and other members of the *HER* family play in lung cancer. The consequences of alterations in *EGFR* expression or functionality in regard to lung cancer therapy are discussed in a separate chapter.

Activated proto-oncogenes contribute to carcinogenesis by driving the cell toward neoplasia. Conversely, TSGs are sequences, which contribute to neoplasia, when their normal functionality is lost. It is generally more difficult pharmacologically to replace a missing or defective protein than to inhibit an inappropriately active molecule. Hence, strategies to therapeutically exploit the loss of TSG function are more complex and to date have been less successful than those targeting somatically activated oncogenes. Unlike the proto-oncogenes, where mutation of just one allele can lead to tumorigenesis, both alleles of a TSG must generally be mutated or deleted before an effect is present (two-hit hypothesis). This is due to the fact that one allele is usually sufficient to produce the functional TSG product. A notable exception is *TP53,* where mutation of one allele already is of biological significance. The *TP53* gene and its product p53 have been described as "the guardian of the genome." Following DNA-damage, wild-type p53 initiates a G1/S checkpoint cell cycle arrest, following which either DNA repair occurs, or, in the case of irreparable damage, apoptosis is triggered. After chronic exposure to tobacco-related carcinogens, *TP53* gene mutation within the bronchial epithelium is relatively common, leading to impaired function of the p53 protein (24). The p53 protein has three domains: one that activates transcription factors, a core domain that recognizes specific DNA sequences, and a domain, which is responsible for protein tetramerization. Most inactivating mutations in p53 occur in the core domain, but, unlike *KRAS*, there are no specifically mutated codons. In an attempt to restore the function of p53 in NSCLC with *TP53* mutations, adenoviral vectors containing the wild-type *TP53* gene (*Adv-p53*) have been constructed and injected intratumorally, with some clinical success (25). Further progress in gene therapy is slowed by the low in vivo infection rate of adenoviral vectors and difficulties in the development of new vectors that are more efficient yet still safe.

Other TSGs frequently inactivated in lung cancer are retinoblastoma 1 (*RB1*) and *CDKN2A* (Table 2) (26). *RB1* was the first TSG discovered after cytogenetic data suggested the position of a disease locus and Knudson proposed the two-hit hypothesis to explain the molecular mechanism responsible for the incidence patterns of hereditary and nonhereditary retinoblastoma in 1971. The gene was subsequently cloned in Weiberg's laboratory in 1986. The active hypophosphorylated gene product, pRb, blocks the cell cycle at the G1/S transition. When progress through the cell cycle is triggered, pRb is hyperphosphorylated by specific kinases such as the CCND1/CDK4 complex. This allows the release of bound transcription factors and cell cycle progression. Recent data suggest that pRb also acts as a tumor survival factor. The *CDKN2A* gene product p16 inhibits CDK4 and

Table 2   Inactivated Tumor Suppressor Genes in Lung Cancer

Gene	Chromosome	Mode of inactivation	Frequency in SCLC (%)	Frequency in NSCLC (%)
TP53	17p13	LOH, mutation	90	50
RB1	13q14	LOH, mutation	90	15
CDKN2A	9p21	Homozygous deletion, methylation, LOH, mutation	<10	60–70
SMAD2	18q21	LOH, mutation	<10	<10
SMAD4	18q21	LOH, mutation	<10	<10
PTEN	10q23	Homozygous deletion, LOH, mutation	10	<10
FHIT	3p14	Homozygous deletion, aberrant splicing	75	75
RASSF1	3p21	Methylation	80	30–40

Note: Frequently inactivated tumor suppressor genes and the mechanisms of inactivation in small cell lung cancer and non–small cell lung cancer.
Abbreviations: LOH, loss of heterozygosity; NSCLC, non–small cell lung cancer; SCLC, small cell lung cancer.
Source: From Ref. 8.

stabilizes p53. The frequency of inactivation of *RB1* or *CDKN2A*, either of which may lead to uncontrolled cell cycle progression, varies among histopathological subtypes of lung cancer. *RB1*, for example, is inactivated in almost all SCLCs, but uncommonly in NSCLC (Table 2).

A large effort has been undertaken to identify additional TSGs in a region on the short arm of chromosome 3 (3p), which is deleted in up to 90% of both NSCLC and SCLC (27). The observation that 3p deletion is frequent in both NSCLC and SCLC has raised the hypothesis of a common genetic alteration in the carcinogenesis of different lung cancer types. A number of genes on 3p were subsequently identified that exhibit characteristics consistent with a TSG, including fragile histidine triad (*FHIT*) gene, ras association domain 1A (*RASSF1A*), semaphorin3B (*SEMA3B*), and retinoic acid receptor-β (*RAR-β*). These genes appear to exert their effect in a coordinated way and their role in lung carcinogenesis is currently being investigated.

Telomeres consist of 2 to 30 kilobases of noncoding *TTAGGG* repeats at the end of chromosome arms, protecting those ends from degradation (28). In differentiated cells, telomerase activity is lost and telomeres gradually become shorter with each cell division, a characteristic sign and a possible cause of cellular ageing. In human germ cells and certain stem cells, telomeres are maintained by the telomerase complex, which is composed of the template-RNA (hTR), the reverse transcriptase subunit (hTERT), and additional proteins. In lung cancer, telomere length is maintained by active telomerase or alternative mechanisms, and expression of hTERT is associated with poor differentiation and a poor prognosis (29,30). Smoking has been shown to result in increased telomerase activity in bronchial cells (31). These results led to the hypotheses that telomerase expression may be one of the molecular events that strongly differentiate between tumor and normal tissue and, therefore, that inhibition of telomerase activity may have therapeutic potential. GRN163L, an oligonucleotide complementary to hTR, and BIBR1532, a small molecule inhibitor of hTERT, have shown preclinical activity against lung cancer cells (32,33). Early clinical trials with telomerase inhibitors are planned or ongoing.

Despite these and other recent advances, lung carcinogenesis remains a complex and incompletely understood process at the genetic level. Introduction of multiple oncogenic changes in human bronchial epithelial cells, including mutant *KRAS*, *TP53* knockdown, mutant *EGFR*, p16 bypass, and telomerase, appears insufficient to confer a full malignant phenotype (34). The formulation of a genetic multistep model of lung carcinogenesis is ongoing, but remains a work in progress (Fig. 1) (35,36). Further research efforts in this area must account for the following: (*i*) different combinations of mutations leading to the same phenotype, (*ii*) one phenotype comprising multiple genotypes with different biological and clinical characteristics, (*iii*) individual lung cancers harboring multiple, genetically different subclones, and (*iv*) individual lung cancers harboring multiple distinct histological subtypes.

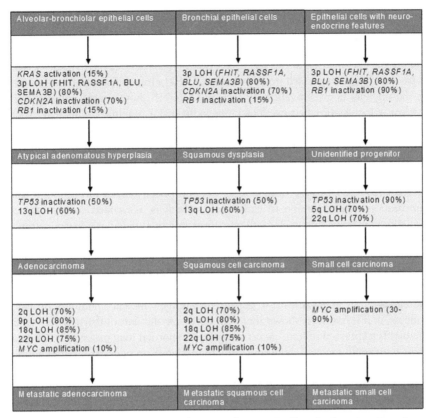

Figure 1 Genetic multistep model of lung carcinogenesis. Genetic alterations in each proposed step of lung carcinogenesis are shown. *Abbreviation*: LOH, loss of heterozygosity. *Source*: From Ref. 8.

GENETIC PREDISPOSITION TO LUNG CANCER

Only a relatively low percentage (10–20%) of smokers develop lung cancer, suggesting the presence of genetic factors that modify individual susceptibilities to various carcinogens. The aforementioned *TP53* is frequently somatically mutated in lung cancer, but lung cancer only occasionally occurs in families with the Li–Fraumeni syndrome (the majority of which are segregating constitutional *TP53* mutations), suggesting that *TP53* is not a high penetrance lung cancer susceptibility gene (37). On the other hand, several low penetrance single nucleotide polymorphisms (SNPs) of genes involved in DNA repair and detoxification have been shown to alter lung cancer risk in smokers, including the cytochrome, glutathione S-transferase and nicotinamide adenine dinucleotide (NADH)-transferase genes, *MGMT*, *XPD*, and *XRCC1* (38). SNPs of genes involved in cell cycle control and mitosis have also been reported in this context. The *CCND1 A870G* gene polymorphism has been correlated with the early onset of lung cancer, as described in our work on smoking-induced lung cancer risk (39). The *CCND1* polymorphism modulates alternative splicing of the primary *CCND1* transcript, which leads, on translation, to two different CCND1 proteins (CCND1a and CCND1b) (40). *CCND1* is frequently overexpressed in tumor cells. CCND1a transfers from the cytoplasm to the nucleus upon activation by CDKs. CCND1b, however, is constitutively nuclear in localization because it lacks a residue that is required for nuclear export (41). As demonstrated in model systems, CCND1b has increased oncogenic potential and this may explain why the *A870G* genotype modifies disease risk and/or clinical outcome across a range of malignancies, including lung cancer.

Another cell cycle gene polymorphism associated with cancer risk is the *AURKA (STK15)* T+91A variant. This polymorphism results in an amino acid substitution (phenylalanine to isoleucine), which is associated with increased aneuploidy in colon tumors and cell transformation in vitro and is a low penetrance lung cancer susceptibility gene (42). The results of this report are very meaningful because the reported variant affected the risk for multiple cancer types in large, ethnically diverse groups. *AURKA* encodes a protein that belongs to the aurora family of mitotic kinases, which control chromosome segregation during mitosis. Deregulation of *AURKA* leads to genetic instability, which is a hallmark of many cancers, and it has been shown that both aurora A and aurora B (*AURKB*) genes are highly expressed in lung cancer compared to normal lung tissue (43). Clinical trials with small molecule inhibitors of aurora kinases in lung cancer are ongoing (44). It will be important to assess the functional characteristics of the *AURKA* T+91A variant, to also consider whether variants in *AURKB* have clinical significance, and to assess whether genetic instability and deregulation of aurora kinases is a cause or consequence of malignant transformation.

EPIGENETIC ALTERATIONS

Epigenetic alterations are commonly defined as reversible chemical modifications of chromatin (DNA and histones) that change gene expression without changing the primary DNA sequence (45). Epigenetic modifications may be heritable, act as a long-term memory of silenced genes, and can be a mechanism for chromosome stabilization. A variety of proteins are involved in the epigenetic process, including DNA-methyltransferases (DNMTs), methyl-CpG binding proteins, histone-modifying enzymes, and chromatin remodeling factors. In lung cancer, aberrant promoter hypermethylation and histone-deacetylation are among the best described epigenetic alterations (Fig. 2). CpG islands are short stretches of DNA in which the frequency of the CG nucleotide sequence is higher than in other regions (46). CpG islands located in the gene promoter regions of many TSGs have been found to be hypermethylated by DNMT in lung cancer, leading to reduced binding of transcription factors and reduced expression of the TSG. Subsequent deacetylation of histones by histone deacetylase (HDAC) results in chromatin condensation and further restriction of access of the transcription-machinery to the DNA. DNA-methylation can be studied by methods that are based

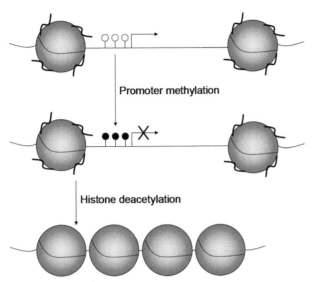

Figure 2 Epigenetic alterations and gene transcription. Gene transcription (*horizontal arrow*) is stopped by methylation of CpG islands (*circles*) in the gene promoter region (by DNA methyl-transferases) and histone deacetylation (by histone deacetylases). These modifications prevent binding of transcription factors and result in condensation of chromatin. Epigenetic silencing of genes that have tumor suppressor function is a common phenomenon in lung cancer.

on the ability of sodium bisulfite to convert unmethylated (but not methylated) cytosine to uracil. Untreated and bisulfite treated DNA can then be compared by polymerase chain reaction (PCR), microarrays, and sequencing, in order to detect specific methylation sites. Using bisulfite-based methods, it has been demonstrated that promoter-hypermethylation frequently inhibits transcription of a variety of different TSGs in lung cancer, including adenomatous polyposis coli, *CDKN2A*, *FHIT*, phosphatase and tensin homolog, *RAR*-β, and *RASSF1A* (47). Promoter-hypermethylation of *CDKN2A* has been reported to be associated with poor prognosis, and different histopathological types of lung cancer have shown distinct methylation profiles for certain genes (48). The mismatch repair genes *MLH1* and *MSH2* are hypermethylated and their protein expression is altered in 65% and 30% of NSCLC, respectively; these abnormalities are associated with poor prognosis in nonsmoking patients (49).

Based on these observations, inhibitors of DNMT such as 5-azacytidine and 5-aza-2-deoxycytidine (decitabine) have been tested in clinical trials (50). These agents have shown limited activity in solid tumor patients, and it has been hypothesized that they may paradoxically induce the transcription of genes that promote cancer cell proliferation and survival. Ongoing studies in this area focus on the development of novel inhibitors of DNMT and HDAC and on the role of DNA-hypomethylation in cancer (51). Some of these inhibitors have demonstrated single-agent clinical activity and are now being studied in combination with chemotherapy. For example, a phase-I trial of the HDAC inhibitor suberoylanilide hydroxamic acid with paclitaxel/carboplatin has been completed and a phase-II study of this regimen is under development for advanced stage NSCLC. To obtain a more comprehensive view, microarrays may be used to study DNA-methylation (CpG island microarrays) and histone-acetylation (chromatin-landscaping microarrays) at a large number of loci simultaneously. Using CpG island microarrays, histological types of lung cancer can be distinguished from normal tissue based on the methylation profiles of specific genes, some of which have not previously been implicated in the disease (52).

ALTERATIONS AT THE RNA LEVEL

Alterations of gene expression at the RNA level in lung cancer have been extensively studied with microarrays in recent years (53). The use of this technology has led to the collection of an enormous amount of data, which are readily accessible (54). For the common two-channel microarray gene expression analysis, mRNA is isolated from cancer and adjacent normal tissue and converted into cDNA by reverse transcriptase (Fig. 3). Two fluorescent dyes are used to label the cDNA from normal

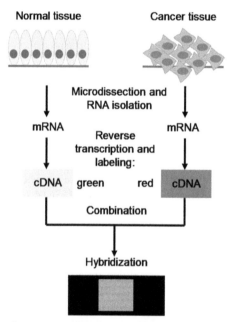

Figure 3   Gene expression microarray. Dual-channel microarrays are frequently used to compare expression levels of thousands of genes in cancer and normal tissue. The mRNA from cancer and normal tissue is extracted, transcribed into cDNA, and labeled with separate fluorescent dyes. The cDNA products are mixed and hybridized to a chip carrying defined sets of gene probes. Scanning of the chip allows determination of relative gene expression levels in tumor compared with normal tissue.

and cancer tissue differently. The labeled cDNA is added to a chip, which may contain up to 390,000 probes that are fixed on glass, plastic, or silicon. These probes represent the genes of interest that will hybridize to complementary cDNA. Nonhybridized cDNA is removed, the fluorescent dye in the hybridized cDNA glows upon laser scanning, and the color and intensity is used to determine the origin and relative expression level of the cDNA. One study compared the expression of 47,650 gene transcripts in resected NSCLC and adjacent normal tissue from 39 patients (55). Approximately 11,000 transcripts were differentially expressed at least twofold. Of these, 96 transcripts were scored as overrepresented fourfold or more in tumors and 30 transcripts were overrepresented 16-fold or more in tumors. Further analysis of the overrepresented genes showed that two of the most dramatically overrepresented transcripts in NSCLC, maspin (*SERPINB5*) and *S100A2*, were strongly expressed at the protein level in cancer and preneoplastic lesions (56,57). The possible role of these genes in the etiology and therapy of lung cancer is now being assessed. Another microarray study reported on the effect of smoking on gene expression in normal bronchial epithelial samples from 75 individuals without cancer (58). Differential analysis of 7119 transcripts revealed that smoking induced the transcription of several putative oncogenes and reduced transcription of several putative TSGs. Importantly, the study indicated, which changes were irreversible after cessation of smoking. Thirteen gene transcripts did not return to normal levels in former smokers, even in those who had discontinued smoking 20 years before testing. For example, transcript expression of carcinoembryonic antigen (CEA)-related cell adhesion molecule 6 and *HN1* (a member of the human Notch family) was permanently increased, whereas expression of *TU3A* (a gene previously isolated from renal cell cancer) and *CX3CL1* (a chemokine ligand) was permanently decreased. These results are interesting, because these genes were not previously associated with lung carcinogenesis. Gene expression microarrays are also being developed to predict lung cancer histology and outcome (59). A panel of 50 transcripts, including *HER2* and vascular endothelial growth factor (*VEGF*) mRNA, was reported to separate patients with early stage lung adenocarcinoma into two groups with different prognosis (60). The National Cancer Institute (NCI) is currently testing the prognostic value of this transcript panel in stages I to II adenocarcinoma patients.

As discussed in the section on *CCND1*, splicing is an important regulatory mechanism that can vary the primary mRNA structure and therefore the encoded protein from a given gene. Another regulatory mechanism at the RNA level has been discovered recently. MicroRNAs (miRs) are noncoding RNA fragments which specifically hybridize to and prevent the translation of coding mRNA (Fig. 4) (61). The human genome encodes approximately 350 miRs, produced as long precursors, which are cleaved into 20 to 25 nucleotide long oligomers that are bound into an active miR-induced silencing complex. These complexes have important functions in normal and cancer cells. For example, translation of the mRNA of the *RAS* proto-oncogene is repressed by the let-7 miR-complexes in normal cells (62). In lung cancer, let-7 miRs are downregulated, which is associated with poor prognosis (63). Downregulation of let-7 in lung cancer was confirmed by

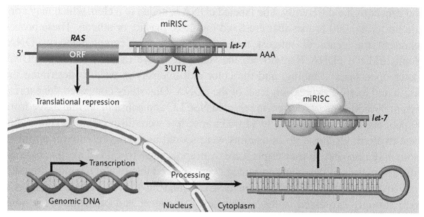

Figure 4 Function of the let-7 microRNA. MicroRNAs are produced as long precursors, which are cleaved into oligomers that are bound into the active miRISC. Translation of the RAS mRNA is repressed by the let-7 miRISC in normal cells. In lung cancer cells, let-7 is downregulated, leading of increased production of potentially oncogenic RAS protein. *Abbreviations*: miRISC, microRNA-induced silencing complex; RAS, rat sarcoma viral oncogene homolog. *Source*: From Ref. 69.

miR-microarray analysis, which could also discriminate lung cancer from normal tissue, define profiles that differ in cancer histology, and show that the level of another miR, miR-155, is frequently increased in lung cancer (64). Two of the potential targets, miR-155 are *SEMA5A* and *TP53*-induced protein 1, both have a tumor suppressor function (65). Interestingly, it is known that viruses use miR for gene regulation in host cells and increased expression of miR-155 is found in Epstein–Barr virus–transformed lymphoblastoid cells (66). A viral cause of human lung cancer has been suggested in the past and although this hypothesis is highly speculative, miR may be the key that could lead to further advances in this field. Other miRs, which are associated with lung cancer, are the miR-17-92 cluster (seven miRs which are overexpressed in SCLC), miR-17-5p, miR-21, miR-128b, miR-191, and miR-199a-1 (67,68). The predicted targets of these miRs are significantly enriched for proto-oncogenes and TSGs, suggesting that a large number of miRs are dominant or recessive lung cancer genes. The discovery of miR may have implications for lung cancer therapy. It was speculated that augmentation of let-7 miR may benefit lung cancer patients, but pharmacological delivery of miR may be challenging and inhibition of overexpressed miRs could be more efficient (69). Antagomirs, cholesterol-conjugated single-stranded RNA analogues, are efficient and specific inhibitors of endogenous miRs in mice, and the safety and activity of these compounds in cancer patients must now be tested (70).

ALTERATIONS AT THE PROTEIN LEVEL

Proteins can be classified, according to their functional properties, as ligand binders or carriers, nucleic-acid binders, enzymes, transporters, storage proteins, structural proteins, signal transducers, motor proteins, and proteins of unknown function. Large-scale technologies (proteomics) are being developed to broadly measure changes at the protein level in lung cancer (71). The therapeutic implications of proteomics research are considerable, because mRNA and protein levels can be discordant and this approach allows the study of posttranslational protein modifications. Two-dimensional gel electrophoresis or protein microarrays can separate complex protein mixtures and individual proteins can then be identified by mass spectrometry. More recently, chromatography has been added to these methods in order to measure changes at the enzyme substrate level (metabolomics) (72). The advantage of metabolomics is that the consequences of protein function and drug treatment can be observed. At present, the reproducibility and global measurement capability of both proteomics and metabolomics are not as high as with genomics, in part because of the additional technical complexity involved in measurement, in part due to the lack of a specific amplification system similar to the PCR.

For the moment, only restricted classes of proteins are considered to be targetable by small molecule inhibitors. Research on one such class, the protein kinases (PKs), has yielded significant success in lung cancer therapy. The PKs were discovered by Krebs and Fischer at the University of Washington in Seattle in the 1950s and 1960s (73). Today, it is known that the human genome contains approximately 500 genes, which encode PKs. PKs transfer phosphate groups from high-energy donor molecules such as adenosine triphosphate (ATP) to target proteins. The phosphate group is covalently attached to a Tyrosine (Tyr, Y), Serine (Ser, S), or Threonine (Thr, T) on the target protein. Many PKs act on Ser/Thr, others act only on Tyr, and a number act on Ser/Thr and Tyr (dual-specificity kinases) (Table 3). Phosphorylation may change the activity and/or subcellular localization of the target protein, or its association with other proteins, thereby regulating the majority of intracellular signal transduction pathways (Fig. 5). Because of this central role, PKs are tightly controlled by many mechanisms, including phosphorylation (sometimes by the PK itself, referred to as autophosphorylation), binding of regulatory proteins, control of their localization in the cell relative to their substrates, and removal of phosphate groups from target proteins by their functional antagonists, the protein phosphatases (74). Activation of PKs is frequent in cancer and new drugs, which inhibit specific kinases, are discussed elsewhere in this book (75).

The three-dimensional (3-D) structure of a protein is an important determinant of its interaction with other molecules, but the process of protein folding is not well understood. Methods of analysis include X-ray diffraction, nuclear magnetic resonance, and prediction by comparison of the amino acid sequence with proteins of known structure and similar sequence. Recent studies in this field revealed the structural features of HER family dimerization (76). It was shown that these receptors, which are produced as inactive monomers, could switch between a tethered and an extended conformation (Fig. 6). Only the extended conformation of the monomer can undergo dimerization with another HER family member. In the case of EGFR, binding of the ligand leads to the receptor adopting the extended conformation, resulting in dimerization and activation of the receptor

Table 3 Protein Kinases

Type	Name	Main function and molecular target	Alteration in lung cancer
Serine/threonine kinase	Phosphorylase kinases	Glycogen storage and muscle function	Not well characterized
	PKA	Glycogen, lipid, and sugar metabolization	Overexpression by gene amplification
	Akt (PKB)	Survival (Bcl-2, survivin)	Activation by PI3K
	PKC (10 isoforms)	Proliferation (MAPK, IKB, RAF, and EGFR)	Overexpression partly by gene amplification
	Calmodulin kinases	Muscle contraction (myosin)	Not well characterized
	MAP kinases	Proliferation and survival (ERK)	Activation by RAS/RAF
	RAF/RAS	Proliferation and survival (MAPK)	Activation by mutation, *EGFR*, and Src/FAK
	GSK3-beta	Glycogen synthesis, proliferation, and differentiation (Wnt-pathway)	Inhibition by PI3K/Akt
	CDK	Cell cycle progression (cyclins)	Overexpression
	CHK1, CHK2	Checkpoint regulation	Activation by DNA damage
	PI3K	Survival (Akt)	Activation by *EGFR*
	Aurora A, Aurora B, Aurora C	Mitosis	Overexpression (A and B)
Dual-specific kinase	Polo-like kinases	Mitosis	Overexpression and mutation
Receptor TK	EGFR	Proliferation	Overexpression by gene amplification, activation by mutation in NSCLC
	PDGFR	Proliferation	Overexpression
	Kit	Proliferation	Overexpression in SCLC
	Met	Proliferation	Mutation in SCLC
Nonreceptor TK	Src	Adhesion (FAK), proliferation (MAPK), angiogenesis	Overexpression
	Abl	Unknown	Overexpression
	JAK	Cytokine signaling and inflammation (STATs)	Overexpression and activation

Note: A selection of human PKs and their role in normal cells and lung cancer are shown (see also Fig. 5).
Abbreviations: CDK, cyclin-dependent kinase; CHK, checkpoint kinase; EGFR, epidermal growth factor receptor; GSK, glycogen synthetase kinase; JAK, Janus kinase; MAPK, mitogen-activated protein kinase(s); NSCLC, non–small cell lung cancer; PDGFR, platelet-derived growth factor receptor; PK, protein kinase; PI3K, phosphatidyl-inositol-3 kinase; Abl, Abelson kinase; SCLC, small-cell lung cancer; TK, tyrosine kinase.

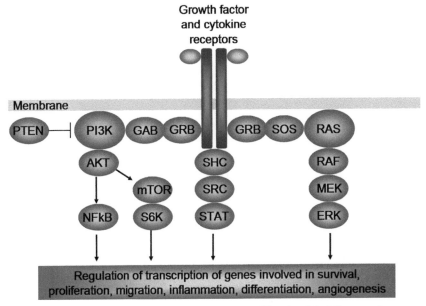

Figure 5 Intracellular signal transduction pathways. The simplified diagram shows some of the most important pathways in human lung cancer cells, including the PI3K-AKT pathway, the SRC pathway, and the RAS-RAF-MEK pathway. These pathways activate particular transcription factors (NFkB, S6K, STAT, ERK, and others), which in turn activate the transcription of genes involved in proliferation, survival, migration, and angiogenesis (Table 3).

kinase. Cetuximab, an EGFR-targeted therapeutic monoclonal antibody, inhibits this process, both blocking ligand binding and also sterically preventing the receptor from adopting the extended conformation necessary for dimerization (77). These results show that proteins can undergo dynamic conformational changes that are functionally and therapeutically relevant.

Knowledge of 3-D protein structure was also important for the discovery of the proteasome, its function, and subsequent development of proteasome inhibitors (78). Proteasomes are intracellular, barrel-shaped macromolecules that specifically digest other proteins into short polypeptides and amino acids. Target proteins are recognized by the proteasome based on a ubiquitin tag, which is added by the ubiquitin ligases. The proteasome removes the ubiquitin tag and degrades the target protein in an ATP-dependent process. Many important proteins involved in cell cycling and apoptosis are degraded by the proteasome complex, including the cyclins and IKB. The elucidation of this system led to the development of the proteasome inhibitor bortezomib (Velcade, PS-341), which is clinically active as a single agent and in combination with cytotoxic drugs in many tumor types, including lung cancer (79,80). The proposed mechanism of action of bortezomib in lung cancer cells rests on the induction of G2-M arrest and apoptosis.

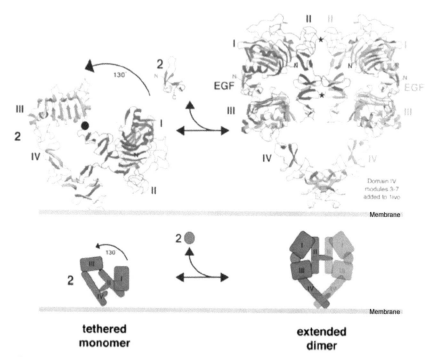

Figure 6   Model of conformational changes of EGFR. Transition between two EGFR structures is shown in both ribbons and cartoon representation. The inactive, tethered structure is shown on the left. A model of the EGF-induced dimer is shown on the right. The speculated position of the plasma membrane is depicted as a gray bar. EGF binding is proposed to induce a 130° rotation of a rigid receptor body containing domains I and II, about the axis represented by a filled black circle (at the domain II/III junction). This exposes the dimerization arm and allows dimerization of EGFR, as depicted on the right. *Abbreviation*: EGF, epidermal growth factor. *Source*: From Ref. 76.

Large clinical trials are ongoing to define optimal administration schedules of bortezomib and combinations with cytotoxic drugs in patients with NSCLC and SCLC.

HISTOPATHOLOGY

Histopathologic subtyping is becoming increasingly important for lung cancer therapy, especially with the advent of molecular targeted therapies, which have been shown to convey different risks and benefits in histologic subtypes of NSCLC. NSCLC (80% of lung cancers) can be divided into several subtypes, including squamous cell carcinoma, adenocarcinoma, large-cell carcinoma, adenosquamous carcinoma, and carcinoma with pleomorphic, sarcomatoid, or sarcomatous elements (81). Large-cell carcinoma and adenocarcinoma are typically located in the periphery of the lung, whereas squamous cell carcinoma often presents as a central tumor with necrosis and endobronchial growth. Squamous cell carcinoma tends to grow more slowly and has a slightly better prognosis than adenocarcinoma and large-cell carcinoma. Squamous cell carcinoma is often necrotic and may invade large blood vessels. The therapeutic consequence of this characteristic is that squamous carcinoma is significantly associated with fatal tumor bleeding in patients treated with the anti-VEGF antibody bevacizumab (82).

Bronchioloalveolar carcinoma (BAC) is another histopathological diagnosis of interest. Despite the World Health Organization designation of this disease as a subtype of adenocarcinoma, BAC has features that are distinct, such as relatively slow and multifocal growth (83). On the genetic level, BAC harbors a high rate of activating *EGFR* mutations (30–60% compared with 5–10% in all NSCLC combined), especially among patients of Asian ethnicity (84). BAC also frequently shows increased copy numbers of the EGFR gene and both genetic alterations increase the sensitivity of the tumor to tyrosine kinase inhibitors (9–19% of BAC vs. 5–10% of all NSCLC combined) (18,85). Interestingly, the *T790M* mutation, which is associated with resistance of EGFR tyrosine kinase inhibitors, was found in the germ line of a family with multiple cases of adenocarcinoma/BAC, strongly suggesting that this mutation predisposes carriers to hereditary lung cancer (86).

SCLC (20% of lung cancers) comprises an aggressive cell type characterized by neuroendocrine differentiation, central location, rapid growth, and high metastatic potential. SCLC belongs to the class of neuroendocrine tumors, which also includes typical carcinoid, atypical carcinoid, and large-cell neuroendocrine carcinoma (87). Although the proto-oncogene *KIT* (stem cell factor receptor) is expressed and activated in 70% to 90% of SCLC and can be blocked with the small molecule inhibitor imatinib, clinical trials failed to show activity of imatinib in SCLC (88). Recent data suggest that activating mutations of *KIT* are not common in SCLC, likely explaining the lack of clinical activity of imatinib (89). SCLC cells also express multidrug resistance-related protein-1 and p-glycoprotein (encoded by the multidrug resistance gene one), which are ATP-binding cassette transporter proteins that confer resistance by enhancing drug efflux (90). Although inhibitors to these proteins have been developed, clinical studies have met with little success and the concentrations required to block multidrug resistance proteins in humans may not have been reached (91). As an alternative resistance mechanism, SCLC cells exposed to cisplatin upregulate survival pathways that directly protect them from cell death. Expression of such antiapoptotic factors, including Bcl-2 and survivin, is induced by phosphatidyl-inositol-3 kinase (PI3K)/Akt (92). Several small molecule inhibitors of PI3K and Akt are currently being tested in clinical trials.

DEVELOPMENT OF PROGNOSTIC AND PREDICTIVE BIOMARKERS

The identification and validation of biomarkers for cancer diagnosis, staging, prognosis, and treatment selection is one of the aims of translational/correlative science. Markers can be prognostic for patient outcome (general effect which is independent of treatment), or predictive for response to a certain therapy, or, conceivably, informative in both respects. Several prognostic biomarkers have been reported for lung cancer, including expression levels of cyclin E, cyclin B1, p16, p21, p27, ERCC1, EGFR, survivin, collagen XVIII, and VEGF (93). Biomarkers reported to be predictive for response to cytotoxic drugs include alterations of ERCC1 (cisplatin), TUBB3 (taxanes), and RRM1 (antimetabolites) (94). Other markers have been isolated from patient sputum and peripheral blood and were associated with lung cancer diagnosis and outcome (95). Interpretation of these preliminary studies has often been limited by small sample size and lack of validation, with the consequence that there is at present no Food and Drug Administration–approved biomarker specific for lung cancer.

One biomarker of interest is the uridine diphosphate (UDP)-glucuronosyl-transferase isoform 1A1 (*UGT1A1*) gene polymorphism, which has been associated both with cancer risk and also toxicity, time to progression, and survival in patients treated with irinotecan (96). Irinotecan is a prodrug, which is converted into its active metabolite SN-38 by the UDP-glucuronosyltransferases in the liver. The presence of seven thymidine-adenine repeats instead of the normal six repeats in the *UGT1A1* promoter results in the variant allele *28, which is associated with reduced enzyme activity in homozygous individuals (about 10% of the U.S. population). Of interest, the incidence of the 7/7 genotype is approximately 2% in Asian populations, compared with 10% to 20% in other racial and ethnic groups (97). A previously reported randomized trial demonstrated improved survival in Japanese patients treated with irinotecan/cisplatin versus etoposide/cisplatin (98). An ongoing phase-III trial of the Southwest Oncology Group is attempting to reproduce these data, while also studying the potential of *UGT1A1* genotyping as a predictive biomarker.

The observation that the *EGFR* tyrosine kinase inhibitors, gefitinib or erlotinib, show dramatic responses in a small subset of NSCLC patients and that *EGFR* mutation status and gene copy number are predictive of clinical benefit has been pivotal to current efforts to develop methods for prospective patient selection for treatment with these agents (19,99,100). These data are now being incorporated into clinical trial design in advanced stage NSCLC, exemplified by trials using molecular screening to identify patients appropriate for randomization to front line erlotinib or chemotherapy.

Other targeted agents are emerging and two different strategies have been developed to predict the sensitivity of tumors to these novel agents: (*i*) hypothesis-driven analyses of the target and a limited number of associated molecules; and (*ii*) large-scale gene expression microarrays to determine the type of deregulated oncogenic pathway in a given tumor (101,102). Both strategies hold the promise that more precise matching of the molecular profile of an individual patient's tumor with potential therapeutic alternatives will improve the success rate of targeted therapies. This process is supported by the NCI, which has awarded six grants to collaborative research groups to explore how information derived from comprehensive molecular analyses can be used to impact the care of cancer patients and ultimately improve outcome. The Strategic Partnering to Evaluate Cancer Signatures program in lung cancer will thus facilitate the development of robust and reproducible assays for specific molecular signatures that can be tested in clinical trials.

CONCLUSION

This chapter describes only selected topics regarding the therapeutic implications of lung cancer biology. We encourage the reader to take advantage of advances in other areas as well (103–106). The following chapters will discuss specific examples translating this increased knowledge to the clinic. Despite these advances, lung cancer remains a multimolecular and heterogeneous disease, both in the laboratory environment and in the clinic. It is likely that additional new technologies and new clinical trial designs capable of integrating this complexity into the treatment decision making process will be required to make further progress in this malignancy.

"The important thing in science is not so much to obtain new facts as to discover new ways of thinking about them." (William Henry Bragg, Nobel Prize in Physics 1915 with his son Lawrence, for their analysis of crystal structure by X-rays).

ACKNOWLEDGMENT

Oliver Gautschi is supported by the Swiss National Science Foundation and the Swiss Cancer League.

REFERENCES

1. Hardy PA, Zacharias H. Reappraisal of the Hansemann–Boveri hypothesis on the origin of tumors. Cell Biol Int 2005; 29(12):983–992.
2. Hecht SS. Tobacco smoke carcinogens and lung cancer. J Natl Cancer Inst 1999; 91(14):1194–1210.
3. Shields PG. Molecular epidemiology of smoking and lung cancer. Oncogene 2002; 21(45):6870–6876.
4. Martin GS. The road to Src. Oncogene 2004; 23(48):7910–7917.
5. Summy JM, Gallick GE. Treatment for advanced tumors: SRC reclaims center stage. Clin Cancer Res 2006; 12(5):1398–1401.
6. Lee D, Gautschi O. Clinical development of Src kinase inhibitors in cancer. Clin Lung Cancer 2006; 7(6):381–384.
7. Yokota J, Kohno T. Molecular footprints of human lung cancer progression. Cancer Sci 2004; 95(3):197–204.
8. Gautschi O, Gumerlock PH. Recent developments in the biology of lung cancer. In: Hansen HH, ed. Lung Cancer Therapy. 5th. ed. New York: Taylor and Francis, 2006.
9. Johnson BE, Ihde DC, Makuch RW, et al. Myc family oncogene amplification in tumor cell lines established from small cell lung cancer patients and its relationship to clinical status and course. J Clin Invest 1987; 79(6):1629–1634.

10. Berg T, Cohen SB, Desharnais J, et al. Small-molecule antagonists of *Myc*/Max dimerization inhibit *Myc*-induced transformation of chicken embryo fibroblasts. Proc Natl Acad Sci USA 2002; 99(6):3830–3835.
11. Friday BB, Adjei AA. K-ras as a target for cancer therapy. Biochim Biophys Acta 2005; 1756(2):127–144.
12. Le Calvez F, Mukeria A, Hunt JD, et al. TP53 and KRAS mutation load and types in lung cancers in relation to tobacco smoke: distinct patterns in never, former, and current smokers. Cancer Res 2005; 65(12):5076–5083.
13. Kim CF, Jackson EL, Woolfenden AE, et al. Identification of bronchioalveolar stem cells in normal lung and lung cancer. Cell 2005; 121(6):823–835.
14. Kim ES, Kies MS, Fossella FV, Tighiouart M, Rogatko A, Khuri FR. Phase II study of the farnesyltransferase inhibitor lonafarnib with paclitaxel in patients with taxane-refractory/resistant nonsmall cell lung carcinoma. Cancer 2005; 104(3):561–569.
15. Pincus MR. Development of new anti-cancer peptides from conformational energy analysis of the oncogenic ras-p21 protein and its complexes with target proteins. Front Biosci 2004; 9:3486–3509.
16. Hynes NE, Lane HA. ERBB receptors and cancer: the complexity of targeted inhibitors. Nat Rev Cancer 2005; 5(5):341–354.
17. Franklin WA, Veve R, Hirsch FR, et al. Epidermal growth factor receptor family in lung cancer and premalignancy. Semin Oncol 2002; 29(1 suppl 4):3–14.
18. Piyathilake CJ, Frost AR, Manne U, et al. Differential expression of growth factors in squamous cell carcinoma and precancerous lesions of the lung. Clin Cancer Res 2002; 8(3):734–744.
19. Hirsch FR, Varella-Garcia M, McCoy J, et al. Southwest Oncology Group. Increased epidermal growth factor receptor gene copy number detected by fluorescence in situ hybridization associates with increased sensitivity to gefitinib in patients with bronchioloalveolar carcinoma subtypes: a Southwest Oncology Group Study. J Clin Oncol 2005; 23(28):6838–6845.
20. Shigematsu H, Takahashi T, Nomura M, et al. Somatic mutations of the *HER2* kinase domain in lung adenocarcinomas. Cancer Res 2005; 65(5):1642–1646.
21. Tang X, Shigematsu H, Bekele BN, et al. EGFR tyrosine kinase domain mutations are detected in histologically normal respiratory epithelium in lung cancer patients. Cancer Res 2005; 65(17):7568–7572.
22. Greulich H, Chen TH, Feng W, et al. Oncogenic transformation by inhibitor-sensitive and -resistant EGFR mutants. PLoS Med 2005; 2(11):e313.
23. Sordella R, Bell DW, Haber DA, et al. Gefitinib-sensitizing EGFR mutations in lung cancer activate anti-apoptotic pathways. Science 2004; 305(5687):1163–1167.
24. Toyooka S, Tsuda T, Gazdar AF. The *TP53* gene, tobacco exposure, and lung cancer. Hum Mutat 2003; 21(3):229–239.
25. Poulsen TT, Pedersen N, Poulsen HS. Replacement and suicide gene therapy for targeted treatment of lung cancer. Clin Lung Cancer 2005; 6(4):227–236.
26. Kohno T, Yokota J. How many tumor suppressor genes are involved in human lung carcinogenesis? Carcinogenesis 1999; 20(8):1403–1410.
27. Zaborowski ER, Lerman MI, Minna JD. Chromosome 3 abnormalities in lung cancer. In: Pass HI, Carbone DP, Johnson DH, Minna JD, Turrisi AT, eds. Lung Cancer. 3rd ed. Philadelphia: Lippincott, Williams and Wilkins, 2005:118–134.
28. Cech TR. Beginning to understand the end of the chromosome. Cell 2004; 116(2):273–279.

29. Hiyama K, Hiyama E, Ishioka S, Yamakido M, Inai K, Gazdar AF, Piatyszek MA, Shay JW. Telomerase activity in small-cell and non–small-cell lung cancers. J Natl Cancer Inst 1995; 87(12):895–902.
30. Komiya T, Kawase I, Nitta T, et al. Prognostic significance of hTERT expression in non-small cell lung cancer. Int J Oncol 2000; 16(6):1173–1177.
31. Yim HW, Slebos RJ, Randell SH, et al. Smoking is associated with increased telomerase activity in short-term cultures of human bronchial epithelial cells. Cancer Lett 2006; 3(Epub ahead of print).
32. Damm K, Hemmann U, Garin-Chesa P, et al. A highly selective telomerase inhibitor limiting human cancer cell proliferation. EMBO J 2001; 20(24):6958–6968.
33. Dikmen ZG, Gellert GC, Jackson S, et al. In vivo inhibition of lung cancer by GRN163L: a novel human telomerase inhibitor. Cancer Res 2005; 65(17):7866–7873.
34. Sato M, Vaughan MB, Girard L, et al. Multiple oncogenic changes (K-RAS(V12), p53 knockdown, mutant EGFRs, p16 bypass, telomerase) are not sufficient to confer a full malignant phenotype on human bronchial epithelial cells. Cancer Res 2006; 66(4):2116–2128.
35. Braithwaite KL, Rabbitts PH. Multi-step evolution of lung cancer. Semin Cancer Biol 1999; 9(4):255–265.
36. Miller YE. Pathogenesis of lung cancer: 100 year report. Am J Respir Cell Mol Biol 2005; 33(3):216–223.
37. Kleihues P, Schauble B, zur Hausen A, et al. Tumors associated with p53 germline mutations: a synopsis of 91 families. Am J Pathol 1997; 150(1):1–13.
38. Liu G, Zhou W, Christiani DC. Molecular epidemiology of non–small cell lung cancer. Semin Respir Crit Care Med 2005; 26(3):265–272.
39. Gautschi O, Hugli B, Ziegler A, et al. Cyclin D1 (CCND1) A870G gene polymorphism modulates smoking-induced lung cancer risk and response to platinum-based chemotherapy in non–small cell lung cancer (NSCLC) patients. Lung Cancer 2006; 51(3):303–311.
40. Betticher DC, Thatcher N, Altermatt HJ, et al. Alternate splicing produces a novel cyclin D1 transcript. Oncogene 1995; 11(5):1005–1011.
41. Knudsen KE, Diehl, JA, Haiman CA, et al. Cyclin D1: polymorphism, aberrant splicing and cancer risk. Oncogene 2006; 25:1620–1625.
42. Ewart-Toland A, Dai Q, Gao YT, et al. Aurora-A/STK15 T+91A is a general low penetrance cancer susceptibility gene: a meta-analysis of multiple cancer types. Carcinogenesis 2005; 26(8):1368–1373.
43. Smith SL, Bowers NL, Betticher DC, et al. Overexpression of aurora B kinase (*AURKB*) in primary non–small cell lung carcinoma is frequent, generally driven from one allele, and correlates with the level of genetic instability. Br J Cancer 2005; 93(6):719–729.
44. Andrews PD. Aurora kinases: shining lights on the therapeutic horizon? Oncogene 2005; 24(32):5005–5015.
45. Herman JG. Epigenetics in lung cancer: focus on progression and early lesions. Chest 2004; 125(5 suppl):119S–122S.
46. Das PM, Singal R. DNA methylation and cancer. J Clin Oncol 2004; 22(22):4632–4642.
47. Toyooka S, Toyooka KO, Maruyama R, et al. DNA methylation profiles of lung tumors. Mol Cancer Ther 2001; 1(1):61–67.
48. Toyooka S, Suzuki M, Maruyama R, et al. The relationship between aberrant methylation and survival in non–small-cell lung cancers. Br J Cancer 2004; 91(4):771–774.

49. Hsu HS, Wen CK, Tang YA, et al. Promoter hypermethylation is the predominant mechanism in hMLH1 and hMSH2 deregulation and is a poor prognostic factor in nonsmoking lung cancer. Clin Cancer Res 2005; 11(15):5410–5416.

50. Digel W, Lubbert M. DNA methylation disturbances as novel therapeutic target in lung cancer: preclinical and clinical results. Crit Rev Oncol Hematol 2005; 55(1):1–11.

51. Hoffmann MJ, Schulz WA. Causes and consequences of DNA hypomethylation in human cancer. Biochem Cell Biol 2005; 83(3):296–321.

52. Wilson IM, Davies JJ, Weber M, et al. Epigenomics: mapping the methylome. Cell Cycle 2006; 5(2):155–158.

53. Kaminski N, Krupsky M. Gene expression patterns, prognostic and diagnostic markers, and lung cancer biology. Chest 2004; 125(5 suppl):111S–115S.

54. www.oncomine.org

55. Heighway J, Knapp T, Boyce L, et al. Expression profiling of primary non–small cell lung cancer for target identification. Oncogene 2002; 21(50):7749–7763.

56. Smith SL, Watson SG, Ratschiller D, et al. Maspin—the most commonly expressed gene of the 18q21.3 serpin cluster in lung cancer—is strongly expressed in preneoplastic bronchial lesions. Oncogene 2003; 22(54):8677–8687.

57. Smith SL, Gugger M, Hoban P, Ratschiller D, et al. S100A2 is strongly expressed in airway basal cells, preneoplastic bronchial lesions and primary non–small cell lung carcinomas. Br J Cancer 2004; 91(8):1515–1524.

58. Spira A, Beane J, Shah V, Liu G, et al. Effects of cigarette smoke on the human airway epithelial cell transcriptome. Proc Natl Acad Sci USA 2004; 101(27):10143–10148.

59. Parmigiani G, Garrett-Mayer ES, Anbazhagan R, et al. A cross-study comparison of gene expression studies for the molecular classification of lung cancer. Clin Cancer Res 2004; 10(9):2922–2927.

60. Beer DG, Kardia SL, Huang CC, et al. Gene-expression profiles predict survival of patients with lung adenocarcinoma. Nat. Med 2002:8(8):816–824.

61. Croce CM, Calin GA. miRNAs, cancer, and stem cell division. Cell 2005; 122(1):6–7.

62. Johnson SM, Grosshans H, Shingara J, et al. RAS is regulated by the let-7 microRNA family. Cell 2005; 120(5):635–647.

63. Takamizawa J, Konishi H, Yanagisawa K, et al. Reduced expression of the let-7 microRNAs in human lung cancers in association with shortened postoperative survival. Cancer Res 2004; 64(11):3753–3756.

64. Yanaihara N, Caplen N, Bowman E, et al. Unique microRNA molecular profiles in lung cancer diagnosis and prognosis. Cancer Cell 2006; 9(3):189–198.

65. www.microrna.org

66. Jiang J, Lee EJ, Schmittgen TD. Increased expression of microRNA-155 in Epstein–Barr virus transformed lymphoblastoid cell lines. Genes Chromosomes Cancer 2006; 45(1):103–106.

67. Hayashita Y, Osada H, Tatematsu Y, et al. A polycistronic microRNA cluster, miR-17-92, is overexpressed in human lung cancers and enhances cell proliferation. Cancer Res 2005; 65(21):9628–9632.

68. Volinia S, Calin GA, Liu CG, et al. A microRNA expression signature of human solid tumors defines cancer gene targets. Proc Natl Acad Sci USA 2006; 103(7):2257–2261.

69. Eder M, Scherr M. MicroRNA and lung cancer. N Engl J Med 2005; 352(23):2446–2448.

70. Krutzfeldt J, Rajewsky N, Braich R, et al. Silencing of microRNAs in vivo with 'antagomirs'. Nature 2005; 438(7068):685–689.
71. Meyerson M, Carbone D. Genomic and proteomic profiling of lung cancers: lung cancer classification in the age of targeted therapy. J Clin Oncol 2005; 23(14): 3219–3226.
72. Fan TW, Lane AN, Higashi RM. The promise of metabolomics in cancer molecular therapeutics. Curr Opin Mol Ther 2004; 6(6):584–592.
73. Marx J. Medicine: a signal contribution to cell biology. Science 1992; 258(5082): 542–543.
74. Fischer EH, Charbonneau H, Tonks NK. Protein tyrosine phosphatases: a diverse family of intracellular and transmembrane enzymes. Science 1991; 253(5018):401–406.
75. Vlahovic G, Crawford J. Activation of tyrosine kinases in cancer. Oncologist 2003; 8(6):531–538.
76. Burgess AW, Cho HS, Eigenbrot C, et al. An open-and-shut case? Recent insights into the activation of EGF/ErbB receptors. Mol Cell 2003; 12(3):541–552.
77. Li S, Schmitz KR, Jeffrey PD, et al. Structural basis for inhibition of the epidermal growth factor receptor by cetuximab. Cancer Cell 2005; 7(4):301–311.
78. Scagliotti G. Proteasome inhibitors in lung cancer. Crit Rev Oncol Hematol 2006; 58(3):177–189.
79. Lara PN Jr, Bold RJ, Mack PC, et al. Proteasome inhibition in small-cell lung cancer: preclinical rationale and clinical applications. Clin Lung Cancer 2005; 7(suppl 2): S67–S71.
80. Davies AM, Lara PN Jr, Mack PC, et al. Bortezomib-based combinations in the treatment of non–small-cell lung cancer. Clin Lung Cancer 2005; 7(suppl 2):S59–S63.
81. Brambilla E, Travis WD, Colby TV, et al. The new World Health Organization classification of lung tumours. Eur Respir J 2001; 18(6):1059–1068.
82. Johnson DH, Fehrenbacher L, Novotny WF, et al. Randomized phase II trial comparing bevacizumab plus carboplatin and paclitaxel with carboplatin and paclitaxel alone in previously untreated locally advanced or metastatic non–small-cell lung cancer. J Clin Oncol 2004; 22(11):2184–2191.
83. Miller VA, Hirsch FR, Johnson DH. Systemic therapy of advanced bronchioloalveolar cell carcinoma: challenges and opportunities. J Clin Oncol 2005; 23(14):3288–3293.
84. Haneda H, Sasaki H, Lindeman N, et al. A Correlation between EGFR gene mutation status and bronchioloalveolar carcinoma features in Japanese patients with adenocarcinoma. Jpn J Clin Oncol 2006; 36(2):69–75.
85. West H, Franklin WA, Gumerlock PH, et al. Gefitinib (ZD1839) therapy for advanced bronchioloalveolar lung cancer (BAC): Southwest Oncology Group (SWOG) Study S0126. Proc Am Soc Clin Oncol 2004; 23:7014.
86. Bell DW, Gore I, Okimoto RA, et al. Inherited susceptibility to lung cancer may be associated with the T790M drug resistance mutation in EGFR. Nat Genet 2005; 37(12):1315–1316.
87. Asamura H, Kameya T, Matsuno Y, et al. Neuroendocrine neoplasms of the lung: a prognostic spectrum. J Clin Oncol 2006; 24(1):70–76.
88. Krug LM, Crapanzano JP, Azzoli CG, et al. Imatinib mesylate lacks activity in small cell lung carcinoma expressing c-kit protein: a phase II clinical trial. Cancer 2005; 103(10):2128–2131.
89. Boldrini L, Ursino S, Gisfredi S, et al. Expression and mutational status of c-kit in small-cell lung cancer: prognostic relevance. Clin Cancer Res 2004; 10(12 Pt 1):4101–4108.

90. Yeh JJ, Hsu NY, Hsu WH, et al. Comparison of chemotherapy response with P-glyco-protein, multidrug resistance-related protein-1, and lung resistance-related protein expression in untreated small cell lung cancer. Lung 2005; 183(3):177–183.

91. Ozben T. Mechanisms and strategies to overcome multiple drug resistance in cancer. FEBS Lett 2006 (Epub).

92. Belyanskaya LL, Hopkins-Donaldson S, Kurtz S, et al. Cisplatin activates Akt in small cell lung cancer cells and attenuates apoptosis by survivin upregulation. Int J Cancer 2005; 117(5):755–763.

93. Singhal S, Vachani A, Antin-Ozerkis D, et al. Prognostic implications of cell cycle, apoptosis, and angiogenesis biomarkers in non–small cell lung cancer: a review. Clin Cancer Res 2005; 11(11):3974–3986.

94. Davies AM, Mack PC, Lara PN, et al. Predictive molecular markers: Has the time come for routine use in lung cancer. J Natl Comp Cancer Net 2004; 2(2):125–131.

95. Bremnes RM, Sirera R, Camps C. Circulating tumour-derived DNA and RNA markers in blood: a tool for early detection, diagnostics, and follow-up? Lung Cancer 2005; 49(1):1–12.

96. Ando M, Hasegawa Y, Ando Y. Pharmacogenetics of irinotecan: a promoter polymorphism of UGT1A1 gene and severe adverse reactions to irinotecan. Invest New Drugs 2005; 23(6):539–545.

97. Beutler E, Gelbart T, Demina A. Racial variability in the UDP-glucuronosyltransferase 1 (UGT1A1) promoter: a balanced polymorphism for regulation of bilirubin metabolism? Proc Natl Acad Sci USA 1998; 95(14):8170–8174.

98. Noda K, Nishiwaki Y, Kawahara M, et al; Japan Clinical Oncology Group. Irinotecan plus cisplatin compared with etoposide plus cisplatin for extensive small-cell lung cancer. N Engl J Med 2002; 346(2):85–91.

99. Paez JG, Janne PA, Lee JC, et al. EGFR mutations in lung cancer: correlation with clinical response to gefitinib therapy. Science 2004; 304(5676):1497–1500.

100. Lynch TJ, Bell DW, Sordella R, et al. Activating mutations in the epidermal growth factor receptor underlying responsiveness of non–small-cell lung cancer to gefitinib. N Engl J Med 2004; 350(21):2129–2139.

101. Solit DB, Garraway LA, Pratilas CA, et al. BRAF mutation predicts sensitivity to MEK inhibition. Nature 2006; 439(7074):358–362.

102. Bild AH, Yao G, Chang JT, et al. Oncogenic pathway signatures in human cancers as a guide to targeted therapies. Nature 2006; 439(7074):353–357.

103. Whitesell L, Lindquist SL. HSP90 and the chaperoning of cancer. Nat Rev Cancer 2005; 5(10):761–772.

104. Silva CM. Role of STATs as downstream signal transducers in Src family kinase-mediated tumorigenesis. Oncogene 2004; 23(48):8017–8023.

105. Dasari V, Gallup M, Lemjabbar H, Maltseva I, McNamara N. Epithelial-mesenchymal transition in lung cancer: is tobacco the "Smoking Gun"? Am J Respir Cell Mol Biol 2006; 35(1):3–9.

106. Polyak K, Hahn WC. Roots and stems: stem cells in cancer. Nat Med 2006; 12(3):296–300.

2

Early Clinical Trial Design Issues: Patient Populations, End Points, and Barriers

Janet E. Dancey

Division of Cancer Treatment and Diagnosis, National Cancer Institute, Rockville, Maryland, U.S.A.

INTRODUCTION

Considerable research efforts within the basic, translational, and clinical fields have contributed greatly in defining how specific alterations in normal cellular functions lead to the development and progression of cancer phenotype. These insights have led to the subsequent identification and the development of effective cancer therapies. However, developing agents that inhibit specific abnormalities within the cancer cell may add complexity to therapeutics development compared to traditional cancer chemotherapy: the optimal dose may not be the most toxic, tumor regression may not occur, reliable surrogate biomarkers of true clinical benefit are not available, and benefit may be limited to a small percentage of patients (1). Thus, while there have been significant advances in understanding cancer biology and potential targets for therapeutics development, there remain significant challenges to efficiently developing cancer target–specific agents. The purpose of this chapter is to highlight the strengths and limitations of the clinical trial strategies used to develop targeted cancer therapies to date and to provide alternatives strategies for future research endeavors.

EARLY PHASE TRIALS OF CANCER THERAPEUTICS

Phase-1 Clinical Trials of Targeted Agents

The primary goal of phase-1 first-in-man studies is to define the recommended dose of a new drug in the schedule(s) tested for subsequent study (2–4). Secondary goals of these trials include the following: (*i*) description of the type, severity, reversibility, and dose dependency of the adverse effects of the agent; (*ii*) determination of the pharmacokinetics (PK) of the drug; (*iii*) description of any observed objective antitumor effects; and (*iv*) assessment of dose-related (or PK-related) pharmacodynamic (PD) effects in normal tissue and tumor by a number of measures. For cytotoxic drugs, the recommended dose corresponds to the highest dose associated with an acceptable level of toxicity and is derived from clinical data and preclinical dose–toxicity and dose–activity studies. However, targeted, so-called "noncytotoxic" therapies as anticancer agents may challenge the traditional phase-1 study paradigm in a variety of ways (2–6). Alternatives to toxicity as an end point for phase-1 dose-escalation trials evaluating noncytotoxic therapies can include measurement of target inhibition and/or PK analysis.

Although there are a variety of designs used to conduct first-in-man phase-1 trials (2,5–7), they have in common several features: selection of a "safe" starting dose, sequential dose escalation in cohorts of patients, and determination of a recommended dose based on a prespecified primary end point. Good phase-1 designs lead to a relatively accurate determination of the recommended dose in a manner that is both safe and efficient: minimal numbers of patients are exposed to doses of drug that are likely to be excessively toxic or subtherapeutic. Once the dose/schedule of interest is preliminarily identified, this dose or doses may be evaluated in an expanded cohort of patients representative of those likely to receive the drug in phase-2 trials. This expanded cohort allows for increased confidence in the safety and appropriateness of the final recommended dose.

Normally, cancer patients for whom no curative or standard therapy remains are enrolled in first-in-man phase-1 trials of new anticancer agents. Toxicity is often the primary end point of these studies and doses are escalated from what is thought to be minimally toxic dose to the maximum tolerated dose (MTD), that is, one that is associated with significant but reversible toxicity. Targeted agents that are minimally toxic provide for some opportunities and challenges to the traditional study population and end points of phase-1 cancer drug trials (1). Because the MTD may not be achieved with these agents, there has been a greater utilization of different study populations, and a greater emphasis on PK and PD end points in phase-1 studies of these agents.

First-in-man studies of targeted agents that are predicted to be minimally or nontoxic may be tested in healthy volunteers. This strategy has been used for some cancer drugs such as certain hormonal agents epidermal growth factor receptor (EGFR) inhibitors, and metalloproteinase inhibitors (MMPI) (8–10). Such agents have either a known spectrum of toxicity that is minimal and reversible and/or preclinical toxicology evaluations that indicate that there are limited adverse effects and thus the agents are unlikely to be harmful in healthy volunteers. Healthy volunteer studies start at lower doses than might be used in cancer patients (usually a fraction of the dose in animals associated with no obvious adverse effects rather than 1/10 the murine lethal dose in 10% of animals) and involve only limited dosing in subjects to limit risk of adverse effects. The primary goal of such studies may be to determine preliminarily the pharmacology of the agent prior to finalizing the initial dose/schedule for more protracted phase-1 trials in cancer patient, which would be conducted to determine a recommended dose.

Normal volunteer studies provide some information relating to PK and safety that may assist in dose/schedule selection; however, these studies alone may not be sufficient to determine recommended doses for phase-2 cancer trials. The degree of toxicity considered "acceptable" or "tolerable" varies between cancer patients and normal volunteers. In addition, PK may be different between healthy volunteers and cancer patients as was seen with MMPI marimastat (9,10). Thus, phase-1 studies in healthy volunteers may precede a phase-1 study in cancer patients that could explore higher doses and dosing of a longer duration, but they are not an alternative for phase-1 study of a new agent in cancer patients as a higher level of toxicity may be considered acceptable and PK may be different.

The purpose of phase-1 trial is to identify a dose/schedule for further evaluation; thus, the end points of the trial should determine decisions about dose escalation and dose recommendation. Toxicity, PK, and PD may all be useful end points to making these decisions. PKs of a drug are "what the body does to the drug" and include assessing concentration, exposure, volume of distribution, and clearance. PD effects are "what the drug does to the body," so these can include things such as toxic effects and clinical antitumor effects (11). For targeted agents, assays and technologies to determine the molecular and imaging changes in tissues are increasingly being used to assess effect of drug on target and, as a result, these types of studies are often referred to as "pharmacodynamic measures." While not all phase-1 first-in-man studies include such PD measures, these end points may be used in trials of targeted, noncytotoxic agents (12). Such assays of drug effects on purported target in normal or tumor tissues may assist in the selection of a biologically active dose/schedule. Ideally, phase-1 clinical trials of agents that inhibit tumor targets, which may be minimally toxic and cytostatic, would be designed to identify a dose/schedule that is associated with acceptable toxicity and appropriate target modulation in tumor.

Although there has been a greater emphasis in developing assays to assess PD effects in tissues, toxicity remains one of the most important and commonly used end points in phase-1 cancer drug trials. Similar to traditional cytotoxic agents, it is clear that targeted agents may induce target-specific toxic effects that correlate with dose-related inhibition of target in normal tissues. Such effects are likely to also correlate with target inhibition in tumor and, subsequently, antitumor effects. If target inhibition is associated with a target-specific toxicity such as has been seen with rash, EGFR (13), hypertension, and vascular endothelial growth factor receptor (14) inhibitors, toxicity remains a relevant PD effect of target modulation and may be utilized as an end point to support the selection of an appropriate dose.

The assessment of the dose and/or PK-dependent effects of the agent on target in tissue and by functional imaging provide proof of principle for the agent/target and measure of assurance that appropriate doses/schedules are carried forward for further clinical trial evaluations. Such PD biomarkers may be particularly useful if there is a known target for the agent, a robust assay for the target and its modulation, no toxicity, toxicity that is related to nontarget effects such that the degree of target modulation is uncertain, or if there is a particular need to dose to a specified level of functional inhibition of target but not exceed it to avoid severe toxicity. The requirements for biomarker studies in phase-1 trials are summarized in Table 1.

Although the rationale for utilizing PD biomarkers to assess target modulation by agent is compelling, in trials of targeted agents conducted to date, toxicity and PK continue to be the major determinants of dose escalation and dose recommendation (19). Attempts to assess other measures have clearly been made in many trials, and results from these tests frequently have supported the dose recommendation made on the basis of toxicity and/or PK.

There are a number of reason why PD biomarkers have not been used despite the compelling rationale for selecting dose/schedule based on the demonstration of target inhibition. First, the development of assays/technologies to assess the PD effects on target is often slower than the development of the agent. Thus, few targeted agents have been developed utilizing well-characterized and robust assays to measure PD effects of the agent. Second, there are practical constraints to repeated sampling of tumors and normal tissue or in conducting expensive imaging evaluations (20,21). Finally, assessment of toxicity must be

Table 1   Phase-1 Trial Requirements for Target Modulation Biomarker

Parameter	Requirements
Agent	Acceptable preclinical activity, toxicology, pharmacology, known target
Assay	Well-characterized assay
	% change in target or target level associated with efficacy
	Concentration/exposure required for target effect
	Time course for effect on target, duration, recovery
	Threshold of detection and coefficient of variability of target measurements
	Target effect on tumor vs. other surrogate tissues
Specimens	Collection, processing, shipping, storage effects known/optimized
Patients	Tissues have relevant target and are amenable to repeated sampling
Examples	Methyl guanine methyl transferase activity and O^6-Benzylquanine (15)
	20S Proteasome activity and Bortezomib (16,17)
	Dynamic contrast-enhanced magnetic resonance imaging and PTK787/ZK (valatanib) (18)

done as part of first-in-man studies, it is a familiar end point to clinical investigators, and toxicity may be related to target inhibition. Given the above, it is not surprising that the standard primary end point for phase-1 trials of targeted agents remains toxicity. To administer the drug in the highest tolerable dose in subsequent phase-2 and phase-3 studies also ensures that it is unlikely that antitumor activity would be missed, since it is unlikely that higher but tolerable doses would be less effective than lower doses (19).

If there is no known target-specific assay or specific toxicity, or if toxicity is related to nontarget effects, alternative means need to be used to determine recommended dose for further studies. One parameter that is frequently utilized is the achievement of specific plasma concentrations or exposures that correlate with activity in preclinical models. However, differences between in vitro and animal model pharmacology, plasma protein binding, and tissue sensitivity compared to that of humans may lead to erroneous assumptions regarding the desired concentration/exposures that are biologically relevant in cancer patients (22). The limitations in extrapolating from preclinical nonhuman models to humans are such that the absence of having robust assays to assess effects of agent on purported target in tumor specimens in phase 1 may lead to drugs failing simply through lack of optimization of dose and schedule to achieve biologically relevant target inhibition.

One phase-1 study design used for relatively nontoxic-targeted agents is to establish a dosing range using toxicity (or measures of blood levels, if toxic effects do not occur) in a standard phase 1 rules for cohort sizes and dose-escalation steps (23). Once the desired dose/dose range is established, an expanded cohort or subsequent phase-1B trial(s) in more homogenous group of patients would be conducted to assess small range of doses, for example, the toxicity-recommended dose and one or two levels below it that fall within the presumed biologically active dose range. In this second study or expanded cohort of patients, molecular effects on normal or malignant tumor lesions could be measured or functional imaging undertaken and PK studies done to narrow down the dose based on assessment of the PD and their relationship to PK measures (19). This approach is illustrated in Figure 1.

The prerequisites for a phase-1 trial that incorporates assessment of the effect of agent on target are greater than for traditional phase-1 study. Additional preclinical experiments are needed for optimization of target assay(s) to ensure accuracy, reliability, to define the degree of target modulation of interest, and to demonstrate the correlation between target effect and tumor activity. The number of patients required for such a phase-1 study would be greater and the patient population may be restricted to those who have tissues or tumor features to assess PD effects (19). The numbers and types of samples and dosing schema may vary with the specific agent, PD end point, desired target effect of interest, and assay variability. Efficiency in the execution of the study may be improved if assessment of biomarkers in tumor is initiated after reaching doses associated with drug

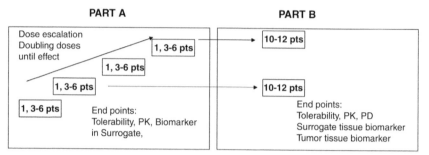

Figure 1 Phase-1 first-in-human study of a novel-targeted agent. Considerations in the design of the phase-1 study should include: (*i*) whether the agent is likely to cause dose-limiting toxicity and whether toxicity is directly related to target inhibition; (*ii*) whether pharmacokinetics (PKs) from preclinical models may be used to determine concentration/ exposure that may be biologically active; and (*iii*) whether there is a pharmacodynamic (PD) marker that may be used to assess target modulation surrogate and/or tumor tissue. Phase 1A of the study includes dose escalation to define dosing range. During the initial dose escalations, an accelerated titration design with one patient or three cohorts could be used until an effect of interest is noted. This effect might be toxicity, PK, or PD effect in either surrogate or tumor tissues. Once the effect of interest is identified, larger cohorts of patients (three to six or more) per dose level could be accrued to refine the effect of dose on these endpoints. Phase-1B evaluations with expanded cohorts would refine dose(s)/ schedule(s) that are of interest and more comprehensively assess biomarker assays, PK, and toxicity. If more than one dose/schedule is assessed, patients may be randomized between selected doses and schedules. *Source*: From Ref. 23.

concentrations/exposures that are consistent with efficacious levels in preclinical models and modulation is seen in more readily assessable surrogate tissue samples. If target toxicity is anticipated, dose-escalation decisions may be determined based on this end point and biomarker effects can provide support for proof of concept and go/no go decisions. Whether PD biomarkers provide primary or supportive data for decisions depends on the level of confidence in the measurement of target effect and the correlation between effect and drug activity.

In summary, the end points of phase-1 dose-escalation studies of targeted agents include not only the traditional end points of identifying an appropriate dose/schedule, safety, and PK, but also the demonstration of achieving concentrations/exposures consistent with antitumor efficacy in preclinical models and, when feasible, appropriate target modulation in surrogate or, preferably, tumor tissue. These evaluations in initial phase-1 trials provide assurance that a biologically active dose/schedule is identified for subsequent trials designed to evaluate the agent's antitumor activity. If there is uncertainty about the validity of the PD biomarker end points, the observation of toxic effects, particularly those that may be due to a target-specific effect of the drug in normal tissue, can allow a reasonable means of making dose decisions. Dosing to toxicity makes it unlikely that the doses selected will be too low. Other measures such as imaging changes, blood levels of drug, and molecular changes in sampled tissues provide proof of principle that the drug does what it was intended to do and provide supportive data for dosing decisions.

Phase-2 Clinical Trials

Phase-2 clinical trials of cancer therapies are designed to preliminarily assess antitumor activity and to more thoroughly define the nature of toxicities in a selected cancer patient population (24–32). There are four key aspects to consider in the design of a phase-2 cancer clinical trial: (*i*) the selection of end points; (*ii*) the patient population for evaluation; (*iii*) the determination of a level of activity that would justify a phase-3 trial; and (*iv*) the level of certainty around the outcome, that is, the statistical significance and power of the trial to detect the desired level of activity. The sample size required for the study to meet these objectives depends on magnitude of effect of interest and level of certainty that the result is a fairly precise estimate of the "true" effect. The development of targeted agents that are predominately cytostatic, and, perhaps, only active in subsets of patients with tumors that have molecularly defined dependency on the target for growth or survival are two additional considerations that may impact on phase-2 trial design (33,34). To address the former, novel end points that incorporate tumor/disease stability and more modest degrees of tumor regression into end point definitions (35,36), evaluations of sequential measures of time to disease progression in patients (28), novel imaging modalities (37,38), and randomized trials utilizing time to progression end points (27,29,32,39) are more commonly used in phase-2 trials. For the latter, considerable research efforts have been focused on designing trials that identify and enrich the study population for those patients thought most likely to benefit (36).

Traditional cytotoxics induce tumor regression, which is not typically seen in the absence of drug-induced antitumor effects. Because spontaneous regression is rare in cancer patients, trials of cytotoxic agents have used objective tumor response as the primary end point and have not required a concurrent control arm. It has been argued that newer noncytotoxic agents, which will perhaps control tumor growth rather than cause objective response, may need different end points to screen for efficacy in phase-2 trials. Response to treatment in solid tumor criteria (41) were modeled on older objective response criteria where partial responses in particular were identified as a "marker" of agents that might be effective in improving survival. Objective response may not be an applicable outcome measure for new agents that do not cause tumor regression but are able to provide clinical benefit. For example, these criteria do not consider durable modest regressions or prolonged disease stability as activity, even though such activity has been shown to correlate with improved survival with several agents such as erlotinib (42), sorafenib (36,43), and bevacizumab (43). On the other hand, drugs may erroneously be defined as active on the basis of stable disease, since stable disease is a composite outcome consisting of inherent tumor growth kinetics and potential drug effect (35) Although cytostatic agents may provide durable stable disease, such agents do not necessarily require new response criteria. Response criteria simply provide definitions to categorize objective assessments of the change in tumor size over time. The criteria themselves do not declare what level of response, duration of stable disease, or rate of progression-free survival should "signal" that a new agent has activity worth pursuing further. End points in which the composite of response and stable disease of prolonged duration or remaining progression-free for a minimum period of time can continue to be used. Use of these end points does not require new response criteria. Rather, better clinical trial designs and new insights to determine the end point of interest, and frequency of occurrence of the end point to warrant further clinical development of an agent are required (44,45).

Assessments of functional measures of tumor metabolism, blood flow, and other parameters are now possible with positron emission tomography (PET), magnetic resonance imaging, and computer tomography (37,38). Such techniques may supplement, and eventually supplant, measures of change in anatomical tumor size as the preferred means of assessing antitumor activity of an agent. Studies to date suggest that alterations in blood flow or vascular permeability assessed radiologically may assist in the dose selection of vascular agents (18) and fluorodeoxyglucose-PET changes may occur considerably earlier in certain situations such as with imatinib in patients with gastrointestinal stromal tumors (46) than occur with anatomical imaging. While there will remain a place for objective anatomical tumor response as an end point for some time in the future, the added value (or perhaps even the replacement value) of functional changes in tumor metabolism, blood flow, or other functional imaging studies requires further evaluation to standardize the description of results of trials that incorporate these measures and to determine the settings in which these modalities are most useful for drug development and patient care (37,38).

Because cytostatic drugs may be erroneously defined as active on the basis of stable disease rate in an uncontrolled trial, as stable disease may be due to either inherent tumor growth kinetics or potential drug effect (35), there has been a much greater emphases on utilizing randomized controlled trials to evaluate the potential antitumor effects of these agents. Randomized phase-2 studies may be of particular value when an agent is not anticipated to induce tumor regression. To accurately assess rates of disease stabilization or progression-free survival in the study population of interest may require randomizing patients to experimental agent versus placebo. In addition, randomized phase-2 studies may be of value when combining new agents with active therapeutic regimens. Finally, randomized phase-2 studies may assist in selecting different doses/schedules of an agent, different agents, or different regimens that are of potential interest for phase-3 evaluation. In each of these situations, assessing single-agent activity versus placebo using disease stability, assessing addition of the agent to an active regimen, and assessing the activities of multiple agents, doses/schedules, randomization between arms assist in defining the "true" merits of the experimental therapy. However, the phase-2 clinical trial designs differ for each of these situations (Table 2).

Table 2 A Limited Selection of Randomized Phase-2 Trial Designs

Design	Summary	Strengths	Weakness	References
Randomized discontinua-tion design	Patients receive agent of interest for a defined period (run-in period); subsequently those with stable disease are randomized to continue with the agent or placebo (evaluation period) and assessed for the outcome of interest postrandomization	Minimize use of placebo Greater acceptance of random-ization to placebo after run-in period Minimize effect of poor compliance and drop-outs from treatment side effects on sample size Population enriched for end point of interest Number of patients may be less than in the phase-3 trial	Overall number of patients similar to phase-3 trial May classify a drug with short effect as inactive Not appropriate if drug has "carryover" effect Ethical concern of randomizing patients with stable disease Limited value if agent produces objective responses May be difficult to extrapolate effect what may be seen in the general population	(25,44,45,56)
Phase-2 designs with a reference arm	The experimental arm compared against historic controls Reference arm is a "check" to compare to historical data	Relatively small sample size required as the arms are not formally compared	Small sample size has limited power for comparison between arms and may fail to identify an experimental regimen with only moderate improvement over standard therapy If the check "fails," the trial would not be easily interpretable	(46)

(Continued)

Table 2 A Limited Selection of Randomized Phase-2 Trial Designs (*Continued*)

Design	Summary	Strengths	Weakness	References
Phase-2/3 design	The standard + agent vs. standard Results of phase 2 determine continuing to phase 3 To preserve power this design allows 50 probability of continuing under the null hypothesis	Moving from phase 2 to phase 3 within one protocol Patients in phase 2 included in phase-3 analysis	High false-positive allowed for phase 2	(51)
Selection design	Designed to evaluate 2 or more experimental regimens Comparison is to historical control If both regimens are active but only one regimen can be carried forward, the "winner" is chosen by considering response rates, toxicity, cost, quality of life, etc.	Greater comparability of patients than if there were two independent phase-2 trials Useful to prioritize multiple experimental regimens, or doses, schedules of an agent	Comparison against historic controls might be unconvincing Not to be used to compare the standard + agent vs. standard alone, it has a high false-positive rate	(52)
Screening design	Nondefinitive comparison of agent + standard vs. standard False-positive and negative rates are adjusted to limit the sample size Avoid compromising the ability to conduct a definitive phase-3 trial by using a surrogate end point for efficacy, i.e., PFS and ORR	Provides a reasonably accurate assessment of agent + standard vs. standard for surrogate end point	The trial design does not allow a definitive answer regarding benefit due to small size and surrogate end point It may compromise the ability to conduct definitive phase-3 trial	(32)

Abbreviations: ORR, objective response rate; PFS, progression-free survival.

Randomized phase-2 trials are particularly valuable when the single-agent activity is being assessed and end point of interest is a measure of prolonged disease stability, or when the agent is combined with an active therapy regardless of whether the end point of interest is objective response rate or a measure of stable disease. In these two settings, an apparent improvement in tumor response rate or tumor progression in the study population may be related to tumor biology or patient demographic features independent of any additive antitumor effect of the new agent. If there is greater variability in tumor or patient biology on prognosis than the anticancer effect of the agent, the results of uncontrolled phase-2 trials may be misleading when compared to historical controls. Thus, evaluating the effect of an agent in inducing tumor growth arrest or the additional contribution of a new agent to an active regimen compared to historical control may lead to erroneous conclusions in an uncontrolled trial. In these situations, randomized designs between experimental agent (or agent + standard treatment) and control may more accurately define improvements in outcome that are related to the antitumor effect of the agent of interest.

Randomized phase-2 trials with an appropriate control arm may yield a more accurate assessment of the experimental therapies (52). Randomized phase-2 designs may reduce biases that stymie comparisons to historical data and reduce selection bias if multiple agents/regimens of interest need evaluation, increasing confidence in the accuracy of the study results. However, randomized phase-2 studies do not eliminate the risk of a false result as they generally use a surrogate end point for patient benefit and are too small to yield a definitive result (32). Thus, a randomized phase-2 study does not obviate the need for a subsequent phase-3 randomized trial to more definitively assess clinically relevant outcomes.

There are a number of randomized phase-2 designs that have been proposed. Some of the most frequently cited are (*i*) the randomized discontinuation design (29,47,48), (*ii*) the phase-2 design with reference arm (50), (*iii*) the phase-2/3 design, (*iv*) the phase-2 selection design (52), and (*v*) the phase-2 screening design (32). A full discussion of these designs, their applications, strengths, and weakness is beyond the scope of this chapter. However, brief summary of these designs and relevant references are provided in Table 2.

In summary, among the factors to be considered in designing a phase-2 study are (*i*) the anticipated activity of the agent/combination; (*ii*) the patient population of interest; (*iii*) the resources available to support the study; (*iv*) whether the outcome with standard therapy is very well defined such that there is a good historical control database; and (*v*) whether objective response rate is the end point of interest. If the agent is likely to induce objective responses and is being assessed in a setting for which no or limited therapeutic options exist, a conventional single arm phase-2 design is reasonable (53,54). If the agent has substantial activity and can be safely combined with standard therapy, then phase-2 evaluations may not be necessary and a phase-3 clinical trial may be justified. If there are multiple agents, doses/schedules, or regimens that need to be evaluated to determine the best experimental arm for a phase-3 trial, then selection or "pick the winner" phase-2 design may be most efficient. If the comparison of interest is between standard + new agent versus standard, a screening design may be useful. However, for all phase-2 studies, consideration should be given to not only selecting a design that will best define the level of activity, but also one which will define the patient population likely to benefit from the targeted agent.

STRATEGIES TO SELECT PATIENTS FOR PHASE-2 AND PHASE-3 TRIALS OF MOLECULARLY TARGETED THERAPIES

Traditionally, cancer agents have been evaluated for their activity in patients populations that have been selected based on histology and tumor stage. However, targets of newer agents may not be present or relevant within all histologically similar tumors and may well be relevant across tumor histologies (1). As a result, a trial that evaluates the activity of the agent in a patient population defined solely by tumor histology and stage may miss significant clinical benefit to the subset of patients with tumors that are sensitive based on specific molecularly defined abnormalities within the target or target pathway of the agent (34). Thus, benefit to subgroup of patients may be masked by lack of benefit to the larger group.

Defining the features that determine sensitivity and/or resistance to an agent is important for the following reasons: it may improve the efficiency of drug development and it may assist in selecting the right treatment for the right patient. The size of trial to assess the antitumor activity of an agent in patients that are not enriched for the presence of features that may correlate with sensitivity depends on the magnitude of the drug effect and the proportion of patients with tumors "sensitive" to the agent (34). If only a relatively small proportion of patients have tumors that are sensitive to the agent, even a relatively large treatment benefit may be missed (34). Thus, the identification of the patients with tumors sensitive to the agent or elimination of patients with tumors insensitive to the agent may improve both the efficiency of the clinical evaluation and the selection of treatment among various options available to individual patients.

The ability to identify predictive biomarkers that correlate with treatment outcome to an individual agent has been limited. The biomarker of interest must be relevant to the stage of disease and to the agent's mechanism of action and be measurable. Lack of knowledge regarding the target function, the mechanism of action of the agent, and technological difficulties in developing robust assays have all contributed to the limited numbers of predictive markers for targeted agents identified to date. Even with better understanding of molecular biology of the target and mechanism of action of the agent, individual markers may not be perfect predictors of patient benefit as disease and patient-related factors may impair drug action on target and/or tumor responsiveness to target inhibition may be variable. However, several good predictive biomarkers to enrich study populations and to select treatments for patients have been identified and are summarized in Table 3.

Selection of patients likely to benefit (or elimination of those least likely to benefit) for a trial evaluating the activity of a specific agent depends on a number

Table 3 Examples of Predictive Biomarkers

Biomarker	Tumor type	Agent
Validated and used prospectively to select treatments		
Estrogen/progesterone receptor	Breast cancer	Antiestrogen therapies (55,56)
HER2 amplification	Breast cancer	Trastuzumab (57,58), lapatinib (59)
Retrospectively identified		
EGFR polysomy and mutation	Non–small cell lung cancer	Erlotinib, gefitinib (60–62)
Oncotype DX recurrence score	Breast cancer	Chemotherapy (63)
C-kit mutations	Gastrointestinal stromal tumor	Imatinib, sunitinib (64,65)
Bcr-Abl mutations	Chronic myelogenous leukemia	Imatinib, dasatinib (66,67)

a factors, the most important of which is whether there is a candidate biomarker, which can be used to enrich the proposed study population. If there is a predictive biomarker, then the additional factors to consider are (*i*) the treatment effect across patient subsets; (*ii*) the prevalence of the subset of patients with "sensitive" disease; and (*iii*) performance characteristics of the assay (i.e., sensitivity/ specificity/predictive value) that may be used in the proposed clinical trial.

Assuming that there is a candidate biomarker predictive of treatment outcome, clinical trials may be designed to either prospectively or retrospectively evaluate for treatment effects within the biomarker-defined groups. When used prospectively, the biomarker result is determined prior to patients enrolling on the study. The advantages of this approach are that the trial would require the fewest numbers of patients, assuming only patients with tumors that have the biomarker are enrolled, and the trial would be guaranteed to have sufficient power to show treatment effect in marker-defined group. The disadvantages of this approach are readily evident: the biomarker must be known, the assay must be available to select patients, and there must be rapid turnaround for testing for the biomarker to determine patient eligibility. The effects of the agent within biomarker-defined groups may also be determined retrospectively. The advantages of retrospective evaluation are that accrual to the study may proceed more rapidly, the biomarker and assay need not be available at the start of the trial, thus allowing refinement of marker/assay while the trial is ongoing, and antitumor effects of the agent may be readily assessed in patients with tumors that express and do not express the biomarker. The disadvantages of relying on retrospective evaluation are that there may be insufficient numbers within marker group(s) due to significant differences in the prevalence of the biomarker expression within patients, and the collection of samples compromised due to incomplete submission or suboptimal handling of specimens.

There are several factors to be considered for designing phase-2 trials that incorporate a predictive biomarker to enrich study population. If patients are to be preselected, there must be a marker that appears to be predictive of antitumor effect of the agent. The strength of supporting data demonstrating the correlation between biomarker and antitumor activity must therefore be compelling. The prevalence of expression of predictive marker in human cancers should be known. There must be a robust assay to identify the marker of interest, thus assay accuracy and reliability must be understood and, preferably, sensitivity, specificity, and predictive value be known. If treatment benefit is limited to a particular subset of patients, that is relatively uncommon, and the available assay has good sensitivity, specificity, and predictive value, then screening of patients to determine eligibility for a trial of a target agent is an efficient strategy to limit the overall size of the trial and to maximize the chances of a successful outcome. However, if treatment effect within marker-defined subgroups of patients is uncertain, the patient subset is very common, or the assay predictive value is questionable, upfront screening may not be optimal strategy (68).

Assuming the marker expression in human cancers is known, the preclinical and clinical data supporting expression of the marker and antitumor effect of the agent are compelling, and an assay is available, there remain some additional caveats for designing clinical trials to assess treatment effects in biomarker-defined subgroups of cancer patients. Preselection based on the presence of the biomarker of interest defines a subgroup of cancer patients that may have a different prognosis from historical outcome data from trials done in an unselected group (34). For example, human EGFR2 (HER2) amplification in breast cancers corre-lates with a poorer prognosis independent of treatment and also correlates with benefit to monoclonal anti-HER2 antibody trastuzumab (57,58). Thus, historical outcome data from treatment trials that were conducted in all breast cancer patients without identifying HER2 status in tumors overestimate the prognosis of patients with HER2-amplified tumors. An uncontrolled trial of a HER2-targeted agent in the molecularly defined group might lead to a result, which appears unfavorable compared to the historical outcome data in patients for whom tumor HER2 status is not known when in fact there has been an improvement in outcome from the experiment treatment in the patients with HER2-amplified tumors. The benefit may not be apparent in an uncontrolled trial, if the poor prognosis of the molecu-larly defined group was not previously identified. Conversely, the benefit in this subset may be masked if the trial were conducted in unselected patients because the benefit in the relatively small subset is "buried" in the lack of benefit seen in the overall study population. Thus, if there is limited historical data for the antici-pated outcome in the marker-defined group with standard treatment and, in par-ticular, the outcome of interest is progression-free survival, a randomized phase-2 design should be considered. In addition to understanding and appreciating the prognostic versus predictive impact of the biomarker, the performance character-istics of the assay are also important. If the trial is designed to assess treatment effects in marker+ and/or marker− patients groups, then false-positives will dilute effect in marker+ group and false-negatives will dilute the apparent differences in treatment effect between marker-defined groups. Lastly, if the trial is designed to assess effects in marker+ and marker– groups, the trial sample size may be considerably larger than the size of a conventional phase-2 and phase-3 studies.

One strategy to identify/evaluate predictive markers of drug activity is to evaluate the effect of agent in marker+/– groups in phase-2 trials. Based on the trial results, a decision can be made whether to design a phase-3 study for marker+ group (as the magnitude of antitumor effect seems greatest in this group), both groups (as there may be an antitumor effect in both groups), or not to use the marker (as there is no apparent differential antitumor effect). If tumors are not prospectively tested for markers to determine patient enrollment, the trial needs to have sufficient numbers of patient to have reasonable statistical power for subset analyses to assess treatment outcome by marker effects. The increased patient numbers to assess marker by treatment outcome effects may be achieved by designing multistage trials in which agents that show interesting antitumor effect may continue to accrue additional patients to facilitate subsequent analysis of antitumor effect within subsets. In addition, if the biomarker and treatment effects are consistent across different patient population, evaluation of specimens obtained from patients across multiple trials may be reasonable. These approaches are illustrated in Figure 2.

In summary, the rationale for enriching study populations for patients most likely to benefit from a targeted agent is quite compelling. However, only in rare

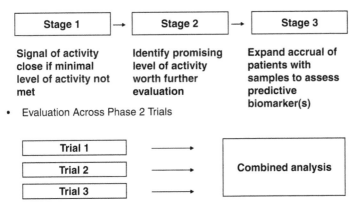

Figure 2 Phase-2 clinical trials to identify predictive biomarkers. The increased patient numbers to assess marker by treatment outcome effects may be achieved by designing multistage trials with such that agents that show interesting antitumor effect may continue to accrue additional patients to facilitate subsequent analysis of antitumor effect within subsets. If the biomarker and treatment effects are consistent across different patient population, evaluation of specimens obtained from patients across multiple trials may be reasonable.

circumstances has there been sufficient knowledge to know what biomarkers may correlate with sensitivity to a particularly agent. The codevelopment of an agent with an assay to select patients that may benefit from the agent requires considerably greater knowledge, resources, and efforts early in development of the drug. There must be a significant coordination of effort to define the relationship between the biomarker of interest and antitumor activity of the agent, to determine the prevalence and relevance of the biomarker in tumors of patients, and to determine an optimal assay to assess the marker in clinical specimens. These efforts significantly increase the cost over "traditional" drug development approaches as both cost of developing the assay and the numbers of patients per trial and cost per patient will be higher. In addition, qualification, standardization, and quality assurance for the biomarker assessment take additional time and resources. However, enrichment strategy may reduce the likelihood of failure in phase-3 studies and may assist with subsequent treatment decisions for individual patients.

CONCLUSIONS

Basic, translational, and clinical research efforts have all played significant roles in the development of targeted agents for the treatment of cancer patients. Basic science endeavors have contributed greatly to the identification and credentialing of targets and the characterization of the biochemical and cellular effects of agents to targets. Clinical research has led to the characterization of expression of normal and mutated targets in human cancers. Drug development has led to the determination of the activity of these targeted agents, of new toxicities, and, to a lesser extent, mechanisms of sensitivity and resistance to the agents. However, the activities within these research spheres have often been conducted in isolation and with limited integration. As a result, there have been significant gaps in the development of biomarkers to assess effects of drug on the target, to predict for sensitivity/ resistance, in our ability to optimize drug combinations, and to predict, prevent, or manage target-specific toxicities.

The decision to use biomarkers to assist in the development of targeted agent must be based on the strength of evidence supporting the correlation between agent, its purported target, and treatment effect, the availability and suitability of assay, and the resources that are available to support the development process. Clearly, it is necessary to understand as much as possible about the agent and its purported target before first-in-human phase-1 study begins, as evaluation of possible markers of target modulation and antitumor activity, tissue toxicity, and the subsequent selection and the development of the assays must occur in parallel with the drug development. Phase-1 study end points of PK, PD, and toxicity (which may be a PD effect) are not necessarily different for targeted agents; however, the emphasis on PD end points to assist in the selection of dose may be greater for agents that do not have target-specific toxicity. Similarly, the goals and end points of phase-2 trials may not have changed for these agents; rather, there has been a greater use of randomized controlled designs to determine whether disease stability reflects drug effect rather than intrinsic tumor growth kinetics and a greater interest in determining biomarkers that correlate with treatment outcome.

Biomarkers may assist with the decisions regarding optimal dose, selection of appropriate patients for clinical trials, and ultimately selecting appropriate treatments for patients. However, the best biomarkers may be different in each of these situations. The specific objectives/goals for biomarker should be carefully considered. Each step in the process of assay development, specimen collection, shipping storage, and analysis should be evaluated and optimized. In the short term, earlier biomarker development may be more expensive and may delay the initiation of phase-3 trials to evaluate the agent; however, in the longer term, the codevelopment of biomarkers with the targeted agents may lead to more cost-effective, efficient drug development and better treatments selection for individual patients. To achieve these goals, collaboration between pharmaceutical companies, academic investigators, biostatisticians, regulatory authorities, and patients will be needed.

REFERENCES

1. Korn EL, Arbuck SG, Pluda JM, Simon R, Kaplan RS, Christian MC. Clinical trial designs for cytostatic agents: are new approaches needed? J Clin Oncol 2001; 19(1):265–272.
2. Ahn C. An evaluation of phase I cancer clinical trial designs. Stat Med 1998; 17(14):1537–1549.
3. Eisenhauer EA, O'Dwyer PJ, Christian M, Humphrey JS. Phase I clinical trial design in cancer drug development. J Clin Oncol 2000; 18(3):684–692.
4. Rosenberger WF, Haines LM. Competing designs for phase I clinical trials: a review. Stat Med 2002; 21(18):2757–2770.
5. Simon R, Freidlin B, Rubinstein L, Arbuck SG, Collins J, Christian MC. Accelerated titration designs for phase I clinical trials in oncology. J Natl Cancer Inst 1997; 89(15):1138–1147.
6. Zohar S, Chevret S. The continual reassessment method: comparison of Bayesian stopping rules for dose-ranging studies. Stat Med 2001; 20(19):2827–2843.
7. Thall PF, Estey EH, Sung HG. A new statistical method for dose-finding based on efficacy and toxicity in early phase clinical trials. Invest New Drugs 1999; 17(2):155–167.
8. Wolf M, Swaisland H, Averbuch S. Development of the novel biologically targeted anticancer agent gefitinib: determining the optimum dose for clinical efficacy. Clin Cancer Res 2004; 10(14):4607–4613.
9. Brown PD. Ongoing trials with matrix metalloproteinase inhibitors. Expert Opin Investig Drugs 2000; 9(9):2167–2177.
10. Wojtowicz-Praga S, Torri J, Johnson M, et al. Phase I trial of Marimastat, a novel matrix metalloproteinase inhibitor, administered orally to patients with advanced lung cancer. J Clin Oncol 1998; 16(6):2150–2156.
11. Yates CR, Pui CH, Evans WE. Pharmacodynamic monitoring of cancer chemotherapy: childhood acute lymphoblastic leukemia as a model. Ther Drug Monit 1998; 20(5):453–458.

12. Lathia CD. Biomarkers and surrogate endpoints: how and when might they impact drug development? Dis Markers 2002; 18(2):83–90.
13. Perez-Soler R, Delord JP, Halpern A, et al. HER1/EGFR inhibitor-associated rash: future directions for management and investigation outcomes from the HER1/EGFR inhibitor rash management forum. Oncologist 2005; 10(5):345–356.
14. Saif MW, Mehra R. Incidence and management of bevacizumab-related toxicities in colorectal cancer. Expert Opin Drug Saf 2006; 5(4):553–566.
15. Parulekar WR, Eisenhauer EA. Phase I trial design for solid tumor studies of targeted, non-cytotoxic agents: theory and practice. J Natl Cancer Inst 2004; 96(13): 990–997.
16. Dowlati A, Haaga J, Remick SC, et al. Sequential tumor biopsies in early phase clinical trials of anticancer agents for pharmacodynamic evaluation. Clin Cancer Res 2001; 7(10):2971–2976.
17. Herbst RS, Lee AT, Tran HT, Abbruzzese JL. Clinical studies of angiogenesis inhibitors: the University of Texas MD Anderson Center trial of human endostatin. Curr Oncol Rep 2001; 3(2):131–140.
18. Thompson J, Stewart CF, Houghton PJ. Animal models for studying the action of topoisomerase I targeted drugs. Biochim Biophys Acta 1998; 1400(1–3):301–319.
19. Hunsberger S, Rubinstein LV, Dancey J, Korn EL. Dose escalation trial designs based on a molecularly targeted endpoint. Stat Med 2005; 24(14):2171–2181.
20. Fazzari M, Heller G, Scher HI. The phase II/III transition. Toward the proof of efficacy in cancer clinical trials. Control Clin Trials 2000; 21(4):360–368.
21. Heitjan DF. Bayesian interim analysis of phase II cancer clinical trials. Stat Med 1997; 16(16):1791–1802.
22. Gray R, Manola J, Saxman S, et al. Phase II clinical trial design: methods in translational research from the Genitourinary Committee at the Eastern Cooperative Oncology Group. Clin Cancer Res 2006; 12(7 Pt 1):1966–1969.
23. Steinberg SM, Venzon DJ. Early selection in a randomized phase II clinical trial. Stat Med 2002; 21(12):1711–1726.
24. Mick R, Crowley JJ, Carroll RJ. Phase II clinical trial design for noncytotoxic anticancer agents for which time to disease progression is the primary endpoint. Control Clin Trials 2000; 21(4):343–359.
25. Kopec JA, Abrahamowicz M, Esdaile JM. Randomized discontinuation trials: utility and efficiency. J Clin Epidemiol 1993; 46(9):959–971.
26. Berry DA. General keynote: clinical trial design. Gynecol Oncol 2003; 88(1 Pt 2): S114–S116; S122–123.
27. Royston P, Parmar MK, Qian W. Novel designs for multi-arm clinical trials with survival outcomes with an application in ovarian cancer. Stat Med 2003; 22(14): 2239–2256.
28. Rubinstein LV, Korn EL, Freidlin B, Hunsberger S, Ivy SP, Smith MA. Design issues of randomized phase II trials and a proposal for phase II screening trials. J Clin Oncol 2005; 23(28):7199–7206.
29. Dancey JE. Predictive factors for epidermal growth factor receptor inhibitors—the bull's-eye hits the arrow. Cancer Cell 2004; 5(5):411–415.
30. Betensky RA, Louis DN, Cairncross JG. Influence of unrecognized molecular heterogeneity on randomized clinical trials. J Clin Oncol 2002; 20(10):2495–2499.
31. Ratain MJ, Eckhardt SG. Phase II studies of modern drugs directed against new targets: if you are fazed, too, then resist RECIST. J Clin Oncol 2004; 22(22): 4442–4445.

32. Ratain MJ, Eisen T, Stadler WM, et al. Phase II placebo-controlled randomized discontinuation trial of sorafenib in patients with metastatic renal cell carcinoma. J Clin Oncol 2006; 24(16):2505–2512.

33. Kelloff GJ, Hoffman JM, Johnson B, et al. Progress and promise of FDG-PET imaging for cancer patient management and oncologic drug development. Clin Cancer Res 2005; 11(8):2785–2808.

34. Kelloff GJ, Krohn KA, Larson SM, et al. The progress and promise of molecular imaging probes in oncologic drug development. Clin Cancer Res 2005; 11(22): 7967–7985.

35. Stadler W. New trial designs to assess antitumor and antiproliferative agents in prostate cancer. Invest New Drugs 2002; 20(2):201–208.

36. Park JW, Kerbel RS, Kelloff GJ, et al. Rationale for biomarkers and surrogate end points in mechanism-driven oncology drug development. Clin Cancer Res 2004; 10(11):3885–3896.

37. Therasse P, Arbuck SG, Eisenhauer EA, et al. New guidelines to evaluate the response to treatment in solid tumors. European Organization for Research and Treatment of Cancer, National Cancer Institute of the United States, National Cancer Institute of Canada. J Natl Cancer Inst 2000; 92(3):205–216.

38. Shepherd FA, Rodrigues Pereira J, et al. Erlotinib in previously treated non-small-cell lung cancer. N Engl J Med 2005; 353(2):123–132.

39. Yang JC, Haworth L, Sherry RM, et al. A randomized trial of bevacizumab, an anti-vascular endothelial growth factor antibody, for metastatic renal cancer. N Engl J Med 2003; 349(5):427–434.

40. Therasse P, Eisenhauer EA, Buyse M. Update in methodology and conduct of cancer clinical trials. Eur J Cancer 2006; 42(10):1322–1330.

41. Therasse P, Eisenhauer EA, Verweij J. RECIST revisited: a review of validation studies on tumour assessment. Eur J Cancer 2006; 42(8):1031–1039.

42. Morgan B, Thomas AL, Drevs J, et al. Dynamic contrast-enhanced magnetic resonance imaging as a biomarker for the pharmacological response of PTK787/ZK 222584, an inhibitor of the vascular endothelial growth factor receptor tyrosine kinases, in patients with advanced colorectal cancer and liver metastases: results from two phase I studies. J Clin Oncol 2003; 21(21):3955–3964.

43. Antoch G, Kanja J, Bauer S, et al. Comparison of PET, CT, and dual-modality PET/CT imaging for monitoring of imatinib (STI571) therapy in patients with gastrointestinal stromal tumors. J Nucl Med 2004; 45(3):357–365.

44. Simon R, Wittes RE, Ellenberg SS. Randomized phase II clinical trials. Cancer Treat Rep 1985; 69(12):1375–1381.

45. Amery W, Dony J. A clinical trial design avoiding undue placebo treatment. J Clin Pharmacol 1975; 15(10):674–679.

46. Rosner GL, Stadler W, Ratain MJ. Randomized discontinuation design: application to cytostatic antineoplastic agents. J Clin Oncol 2002; 20(22): 4478–4484.

47. Herson J, Carter SK. Calibrated phase II clinical trials in oncology. Stat Med 1986; 5(5):441–447.

48. Simon R. Designs for efficient clinical trials. Oncology (Williston Park) 1989; 3(7):43–49; discussion 51–53.

49. Simon R. Optimal two-stage designs for phase II clinical trials. Control Clin Trials 1989; 10(1):1–10.

50. Simon R, Maitournam A. Evaluating the efficiency of targeted designs for randomized clinical trials. Clin Cancer Res 2004; 10(20):6759–6763.
51. Bartlett JM. Pharmacodiagnostic testing in breast cancer: focus on HER2 and trastuzumab therapy. Am J Pharmacogenomics 2005; 5(5):303–315.
52. Pegram MD, Pauletti G, Slamon DJ. HER-2/neu as a predictive marker of response to breast cancer therapy. Breast Cancer Res Treat 1998; 52(1–3):65–77.
53. Friedman HS, Kokkinakis DM, Pluda J, et al. Phase I trial of O6-benzylguanine for patients undergoing surgery for malignant glioma. J Clin Oncol 1998; 16(11): 3570–3575.
54. Lightcap ES, McCormack TA, Pien CS, Chau V, Adams J, Elliott PJ. Proteasome inhibition measurements: clinical application. Clin Chem 2000; 46(5):673–683.
55. Adams J. Development of the proteasome inhibitor PS-341. Oncologist 2002; 7(1):9–16.
56. Freidlin B, Simon R. Evaluation of randomized discontinuation design. J Clin Oncol 2005; 23(22):5094–5098.
57. Ellenberg SS, Eisenberger MA. An efficient design for phase III studies of combination chemotherapies. Cancer Treat Rep 1985; 69(10):1147–1154.
58. Osborne CK, Schiff R, Arpino G, Lee AS, Hilsenbeck VG. Endocrine responsiveness: understanding how progesterone receptor can be used to select endocrine therapy. Breast 2005; 14(6):458–465.
59. Green S. Modulation of oestrogen receptor activity by oestrogens and anti-oestrogens. J Steroid Biochem Mol Biol 1990; 37(6):747–751.
60. Johnston SR, Leary A. Lapatinib: a novel EGFR/HER2 tyrosine kinase inhibitor for cancer. Drugs Today (Barc) 2006; 42(7):441–453.
61. Pao W, Miller VA. Epidermal growth factor receptor mutations, small-molecule kinase inhibitors, and non-small-cell lung cancer: current knowledge and future directions. J Clin Oncol 2005; 23(11):2556–2568.
62. Hirsch FR, Varella-Garcia M, Bunn PA Jr, et al. Molecular predictors of outcome with gefitinib in a phase III placebo-controlled study in advanced non-small-cell lung cancer. J Clin Oncol 2006; 24(31):5034–5042.
63. Tsao MS, Sakurada A, Cutz JC, et al. Erlotinib in lung cancer—molecular and clinical predictors of outcome. N Engl J Med 2005; 353(2):133–144.
64. Paik S, Tang G, Shak S, et al. Gene expression and benefit of chemotherapy in women with node-negative, estrogen receptor-positive breast cancer. J Clin Oncol 2006; 24(23):3726–3734.
65. Prenen H, Cools J, Mentens N, et al. Efficacy of the kinase inhibitor SU11248 against gastrointestinal stromal tumor mutants refractory to imatinib mesylate. Clin Cancer Res 2006; 12(8):2622–2627.
66. Heinrich MC, Corless CL, Blanke CD, et al. Molecular correlates of imatinib resistance in gastrointestinal stromal tumors. J Clin Oncol 2006; 24(29):4764–4774.
67. Talpaz M, Shah NP, Kantarjian H, et al. Dasatinib in imatinib-resistant Philadelphia chromosome-positive leukemias. N Engl J Med 2006; 354(24):2531–2541.
68. Druker BJ. Circumventing resistance to kinase-inhibitor therapy. N Engl J Med 2006; 354(24):2594–2596.

3

Antiangiogenic Therapy for Lung Cancer: Small-Molecule Inhibitors

Nithya Ramnath and Alex A. Adjei

Roswell Park Cancer Institute, Buffalo, New York, U.S.A.

INTRODUCTION

It has been three decades since Folkman described his seminal observations regarding the dependence of tumors on the process of sustained angiogenesis in order to grow and metastasize. There has been a tremendous translational effort in drug development and therapeutics targeting angiogenesis. This has led to advances in previously untreatable conditions such as age-related senile macular degeneration and, more recently, in cancer. This chapter includes a brief discussion on angiogenesis, particularly as it relates to the vascular endothelial growth factor (VEGF) pathway and small-molecule antiangiogenic agents that are in clinical development. A detailed discussion on angiogenesis as it relates to lung cancer is discussed elsewhere in this monograph.

VASCULAR ENDOTHELIAL GROWTH FACTOR

While a number of angiogenesis factors exist, this section focuses on VEGF because of its seminal role in the angiogenic process and its central role in the targeting of antiangiogenic agents. VEGF is a homodimeric heparin-binding glycoprotein (Fig. 1). The VEGF family of angiogenic factors includes six secreted glycoproteins based on the number of amino acids. These are referred to as VEGF-A, VEGF-B, VEGF-C, VEGF-D, VEGF-E, placenta growth factor (PIGF)-1, and PIGF-2 (2). VEGF, unlike other angiogenic factors, is selectively mitogenic for endothelial cells and increases vessel permeability.

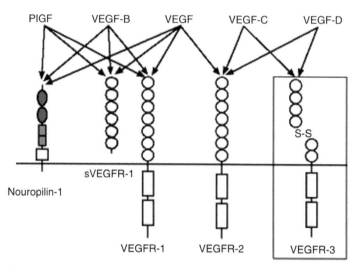

Figure 1   The VEGFs and their receptors. VEGFR-3 (*boxed*) is largely restricted to lymphatic endothelium. The different structural elements of the receptors are illustrated as follows: (*open circle*) immunoglobulin domain; (*shaded box*) tyrosine kinase domain; (*light gray shaded box*), domain homologous to coagulation factors V and VIII; (*gray shaded oval*) CUB domain; and (*open box*) MAM domain. *Abbreviations*: PlGF, placenta growth factor; S-S, disulfide bridge; sVEGFR-1, soluble form of VEGFR-1; VEGF, vascular endothelial growth factor; VEGFR, vascular endothelial growth factor receptor. *Source*: From Ref. 1.

Some VEGF family members are involved in lymphangiogenesis (VEGF-C and -D). VEGF expression can be seen in the vast majority of tumors and is usually elevated above normal tissue levels. As tumors grow, the size outstrips the blood supply, and there is impaired supply of oxygen and nutrients, with resultant accumulation of metabolites within the tumor. This is accompanied by changes in the tumor microenvironment, for example, hypoxia, hypoglycemia, and acidosis, which stimulate the upregulation and release of hypoxia-inducible factor-1α (HIF), VEGF, and other angiogenic factors by the tumor cells.

VEGF Receptors

VEGF exerts its effects by binding to one of its three receptors [VEGF receptor (VEGFR)-1/Flt-1, VEGFR-2/KDR/Flk-1, and VEGFR-3/Flt-4)]. Following ligand binding, the receptor undergoes transautophosphorylation with subsequent activation of a cell type-dependent signaling cascade.

The VEGFRs are tyrosine kinases, having an extracellular immunoglobulin-like domains and an intracellular kinase domain (Fig. 2). These receptors are not present in the endothelial cells of mature blood vessels and the level of receptor expression is felt to be related to the amount of VEGF secreted. Klagsbrun and Soker put forth four postulates that gave evidence for a seminal role for VEGF in

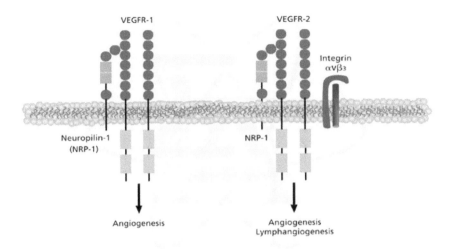

Figure 2 The VEGF receptors shown are VEGFR-1 (Flt-1) and VEGFR-2 (Flk/KDR). *Abbreviations*: VEGF, vascular endothelial growth factor; VEGFR, vascular endothelial growth factor receptor. *Source*: From Refs. 3, 4.

tumor angiogenesis (5): (*i*) VEGF is found in almost every type of human cancer and in high concentrations around tumor blood vessels. In the periphery of tumors, high VEGF levels are seen, possibly as a consequence of hypoxia. Hypoxia is a potent inducer of VEGF. (*ii*) VEGFRs are detected in blood vessels in close proximity to tumors. (*iii*) Monoclonal antibodies to VEGFRs suppress the growth of tumors in VEGF expressing solid tumors in mice, but not in cell culture where angiogenesis is not required (2). (*iv*) VEGF, unlike other angiogenic factors, can induce the extracellular matrix in tumors (6). VEGF secretion is influenced by many factors. Some potent inducers of VEGF include hypoxia, basic fibroblast growth factor (bFGF), and transforming growth factors α and β. Since these inducers all converge on the final common pathway of VEGF/VEGFR, it is rational to direct therapeutic interventions at this pathway.

VEGF levels are also influenced by proto-oncogenes such as *ras* and *met*. Mutant *ras* can increase VEGF levels in tumors (7). Similarly, stimulation of *met* and *erbB-2* pathways can enhance production of VEGF. It has been shown that blocking the receptor tyrosine kinases (RTKs) in these pathways (e.g., *met* and *erbB-2*) or blocking the proteins encoded (e.g., Ras farnesyl transferase inhibitors) can decrease VEGF levels, thereby showing that these therapies can be both antiproliferative and antiangiogenic (8,9). VEGF regulates several endothelial cell functions, including proliferation, differentiation, permeability, vascular tone, and the production of vasoactive molecules. VEGF ligands act through specific binding to three different cell membrane receptors: VEGFR-1 (Flt-1), VEGFR-2 (Flk/KDR), and VEGFR-3 (Flt-4) (10). These receptors consist of an extracellular domain that binds specific VEGF ligands, a transmembrane domain, and an

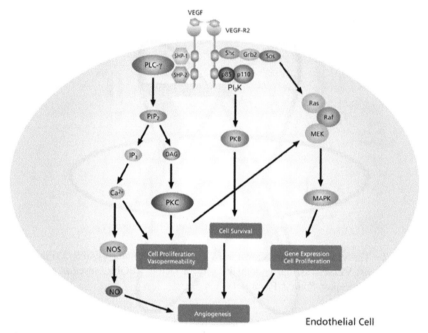

Figure 3   Vascular endothelial growth factor and interactive pathways. *Source*: www. sigmaaldrich.com.

intracellular region that contains a tyrosine kinase domain. In addition, neuropilin 1 (NRP-1) and NRP-2 are coreceptors for specific isoforms of VEGF family members and increase the binding affinity of these ligands to their respective receptors (11).

Of the three receptors, it is VEGFR-2 that mediates the majority of the downstream effects of VEGF-A, including vascular permeability and endothelial cell proliferation.

INHIBITORS OF ANGIOGENESIS

These can be broadly classified into endogenous and exogenous. Endogenous inhibitors may be matrix-derived or non–matrix-derived. Exogenous inhibitors can be either direct or indirect inhibitors. In fact, the first endogenous inhibitor described belongs to the family of tissue inhibitors of metalloproteinases or TIMPs. Called CDI for cartilage-derived inhibitor, the antiangiogenic action is secondary to suppression of proteases involved in endothelial cell migration during the formation of vessel "sprouts" (12). Since then, the list of endogenous inhibitors has grown. A partial list is summarized in Table 1.

Table 1 Endogenous Inhibitors of Angiogenesis

Matrix derived	Nonmatrix derived
Arresten	*Growth factors and cytokines*
Canstatin	Interferons
Collagen fragments	Interleukins
EFC-XV	PEDF
Endorepellin	Platelet factor-4
Endostatin	*Other*
Fibronectin fragments	Angiostatin
Fibulin	Antithrombin III (cleaved)
Thrombospondin-1 and -2	Chondromodulin
Tumstatin	2-Methoxyestradiol
	PEX
	Plasminogen Kringle 5
	Prolactin fragments
	Prothrombin Kringle 2
	sFlt-1
	Tissue inhibitors of metalloproteinases
	Troponin 1
	Vasostatin

Source: From Ref. 13.

Trials of Endogenous Inhibitors of Angiogenesis in Lung Cancer

Angiostatin: Recombinant human angiostatin (rhAngiostatin), a 38 kDa proteo-lytic fragment of plasminogen, is a naturally occurring potent inhibitor of angiogenesis, tumor growth, and metastasis. Angiostatin was discovered during tumor dormancy studies, explaining the process by which primary tumors inhibit growth of remote metastases (14). In vitro rhAngiostatin protein inhibited endo-thelial cell proliferation and migration in response to bFGF. In addition, in vitro, bFGF-induced angiogenesis was also inhibited by rhAngiostatin. Based on phase-I studies and pilot studies in combination with chemotherapy, a phase-II study of two doses of rhAngiostatin was undertaken in advanced non–small cell lung cancer (NSCLC). In this study, all patients received paclitaxel (175 mg/m^2, three-hour infusion) followed by carboplatin [area under the curve (AUC) of 5 mg/mL·minute) administered by intravenous infusion on day 1, and repeated every 21 days, for up to six cycles of treatment. The development of this agent has been halted because of suboptimal efficacy results (15).

Interferons (IFNs): The antiangiogenic effect of IFN was first shown clinically in the treatment of life-threatening hemangiomas of infancy (16) and subsequently also in the treatment of Kaposi's sarcoma (17). At least four randomized trials involving IFN or observation in the adjuvant setting following completion of treatment for limited stage small cell lung cancer (SCLC) have been reported (18–21). Many patients in these trials could not complete the prescribed doses of IFN due to toxicity. The only study to show an improved two-year survival for IFN-treated patients was by Lebeau et al. These patients were in complete remission for their limited stage SCLC at the time of study entry (21). Overall, however, these studies do not support the role of IFN for adjuvant use in SCLC.

Trials of Exogenous Inhibitors of Angiogenesis

These may be direct inhibitors such as TNP-70, a synthetic analogue of fumagillin, a fungus-derived inhibitor of endothelial cell proliferation, the matrix metalloproteinase inhibitors (MMPIs) such as marimastat and batimastat, and Vitamin D3 (mechanism of antiangiogenesis unknown). "Indirect inhibitors" can be considered as those that inhibit angiogenic signaling, such as monoclonal antibodies directed against VEGF isoforms or small-molecule tyrosine kinase inhibitors (TKIs) directed at VEGFRs.

MMPIs in lung cancer: All of the MMPIs that have been extensively studied in lung cancer are summarized in Table 2. In general, these compounds failed to demonstrate any efficacy in the clinic and their development has been halted.

Table 2 Randomized Trials of Matrix Metalloproteinase Inhibitors in Lung Cancer

Drug	Stage	Status
BAY 12-9566	Pharmaceuticals limited SCLC in CR or near CR	Study closed at interim analysis. No benefit; increased thrombocytopenia noted with BAY-12-9566
BMS 275291	Stage III NSCLC; BMS 275291 with and after paclitaxel and carboplatin	Study closed; no benefit
Marimastat, BB2516	Adjuvant therapy in NSCLC	Study completed and closed. Results not reported
Marimastat, BB2516	Limited and extensive SCLC in CR/PR	Two studies completed and closed; no benefit
Prinomastat, AG3340	Stage IIIB and IV NSCLC; prinomastat given with and after paclitaxel and carboplatin	Study closed. No survival benefit
Prinomastat, AG3340	Agouran stage IIIB and IV NSCLC; prinomastat given with and after gemcitabine and cisplatin	Study closed at interim analysis. No survival benefit
Neovastat, AE 941	Stage III NSCLC study open. AE 941 with and after induction chemotherapy, thoracic radiation	Study closed; results awaited

Abbreviations: CR, complete remission; NSCLC, non–small cell lung cancer; SCLC, small cell lung cancer.

TNP-470: It is a synthetic analog of fumagillin that blocks the growth of new blood vessels by inhibiting methionine aminopeptidase, an enzyme that plays a key role in endothelial cell proliferation (22). Preclinical studies support a role for TNP-470, in slowing tumor growth, but not in causing shrinkage of existing tumors (23). However, when used in combination with paclitaxel or other cytotoxic agents, tumor regression, disease stabilization, and improved survival were seen (24). TNP-470 combined with paclitaxel was evaluated in the phase-I setting in several tumor types including 16 patients with NSCLC. Overall this regimen was well tolerated, with minimal pharmacokinetic (PK) interactions between the two drugs. Mild-to-moderate subclinical neurocognitive impairment was seen, but this was reversible. Notably, partial responses were reported in 6/16 NSCLC patients, 60% of whom had been pretreated with chemotherapy (25). The future role of this agent in the therapy of lung cancer is, however, unclear.

Indirect Inhibitors of Angiogenic Signaling

The monoclonal antibodies and decoy protein receptors are covered elsewhere in this book.

Small-molecule TKIs: The TKIs of VEGFRs are low-molecular-weight, adenosine triphosphate (ATP)-mimetic proteins that bind to the ATP-binding catalytic site of the tyrosine kinase domain of VEGFRs, resulting in blockade of intracellular signaling. As each of the known receptors to which the VEGF family bind is relevant in various ways to carcinogenesis, not to mention the role of other proangiogenic factors, methods that selectively curtail either VEGFR-1 or VEGFR-2 effects alone, as exemplified by angiozyme (26), or by the monoclonal antibody to VEGFR-2, are likely insufficient. In contrast, more significant clinical activity can be seen with the group of ATP-competitive small-molecule inhibitors of the VEGFR tyrosine kinase activity. Because of the structural homology among various members of the tyrosine kinase family of proteins, these drugs exhibit promiscuous activity against different target kinases. This property is desirable from the drug efficacy aspect as, like any other cancer, lung cancer is characterized by a complex interaction of multiple intersecting, hierarchical intracellular and intercellular signaling pathways. In addition, these drugs may offer distinct advantages over monoclonal antibodies, such as their oral bioavailability, relatively shorter half-lives, and smaller molecular weights that may facilitate improved tissue penetration. The multistep angiogenic process, exemplified by the transcriptional activation of VEGF, is highly regulated by factors such as HIF-1α, and is modulated by a large number of highly coordinated and interdependent signaling nodes sensitive to inputs from, as well as providing feedback to, a variety of major signaling hubs (27). In the context of current drug development, the most relevant to NSCLC is the synergistic interaction shown in preclinical studies between the combination of an anti-VEGF and antiepidermal growth factor receptor TKIs (28).

Pure Angiogenic Inhibitors

Pazopanib: GW786034 is a novel, orally active small-molecule inhibitor targeting multiple tyrosine kinases including VEGFR-1, VEGFR-2, and VEGFR-3. In addition to its effects on VEGFRs, GW786034 targets additional tyrosine kinases including platelet-derived growth factor (PDGF) receptors (PDGFRs) and c-Kit that have established roles in tumorigenesis (29). Preliminary data from a phase-I study of GW786034 in patients with solid tumors demonstrated early evidence of antitumor activity (30). Among 43 patients enrolled, a minimal response was noted in four patients and stable disease (SD) for more than six months was observed in six additional patients. GW786034 was well tolerated at doses up to 2000 mg daily. A second phase-1 dose-escalation study of orally administered GW786034 has completed enrollment of 63 patients with a variety of solid tumor types. Doses administered ranged from 50 mg three times/week to 2000 mg once daily (QD) (29,31). The maximum tolerated dose (MTD) was not defined in this trial. Tumor shrinkage (one partial and four minimal responses) or SD (two cases) has been observed in all seven patients with renal cell carcinoma (RCC) treated at ≥800 mg QD ($n = 5$) and 300 mg twice daily (bid) ($n = 2$). Tumor shrinkage was also seen in patients with Hurthel cell and neuroendocrine tumors, as well as chondrosarcoma. In all, 15 patients, including those with RCC, Hurthel cell, carcinoid, gastrointestinal stromal tumors (GIST), neuroendocrine, sarcoma, melanoma, and lung cancer, have remained on study for six months or longer. Phase-I/II studies of pazopanib in combination with pemetrexed/erlotinib as well as single agent pazopanib in refractory NSCLC are planned.

AZD2171: The novel indole-ether quinazoline AZD2171 is a highly potent ($IC_{50} < 1$ nmol/L) ATP-competitive inhibitor of recombinant KDR tyrosine kinase in vitro. Concordant with this activity, in human umbilical vein endothelial cells, AZD2171 inhibited VEGF-stimulated proliferation and KDR phosphorylation with IC_{50} values of 0.4 and 0.5 nmol/L, respectively. Once-daily oral administration of AZD2171 ablated experimental (VEGF-induced) angiogenesis in vivo and inhibited endochondral ossification in bone or corpora luteal development in ovary, both physiologic processes that are highly dependent upon neovascularization. The growth of established human tumor xenografts (colon, lung, prostate, breast, and ovary) in athymic mice was inhibited dose dependently by AZD2171, with chronic administration of 1.5 mg/kg/day producing statistically significant inhibition in all models. A histologic analysis of Calu-6 lung tumors treated with AZD2171 revealed a reduction in microvessel density within 52 hours, which became progressively greater with the duration of treatment. These changes are indicative of vascular regression within tumors. Collectively, the data obtained with AZD2171 are consistent with potent inhibition of VEGF signaling, angiogenesis, neovascular survival, and tumor growth (32). In the phase-I study, dose-limiting toxicities (DLTs) were grade-4 cerebral hemorrhage, grade-4 hypoglycemia, and grade-3 hypertension. Following a single dose, the terminal phase half-life ranged from 12.5 to 35.4 hours. Early data showed two unconfirmed partial responses in the 60 mg cohort and three minor responses at lower doses. Continuous once-daily treatment with

45 mg AZD2171 is being developed (33). A phase-II/III study of AZD2171 in advanced NSCLC is underway. Patients will receive intravenous paclitaxel and carboplatin on day 1 and start oral AZD2171 QD from day 2 through 21 of course 1 and on days 1 to 21 of all subsequent courses. Treatment with paclitaxel and carboplatin will repeat every 21 days for up to eight courses in the absence of disease progression or unacceptable toxicity.

Vatalanib: PTK787/ZK222584 is a synthetic, low-molecular-weight, orally bioavailable agent belonging to the chemical class of aminophthalazines. Vatalanib inhibits all three VEGFRs as well as PDGFR and c-Kit at submicromolar concentrations. At higher concentrations, this drug can inhibit epidermal growth factor receptor (EGFR) and fibroblast growth factor 1 or 2 (34). In a human lung adenocarcinoma model, PTK787 significantly reduced the formation of pleural effusion and suppressed vascular hyperpermeability (35). PK results for doses up to 1000 mg/day showed that vatalanib given QD is rapidly adsorbed, with a time to maximum concentration (C_{max}) of 1.5 hours and a terminal half-life ($t_{1/2}$) of about three to six hours (36). In a phase-I dose-escalation study, notable adverse events were grade 3 hypertension (4/26 patients), grade 3 transaminitis (6/26 patients) and lightheadedness (2/3 patients at the 1000 mg dose level), ataxia, and dyspnea (both in 3/22 patients) (37). Promising antitumor activity was observed in patients with metastatic colorectal cancer and led to further studies in colon cancer. An exploratory analysis in patients with pretreatment high serum levels of lactate dehydrogenase (LDH) showed a statistically significant longer progression-free survival (PFS) time in the group treated with vatalanib (38). High pretreatment serum levels of LDH may therefore predict for optimal benefit from vatalanib in inhibiting VEGF. The role of PTK787 in patients with NSCLC is being evaluated in a phase-II study [the growth arrest with oral anti-angiogenic agents in lung cancer (GOAL) Study] in France and Germany.

CEP-7055: This is an orally active pan-VEGFR TKI (RTKI) with potent antiangiogenic activity and antitumor efficacy in preclinical models (39). CEP-7055 is the dimethylglycine ester of CEP-5214, a low-molecular-weight TKI, with nanomolar potency against VEGFRs-1, 2, and 3 (IC_{50} = 4–17 nM). The clinical activity and tolerability of CEP-7055 have been explored in a phase-I study using a conventional MTD design. CEP-7055 was given continuously for 28 days followed by a 14-day washout period (one cycle). Patients were eligible for further cycles subject to tolerability and tumor status. Nineteen patients were treated at doses of 10, 20, 40, 80, and 120 mg, given bid. Adverse events were generally mild and DLTs have not been observed to date. Hypertension was observed in one patient at 120 mg bid. The relationship between dose and plasma exposure for CEP05214 was approximately linear between 10 and 40 mg bid, but appeared to plateau at 80 and 120 mg bid. The C_{max} achieved at 40 to 80 mg bid is greater than that associated with anticancer effects in cancer models and three times daily schedules of both dose levels are being evaluated (40).

Axitinib: AG-013736 is an oral RTKI of all three VEGFRs, PDGF, and c-Kit. In the phase-I study, 36 patients received AG-013736 at doses ranging from

5 to 30 mg by mouth bid. Patients initially received two single test doses of AG-013736 (10 and 30 mg); subsequent dosing was determined by individual PK parameters. The DLTs observed included hypertension, hemoptysis, and stomatitis and were seen primarily at the higher dose levels. AG-013736 was absorbed rapidly, with peak plasma concentrations observed within two to six hours after dosing. The MTD and recommended phase-II dose of AG-013736 was 5 mg bid, administered in the fasting state. No significant drug interaction with antacids was seen. There were three confirmed partial responses. The unique phase-I design in this study allowed early identification of important absorption and metabolic issues critical to orally administered small molecules (41). AG-013736 has also shown a superadditive effect in combination with docetaxel (42). A phase-II study in renal cell cancer demonstrated significant efficacy with a response rate (RR) of 46% (43). AG-013736 is being tested in a phase-II study of 32 patients for refractory NSCLC after failure of more than one previous regimen.

KRN951: This is a highly potent RTKI of the VEGFR; it has antitumor and antivascular properties (44). KRN951 potently inhibited VEGF-induced VEGFR-2 phosphorylation in endothelial cells at in vitro subnanomolar IC_{50} values ($IC_{50} = 0.16$ nmol/L). It also inhibited ligand-induced phosphorylation of PDGFR-β and c-Kit ($IC_{50} = 1.72$ and 1.63 nmol/L, respectively). KRN951 blocked VEGF-dependent, but not VEGF-independent, activation of mitogen-activated protein kinases (MAPK) and proliferation of endothelial cells. KRN951 is currently in phase-I clinical development for the treatment of patients with advanced cancer (44).

Multitargeted Kinase Inhibitors

Dual inhibition of EGFR and VEGFR signaling: Combining inhibitors of EGFR and VEGF signaling might have increased activity over either approach alone by simultaneously targeting tumor growth and preventing the formation of tumor neovasculature. Additionally, the EGFR and VEGFR pathways share common downstream effectors for signaling within the cell. In preclinical studies, both EGFR and VEGF signaling have shown direct influence on tumor cells and also indirect effects on the tumors through their vasculature. For instance, blocking EGFR expression in both tumor and endothelial cells has demonstrated antitumor activity in prostate cancer models (45,46). In other studies, production of VEGF in tumor cells is downregulated by EGFR inhibition (9,47,48), and, conversely, blocking VEGF has been shown to inhibit autocrine signaling through EGFR (47). Therefore, it is rational to postulate that inhibiting both signaling pathways simultaneously, thus affecting tumor cells directly and indirectly through their vasculature, might be a more effective treatment strategy against refractory tumor cells. Targeting both signaling pathways together might result in additive or even synergistic antitumor effects than targeting a single pathway. A number of agents with predominant EGFR and VEGFR inhibition are being studied.

ZD6474: Vandetanib is an anilinoquinazoline that belongs to the same class of drugs as gefitinib. It is a potent, orally available, low-molecular-weight TKI with specificity for VEGFR [inhibitory concentration $(IC)_{50}$ for VEGFR-2—40 nM and VEGFR-3—110 nM], RET $(IC_{50}$ 130 nM), and at higher concentrations, EGFR $(IC_{50} = 500$ nM) tyrosine kinases (49). Statistically significant dose-dependent antitumor activity has been demonstrated in all human tumor xenograft models $(0.15–0.47$ cm^3) including lung cancer $(P < 0.001$ with ≥12.5 mg/kg/day vandetanib in A549 and Calu-6 lung cancer models). Preclinical studies have also attempted to delineate the effects of vandetanib on EGFR signaling either as a single agent or in combination with taxanes (47). Vandetanib inhibited EGFR tyrosine kinase activity in intact tumor cells. It also exhibited synergism in tumor inhibition and apoptosis with both paclitaxel and docetaxel in cell lines that over-expressed human EGFR but not VEGFR-2. Vandetanib has been investigated as a single agent in phase-I studies in the United States, Australia, and Japan (50,51). The MTD of vandetanib was established as 300 mg/day. The most common DLTs were diarrhea, hypertension, and rash. The half-life of vandetanib was 109 hours with the 300 mg/day dose. Steady-state plasma concentrations were achieved after a minimum of 28 days of dosing. No objective responses according to the response evaluation criteria in solid tumors (RECIST) were seen in the 77 patients in this study; however, 44% of the patients receiving vandetanib 300 mg/day had SD. Median time to progression was 1.8 to 7.2 months across all dose levels. A phase-I study in 18 Japanese patients included nine patients with NSCLC; all patients received a single dose of vandetanib 100 to 400 mg followed by a seven-day wash-out period (51). Four of the nine NSCLC patients at the 200 and 300 mg/day doses achieved a partial response (PR) that was maintained following dose reductions. Vandetanib has been evaluated in phase-II studies as a single agent or in combination with chemotherapy in patients with previously treated advanced NSCLC.

Randomized Phase-II Study with Vandetanib Monotherapy

Single agent vandetanib has been compared to gefitinib in a randomized phase-II trial with a crossover design and has demonstrated substantially higher clinical benefit when administered before or after the crossover design (52). The crossover design was intended to investigate the mechanism of action of vandetanib, partic-ularly to gain insight into whether one or both receptors (EGFR and VEGFR) are inhibited. In this trial, patients with advanced NSCLC who had failed first and/or second-line platinum-based chemotherapy were randomized to receive vande-tanib 300 mg or gefitinib 250 mg. The adverse events profile of both agents was considered similar enough to allow for a double-blind study design. The primary end point of the study was PFS and the secondary end points included RRs, over-all survival (OS), and safety. Eighty-three patients were treated with vandetanib and 85 with gefitinib. In the first part of the study, median PFS was significantly improved with vandetanib [11.0 weeks vs. 8.1 weeks with gefitinib, hazard ratio (HR) = 0.69; $P = 0.025$], corresponding to 45% prolongation in PFS. Objective RR was 8% (7/83 patients) with vandetanib and 1% (1/85 patients) with gefitinib. Disease control (lasting >8 weeks) was achieved in 45% (37/83) and 34% (29/85) of patients, respectively. No significant differences were noted between vandetanib and gefitinib in the class effect toxicities of EGFR inhibitors such as grade-3 rash (5% vs. 1%, respectively). However, vandetanib also exhibited the common adverse events observed with antiangiogenic agents (grade-3/4 dizziness/seizures, grade-3/4 hypertension, and grade-3 headaches). These adverse events occurred in less than 5% of the patients in the vandetanib arm and none were seen in the gefitinib arm. QTc-related events were observed in 21% and 5% of patients, respectively (50,53).

Serial CT scans were obtained from the patients every four weeks, and upon disease progression or severe toxicity patients were switched between treatment groups following a washout period of four weeks. In the second part of the study, of the 62 patients alive in the vandetanib arm with progressive disease (PD), 29 switched to gefitinib, and 37 of 73 patients alive with PD in the gefitinib arm switched to vandetanib. Disease control was achieved in 24% of patients (7/29) who switched to gefitinib; this was lower than that seen in the first part of the study and was suggestive of the fact that vandetanib had exerted its EGFR inhibitory properties, thus, exhausting responses with EGFR-targeted therapy in this patient population. A disease control rate of 43% (16/37) was noted in patients who crossed over to vandetanib suggesting a different mechanism of action of vandetanib besides EGFR inhibition, most likely blockade of VEGF signaling. No significant difference was observed in median OS between the treatment arms (6.1 months with vandetanib $\rightarrow$ gefitinib vs. 7.4 months with gefitinib $\rightarrow$ vandetanib, HR = 1.19; P = 0.34). It is possible that several factors including the switch design and adenocarcinoma histology contributed to the lack of significant difference in OS between the treatment arms.

Vandetanib in Combination with Chemotherapy

Although agents directed against EGFR have enhanced clinical benefit in combination with chemotherapeutic agents compared to chemotherapy alone in colorectal and pancreatic cancers (54,55), to date, a significant improvement in OS has not been demonstrated with gefitinib or erlotinib in combination with platinum-based chemotherapy in the treatment of NSCLC in unselected populations (56,57). On the other hand, agents targeting angiogenesis have been combined successfully with platinum-based chemotherapy to substantially improve clinical outcomes in NSCLC (58). Given that vandetanib is a dual inhibitor of EGFR and VEGFR, one question that needed to be addressed in NSCLC was whether vandetanib administered simultaneously with chemotherapy was more beneficial compared to chemotherapy alone and if this combination had a tolerable toxicity profile. A randomized, two-part, phase-II study with vandetanib plus docetaxel as second-line therapy in advanced NSCLC has been conducted. Patients with prior docetaxel therapy were excluded. The run-in phase evaluated the safety of the combination (59). Follow-up results of the second, randomized phase of the study assessing efficacy were recently presented (60). In the randomized phase, a total of 127 patients received vandetanib (100 or 300 mg) daily plus docetaxel 75 mg/m^2 every three weeks, or placebo plus docetaxel on the same schedule. The primary objective was PFS and secondary end points including RR, OS, and safety. The trial was designed to have >75% power to detect 50% prolongation of PFS at significance level of $P = 0.2$.

Docetaxel in combination with low-dose vandetanib gave the most favorable response. The cause for the relative decrease in clinical benefit with increase in dose of vandetanib is not known, but might reflect an antagonistic effect of increased EGFR inhibition at higher doses of vandetanib. Low-dose vandetanib is thought to exert its effects primarily through VEGFR inhibition, which shows synergistic activity with chemotherapy in the clinic. Compared to treatment with docetaxel plus placebo (median PFS: 12 weeks), PFS improved by 57% with vandetanib 100 mg plus docetaxel, and by 21% with vandetanib 300 mg plus docetaxel [median PFS: 18.7 weeks (HR = 0.64; $P = 0.074$) and 17 weeks (HR = 0.83; $P = 0.461$), respectively]. The overall response rate (ORR) was 26% with vandetanib 100 mg plus docetaxel, 18% with vandetanib 300 mg plus docetaxel, and 12% with placebo plus docetaxel.

The addition of vandetanib 100 mg to docetaxel did not improve median OS (13.1 months vs. 13.4 months with placebo plus docetaxel, HR = 0.91; $P = 0.723$), and the addition of vandetanib 300 mg further increased the risk of death by 28% compared to placebo plus docetaxel (HR = 1.28; $P = 0.334$). Six patients (two in each arm) died due to serious adverse events (respiratory distress and hemoptysis in the placebo arm, atrial fibrillation and acute respiratory failure in the vandetanib 100 mg arm, and interstitial pneumonitis with exacerbation of chronic obstructive pulmonary disorder in the vandetanib 300 mg arm).

Vandetanib is being evaluated in previously untreated, stage-IIIB/IV recurrent NSCLC in a phase-II trial (61). An estimated 220 patients will be randomized to single agent vandetanib or vandetanib plus platinum-based chemotherapy or chemotherapy alone. The dose of vandetanib (100 mg/day) that demonstrated maximum clinical benefit with minimal side effects in the phase-II trial is being assessed in a phase-III trial in stage III/IV NSCLC as second-line therapy in combination with docetaxel compared to placebo plus docetaxel (62). The targeted accrual for this trial is 1240 patients. Lastly, a phase-III study with a target accrual of 1150 patients is comparing the efficacy of vandetanib versus erlotinib as second- or third-line therapy for the treatment of advanced NSCLC (62).

AEE788: AEE788 is an orally active, small-molecule, multitargeted kinase inhibitor with potent inhibitory activity against multiple tyrosine kinases, including EGFR, HER2, and VEGFR-2. The phase-I study was conducted to assess its safety, PK, PD, MTD, and optimal biologic dose in patients with advanced solid tumors. AEE788 was given by mouth (PO) at 25, 50, 100, 150, 225, 300, 400, 450, 500, and 550 mg/day in 28-day cycles to 3 to 6 patient cohorts. Twenty-four-hour PK profiles were performed on days 1, 15, 28. PK parameters of AEE788 and AQM674 (active metabolite) were computed by model-independent methods. PD markers were analyzed in skin and tumor biopsies pre- and posttreatment. Sixty-nine patients were treated with a median of two cycles (range < 1–10). AEE788 and AQM674 concentrations varied widely and increased with dose and duration. IC_{50} values were estimated for pEGFR (42 nM), pMAPK (38 nM), Ki67 (7 nM) in SK and pEGFR (28 nM), pMAPK (22 nM) in tumors. A dose-dependent inhibition of EGFR signaling in skin and tumor was observed; profound receptor inhibition is achieved with ≥300 mg/day. As expected, inhibition of endothelial pMAPK and Ki67 occurred at higher doses than EGFR inhibition (≥300 mg). Exposure-dependent effects were observed and estimated IC_{50} corresponded to the preclinical data (63). In addition to inhibiting cutaneous cancer cell growth by blocking EGFR and VEGFR signaling pathways in vitro, AEE788 inhibited in vivo tumor growth by inducing tumor and endothelial cell apoptosis (64).

XL647: This is an orally bioavailable, potent inhibitor of multiple RTKs including EGF, HER2, and VEGF. In addition, XL647 inhibits EphB4, an RTK-promoting angiogenesis that is highly expressed in many human tumors. In a broad array of preclinical tumor models including breast, lung, colon, and prostate cancer, XL647 demonstrated potent inhibition of tumor growth and caused tumor regression. In cell culture models, XL647 retained significant potency against mutant EGFRs that cause resistance to current EGFR inhibitors. In the phase-I study of XL467 in patients with advanced solid tumors, the primary objective of the phase-I dose-escalation trial was to establish an MTD, and to assess safety and tolerability of oral administration of XL647. Secondary objectives included PK analyses and tumor response. The study enrolled patients in successive cohorts to receive XL647 orally as a single dose on day 1, followed by five continuous daily doses starting on day 4. Patients then continued to receive dosing for five continuous days followed by a break with cycles repeated every 14 days. The investigators reported that of 40 evaluable patients, one patient (NSCLC had a PR) and 12 others [NSCLC (3), chordoma (2), adenoid cystic carcinoma (2), adrenocortical carcinoma, colorectal, ovarian, mesothelioma, and head and neck cancer] had prolonged SD (>3.5 months). The first two patients treated at the 7.0 mg/kg dose experienced DLTs of grade-3 diarrhea, which resolved upon a reduction in dose to 4.68 mg/kg. One serious adverse event of grade-4 pulmonary embolism was considered potentially related to study treatment in a patient treated at the 0.28 mg/kg dose. One patient at the 3.12 mg/kg dose had an asymptomatic QTc prolongation on electrocardiogram. Expansion of the 4.68 mg/kg cohort to six patients occurred without further DLTs and this was considered the MTD (65). The primary objectives of the follow-up phase-II study are to determine the RR of subjects with NSCLC treated with XL647 and to evaluate the safety and tolerability of XL647. The trial will be conducted in patients with advanced (stage IIIB or IV) NSCLC who have not previously been treated with chemotherapy. In this proof-of-concept trial, participants must meet at least two of the following criteria: Asian, female, nonsmoker, or a patient of adeno-carcinoma. Secondary objectives include assessment of PFS, duration of response, OS, and characterization of PK and PD parameters.

Sunitinib: This is an orally administered TKI of the VEGFR, PDGFR, and RET, Kit, and Flt-3 targets neovascular endothelium, pericytes as well as tumor cells (66). In mouse xenograft models, sunitinib exhibited potent antitumor activity causing regression or reduced growth of various established xenografts derived from human or rat tumor cell lines (67). In phase-I clinical studies, the recommended dose of sunitinib was found to be 50 mg orally, QD for four weeks, followed by two weeks off, in a repeated six-week cycle (68). PK data indicated good oral absorption and a long $t_{1/2}$ of 40 hours. It was recently approved by the U.S. Food and Drug Administration (FDA) for treatment of advanced RCC and imatinib-resistant gastrointestinal stromal tumors. Since sunitinib targets the signaling pathways implicated in NSCLC, clinical trials of single agent sunitinib as well as sunitinib in combination with chemotherapy were launched to study the efficacy and tolerability of this agent in NSCLC (69). Results from a single arm multicenter phase-II trial of sunitinib in previously treated advanced NSCLC were presented (69). Patients with histologically proven stage IIIB (with pleural effusion) or stage IV refractory NSCLC, an Eastern Cooperative Oncology Group performance status (PS) of 0 or 1, and disease progression on at least one prior platinum-containing systemic regimen were eligible. Patients with a recent grade-3 hemorrhage or gross hemoptysis, uncontrolled hypertension, brain metastases, history of cardiac disease, cerebrovascular accident, or pulmonary embolism were not eligible to participate in the study. Prior treatment with angiogenesis inhibitors was not permitted. Sixty-three eligible patients received sunitinib 50 mg/day for four of six weeks until disease progression or unacceptable toxicity. The primary objective was confirmed ORR. Common histologic subtypes were adenocarcinoma (64%) and squamous cell carcinoma (22%), with only 17% nonsmokers. Fifty-seven percent of patients had received at least two prior regimens and 33% had been treated with an EGFR inhibitor. Dose interruptions and dose reductions were required in 27% and 21% of patients, respectively. Treatment discontinuation due to adverse events was needed in 38% of patients. An ORR of 9.5% (6/63 patients, all partial responses) was achieved. The median duration of response was 12.2 weeks (4.3–30.3+ weeks). SD was reported in 27 (42.9%) patients. The median PFS was 11.3 weeks. The median OS was 23.9 weeks. Three hemorrhage-related (two pulmonary and one cerebral) deaths were reported. Grade-3/4 neutropenia and thrombocytopenia occurred in 5% of patients each. Grade-3/4 nonhematologic toxicities reported in 10% of patients or more were fatigue/asthenia (27%) and pain/myalgia (17%). Other grade-3 toxicities were nausea/vomiting (10%), dyspnea (13%), and hypertension (5%). The incidence of fatal hemorrhages, reminiscent of data with bevacizumab, needs to be carefully monitored during sunitinib therapy in NSCLC. Other drug-related toxicities were typical of those seen with any targeted agent in this category. The expansion phase of this trial has already enrolled 47 patients to test the continuous dosing schedule of sunitinib at 37.5 mg/day. To further explore the role of sunitinib in NSCLC, a phase-II trial has been initiated to test the efficacy and safety of sunitinib in combination with erlotinib in advanced NSCLC (70).

AMG 706: This is an oral, multikinase inhibitor with both antiangiogenic and direct antitumor activity achieved by targeting VEGFRs, PDGFR, and Kit.

By inhibiting multiple receptors, AMG 706 potentially may provide more than one mechanism of action in various cancers. A phase-II clinical study evaluating AMG 706 monotherapy in imatinib-resistant GIST has completed enrollment, and a phase-II trial in advanced thyroid cancer is ongoing. AMG 706 is also being developed in combination with multiple chemotherapy regimens, with and without panitumumab (an EGFR TKI), in the treatment of solid tumors. A phase-I study in advanced solid tumor patients was presented (71). Patients with advanced solid tumors, refractory to standard therapy or with no standard therapy available, were enrolled in this study. After establishing the maximum tolerated intermittent dose (21 days of therapy followed by seven days without dosing) in 31 patients, an additional 34 patients were given AMG 706 125 mg QD in a continuous dosing pattern. AMG 706 was generally well tolerated up to 125 mg QD using the intermittent and continuous dosing schedules, with three patients continuing on study for more than one year. Most adverse events were mild-to-moderate in severity and reversible. Across all cohorts, the most frequent medication-related adverse events were hypertension (31%), fatigue (29%), and headache (25%) that were primarily of mild-to-moderate severity. Among 56 evaluable patients, best responses were two (4%) partial responses and 34 (61%) SD (including 17 patients with decreases ranging up to 29% in the sum of the longest diameter of target lesions). A follow-up phase-I open-label, dose-finding study to evaluate the safety and PK of AMG 706 with carboplatin/paclitaxel, AMG 706 with panitumumab, and AMG 706 with panitumumab with carboplatin/paclitaxel in the treatment of subjects with advanced NSCLC has been initiated.

Sorafenib: BAY 43-9006 is a novel bi-aryl urea was initially developed as a specific inhibitor of RAF/MEK/ERK pathway. Subsequent studies have shown this compound to also inhibit several other tyrosine kinases involved in tumor progression, including VEGFRs, PDGFR, Flt-3, and c-Kit (72). Xenograft models of colon, breast, and NSCLC treated with sorafenib demonstrated significant inhibition of tumor angiogenesis, as measured by anti-CD31 immunostaining (73). Phase-I studies of sorafenib, involving 163 patients treated with different continuous oral dosage schedules, identified 400 mg bid as the recommended phase-II dose that targets VEGFR-2. In addition, this agent targets RAF/MEK/ERK as well (74,75). Subsequently, phase-II trials have been carried out in several cancers including renal cell, hepatocellular carcinoma, metastatic melanoma, and NSCLC. The novel, randomized discontinuation design was used in the phase-II trial in RCC (76). The improved RRs and PFS for sorafenib compared with placebo were confirmed in a subsequent phase-III study that led to approval by the FDA for sorafenib in RCC (77). A phase-II study in NSCLC was reported by Gatzeimeir et al. at ASCO, 2006. Fifty-two patients with refractory metastatic NSCLC were enrolled. In this multicenter, open-labeled, single arm phase-II study, sorafenib was given at a dose of 400 mg bid continuously for a 28-day cycle until progression noted by RECIST. No objective responses were seen. SD was noted in 59% of patients. The PFS was 2.7 months and OS 6.8 months. Two patients were continuing therapy at two years. The most common toxicities were diarrhea (40%) and hand foot syndrome (37%). Four patients had a bleeding event (three with epistaxis and one patient with squamous histology and a cavitary lesion who developed fatal pulmonary hemorrhage after radiation, 30 days after stopping sorafenib). Presently, at least two phase-III studies are underway (in Europe and in North America). In addition to studies evaluating single agent sorafenib in refractory NSCLC, there are studies looking at the combination of sorafenib both with chemotherapy and with other targeted agents such as gefitinib. In a phase-I study of sorafenib in combination with gefitinib, the combination of sorafenib at 400 mg PO bid and gefitinib 250 mg PO QD was well tolerated and led to tumor regression in 9/12 patients (78). In addition, there is a large randomized study evaluating sorafenib and chemotherapy versus bevacizumab and chemotherapy in patients with metastatic NSCLC.

CP-547, 632: This is another oral, antiangiogenic small-molecule inhibitor of VEGFR-2 tyrosine kinase activity, which also targets EGFR, PDGFR, and other tyrosine kinases. In vitro CP-547, 632 inhibits endothelial cell proliferation and, in xenografts including NSCLC, retards tumor growth. Early phase-I data suggest an encouraging safety profile and PK parameters (79,80). Phase-II trials have not yet begun.

Some of the agents (described above) and their recommended phase II doses are summarized in Table 3. Select ongoing trials are summarized in Table 4.

Novel Mechanisms

ABT-510: Mimicking the behavior of a natural antiangiogenic protein, thrombospondin-1, ABT-510 is being evaluated to determine its potential to block multiple proangiogenic growth factors including VEGF, bFGF, and interleukin-8. ABT-510 currently is being studied in phase-II clinical trials in various cancers including

Table 3 Selected Agents Exhibiting VEGFR Tyrosine Kinase Inhibitory Activity

Drug	Target	Recommended phase-II dose
AZD2171	VEGFR-1	45 mg/day
PTK787 (vatalanib)	VEGFR-2	1250 mg/day or 750 mg twice/day
GW786034 (pazopanib)	VEGFR-3	800 mg/day
AG013736 (axitinib)	PDGFR-β; c-Kit	5 mg twice/day
BAY 43-9006 (sorafenib)	Raf; VEGFR 2,3; Flt-3; c-Kit	400 mg twice/day
SU11248 (sunitinib)	PDGFR-β; VEGFR 2; Flt-3; c-Kit	50 mg/day 4 wk on/2 wk off
ZD6474 (vandetinib)	EGFR; RET; VEGFR 2,3	100–300 mg/day
AEE788	EGFR; HER2/neu; VEGFR 1,2; c-Abl; c-Src; c-Src	450 mg/day
AMG 706	VEGFR 1,2,3; PDGFR; c-Kit	125 mg/day

Abbreviations: PDGFR, platelet-derived growth factor receptor; VEGFR, vascular endothelial growth factor receptor.

Table 4 Select Ongoing Trials of Antiangiogenic Agents in Advanced Stage Non–Small Cell Lung Cancer

Phase	Regimen	Setting	Number of patients	Sponsor
III	Carboplatin + paclitaxel plus/minus sorafenib	First line	900	Bayer
III	Carboplatin + paclitaxel plus/minus sorafenib followed by sorafenib vs. placebo	First line	600	EORTC
II	Sorafenib vs. placebo	≥2 Previous regimens	311 (after completion of induction sorafenib, days 1–28)	Bayer
I/II	Carboplatin/paclitaxel/sorafenib/bevacizumab	Non–small cell lung cancer		Bayer
II	Sunitinib/erlotinib vs. sunitinib/placebo	1–2 Previous regimens	136 (after initial safety run-in phase of erlotinib/sunitinib)	Pfizer, Inc.
II	Sunitinib	≤2 Previous regimens	104	Pfizer, Inc.
II	Carboplatin + paclitaxel followed by sunitinib	First line	83	Pfizer, Inc.
II	ZD6474 vs. ZD6474 + carboplatin and paclitaxel vs. placebo + carboplatin and paclitaxel	First line	10–220 (10 pts in initial safety study)	NCI
III	Docetaxel ± ZD6474	Second line	1240	AstraZeneca, LP
III	ZD 6474 vs. erlotinib	Second line	1150	AstraZeneca, LP
II/III	AZD2171 + carboplatin and paclitaxel vs. placebo + carboplatin and paclitaxel	First line	750	AstraZeneca, LP
II	VEGF Trap	≥2 Previous regimens	94	Sanofi-Aventis
II	Axitinib	≥1 Previous regimen	32	Pfizer
I/II	AMG 706 + carboplatin and paclitaxel and/or panitumumab	First line		Amgen, Inc.
I/II	AMG 706 + panitumumab + gemcitabine and cisplatin	Advanced cancers		Amgen, Inc.
II	AMG 706 vs. bevacizumab	First line		Amgen, Inc.
III	Erlotinib plus bevacizumab vs. erlotinib plus placebo	Second line	650	Genentech, Inc.
II	Cetuximab, paclitaxel, carboplatin, and bevacizumab in treating patients with advanced non-small cell lung cancer	First line	90	NCI
II	Docetaxel, carboplatin, and bevacizumab	Adjuvant, stage I, II, III	50	NCI
II	Carboplatin, pemetrexed and bevacizumab	First line	50	NCI
II	Docetaxel and thalidomide	Second line	37	NCI

Abbreviations: VEGF, vascular endothelial growth factor; EORTC, European Organization for Research and Treatment of Cancer.

sarcoma, lymphoma, and kidney cancer. ABT-510 was granted an orphan drug designation by the FDA for soft tissue sarcoma. A phase-I study of ABT-510 was conducted in which ABT-510 was administered subcutaneously as a continuous infusion (100 mg/24 hour) and bolus injections (100, 200, and 260 mg QD) in 28-day cycles. Thirty-nine patients received a total of 144 treatment cycles. Administration by continuous infusion was hampered by the onset of painful skin infiltrates at the injection site. In the bolus injection regimens, the most common toxicities observed were mild injection-site reactions and fatigue. MTD was not defined, but 260 mg was defined as the maximum clinically practical dose. Median serum bFGF levels decreased from 14.1 pg/mL (range, 0.5–77.7 pg/mL) at baseline to 3.2 pg/mL (range, 0.2–29.4 pg/mL) after 56 days of treatment ($P = 0.003$). No correlations with time on study or ABT-510 dose or exposure were observed for individual changes in bFGF. SD lasting for six cycles or more was seen in six patients. ABT-510 demonstrated a favorable toxicity profile and linear and time-independent PKs with biologically relevant plasma concentrations (plasma concentrations > 100 ng/mL >3 hr/day). The significant number of patients with prolonged SD and the convenient method of dosing merit further studies with this angiogenesis inhibitor (81). Phase-II studies in NSCLC are planned.

Integrin antagonists: Integrins α versus β 3 and α versus β 5 are important in tumor growth and angiogenesis and have been recently explored as targets for cancer therapy. Examples of integrin antagonists include cilengitide (EMD 121974) in vitro and clonogenic studies demonstrated that cilengitide acted as a radiosensitizer in combination with ionizing radiation with an increase in apoptotic cell death and detached cells (82). Clinical development of this agent is continuing.

Thalidomide: Thalidomide has been shown to have immune-modulating and antiangiogenic effects (83). To examine the efficacy and toxicity of adding thalidomide to the conventional cytotoxic agents, carboplatin and irinotecan, a single-arm phase-II study was conducted in patients with untreated extensive stage small cell lung cancer (SCLC). Four cycles of chemotherapy with carboplatin AUC 5 on day 1 and irinotecan 50 mg/m² IV on days 1 and 8 were planned every 21 days. Thalidomide was initiated on day 1 at 200 mg daily and increased 100 mg weekly to a total dose of 400 mg daily. Six patients were enrolled. Hematologic and nonhematologic toxicities were monitored. Treatment-related, grade-3 adverse events included diarrhea, dizziness, drug reaction, neutropenia, and rash. Partial responses (by RECIST) were identified in two patients. Two grade-3 thrombotic events (bilateral deep venous thromboses/pulmonary embolism and cerebellar stroke) occurred, but the association to thalidomide administration was uncertain. Unfortunately, treatment-related side effects limited the ability of patients not only to titrate thalidomide to the maximum goal but also to continue the medication altogether. The study was therefore suspended (84). Alternative strategies are being explored including the role of maintenance of thalidomide after initial chemotherapy for extensive stage SCLC. A randomized trial of carboplatin/etoposide with or without thalidomide in SCLC is proposed in the United Kingdom.

Vascular-disrupting agents: These agents target the endothelium of existing blood vessels in tumors by both direct and indirect mechanisms, as against other antiangiogenic drugs that target the "neovasculature." The parent compound for this group of drugs was flavone acetic acid, a compound that caused hemorrhagic necrosis of murine tumors. Despite promising preclinical activity, the clinical trials were negative. Working on the structure of flavone acetic acid, researchers in New Zealand developed compounds with greater activity (85). The most active of these compounds is AS1404 (DM-XAA, dimethylxanthenone acetic acid).

Two phase-I studies have been carried out. AS1404 was given at doses ranging from 6 to 4900 mg/m^2 and was well tolerated at low doses. The PK of the drug in human beings, similar to that in mice, was dose-dependent with decreased clearance at higher doses. No myelosupression was observed, but at the maximum dose, dose-limiting toxic effects, although rapidly reversible, included tremors, cognitive impairment, and visual disturbance. Transient, asymptomatic QT prolongation was noted at the two highest doses (85). In a phase-II study in lung cancer (first-line treatment of stage-IIIb/IV NSCLC) combining AS1404 with carboplatin and paclitaxel showed a median survival of 14.0 months in patients receiving AS1404 plus chemotherapy versus 8.8 months in patients receiving chemotherapy alone. These promising results justify further studies of this compound.

Combretastatin A4 phosphate (CA4P): CA4P belongs to the class of microtubule-disrupting agents such as colchicine. It blocks the vascular endothelial-cadherin/B-catenin complex that is required for the endothelial cell–cell adhesion and survival during tumor neovessel formation. This leads to vascular shutdown in experimental tumor models with resultant hemorrhagic necrosis of tumors (86). In the phase-I study, the drug was delivered by a 10 minute weekly infusion × 3 followed by a one-week gap, with intrapatient dose escalation until two instances of grade-2 toxicity occurred. Dose was escalated by doubling until grade-2 toxicity was seen, then by 1.3-fold increase. The starting dose was 5 mg/m^2. CA4P was well tolerated in 11/13 patients at 52 or 68 mg/m^2, and tumor blood flow reduction was reproducibly seen at these doses. DLT was reversible ataxia at 114 mg/m^2, and vasovagal syncope and motor neuropathy at 8 mg/m^2 (87). Phase-II studies in various tumor types are planned.

CONCLUSIONS AND FUTURE DIRECTIONS

In the last decade, there has been a profusion of biologically targeted agents, several of which have shown promise in the treatment of lung cancer. The success with the monoclonal antibody, bevacizumab, validated VEGF as a therapeutic cancer target for lung cancer. This is described in the next chapter of this book. Since then, the small-molecule TKIs have demonstrated initial clinical activity in lung cancer.

However, there are several questions that arise with respect to these compounds. While important, targeting the VEGF pathway alone may not be sufficient to arrest tumor growth. There is cross talk at multiple levels in signal transduction pathways. Additionally, angiogenic pathways independent of VEGF have also been described. The role played by other pathways responsible for tumor growth such as PI3-AKT, met, ras, MAPK, Src family kinases, and epigenetic regulatory mechanisms that contribute to both VEGF-dependent and VEGF-independent angiogenesis cannot be ignored. Indeed, it has been shown that inhibiting RTK pertaining to EGFR or met can have a secondary downstream effect on VEGF levels (88). Similar synergistic or additive angiogenic effects may be the case when chemotherapy is combined with the more traditional antiangiogenic drugs. The effectiveness of such an approach was shown in the bevacizumab trial with carboplatin/paclitaxel. However, this approach has not been effective for all small-molecule TKIs as evidenced by studies with vatalanib and semaxinib. This approach of combining targeted drugs with each other as well as with chemotherapy continues to be explored.

A conceptually attractive approach to targeting multiple signaling pathways is the use of a single agent that is capable of inhibiting multiple targets. Thus single agent studies of sunitinib and sorafenib in refractory NSCLC have demonstrated early clinical activity, equivalent to second-line chemotherapy in this setting with fewer side effects. Other agents such as ZD6474 were effective, albeit at lower doses (than required to block VEGF) in combination with chemotherapy. It may be that at lower doses, "normalization" of tumor blood vessels occurs by virtue of VEGF blockade, allowing better delivery of chemotherapy, in keeping with the hypothesis put forth on pruning and tumor vasculature by Jain et al. (89).

Host factors are also very important. Before an oral agent can interact with its target, the drug has to be absorbed and transported to the tumor microenvironment. Metabolism may occur during this process. Secondly, a number of tumors harbor efflux pumps for which a large number of currently available oral TKIs are substrates. A number of these transporters and metabolic enzymes are polymorphic, thus potentially leading to variable toxicity and efficacy.

With the plethora of kinase inhibitors having overlapping target specificities, therapeutic index and the pharmacology of these agents will be a primary determinant of which agents demonstrate clinical benefit. A number of the newer antiangiogenic agents have been associated with vascular complications such as hypertension and hemorrhage. While rare, these can be serious and sometimes fatal. At the present time, phenotypic characteristics such as squamous histology, presence of brain metastasis, and propensity for bleeding/clotting are used to exclude patients from receiving some of the agents such as bevacizumab. There is potential for the utilization of pharmacogenetics to identify allelic variants that may predict for toxicity.

It is indeed an exciting time in the treatment of lung cancer with the availability and development of several antiangiogenic drugs. However, a multipronged approach would offer the best way of tackling the morbidity and mortality from this terrible disease.

REFERENCES

1. Olofsson B, Jeltsch M, Eriksson U, Alitalo K. Current biology of VEGF-B and VEGF-C. Curr Opin Biotechnol 1999; 10:528–535.
2. Ferrara N, Gerber HP, LeCouter J. The biology of VEGF and its receptors. Nat Med 2003; 9:669–676.
3. Yancopoulos GD, Davis S, Gale NW, Rudge JS, Wiegand SJ, Holash J. Vascular-specific growth factors and blood vessel formation. Nature 2000; 407:242–248.
4. Clauss M. Molecular biology of the VEGF and the VEGF receptor family. Semin Thromb Hemost 2000; 26:561–569.
5. Klagsbrun M, Soker S. VEGF/VPF: the angiogenesis factor found? Curr Biol 1993; 3:699–702.
6. Senger DR, Galli SJ, Dvorak AM, Perruzzi CA, Harvey VS, Dvorak HF. Tumor cells secrete a vascular permeability factor that promotes accumulation of ascites fluid. Science 1983; 219:983–985.
7. Grugel S, Finkenzeller G, Weindel K, Barleon B, Marme D. Both v-Ha-Ras and v-Raf stimulate expression of the vascular endothelial growth factor in NIH 3T3 cells. J Biol Chem 1995; 270:25915–25919.
8. Rak J, Filmus J, Finkenzeller G, Grugel S, Marme D, Kerbel RS. Oncogenes as inducers of tumor angiogenesis. Cancer Metastasis Rev 1995; 14:263–277.
9. Petit AM, Rak J, Hung MC, et al. Neutralizing antibodies against epidermal growth factor and ErbB-2/neu receptor tyrosine kinases down-regulate vascular endothelial growth factor production by tumor cells in vitro and in vivo: angiogenic implications for signal transduction therapy of solid tumors. Am J Pathol 1997; 151:1523–1530.
10. Paavonen K, Puolakkainen P, Jussila L, Jahkola T, Alitalo K. Vascular endothelial growth factor receptor-3 in lymphangiogenesis in wound healing. Am J Pathol 2000; 156:1499–1504.
11. Soker S, Takashima S, Miao HQ, Neufeld G, Klagsbrun M. Neuropilin-1 is expressed by endothelial and tumor cells as an isoform-specific receptor for vascular endothelial growth factor. Cell 1998; 92:735–745.
12. Moses MA, Langer R. Inhibitors of angiogenesis. Biotechnology (NY) 1991; 9:630–634.
13. Nyberg P, Xie L, Kalluri R. Endogenous inhibitors of angiogenesis. Cancer Res 2005; 65:3967–3979.
14. O'Reilly MS, Holmgren L, Shing Y, et al. Angiostatin: a novel angiogenesis inhibitor that mediates the suppression of metastases by a Lewis lung carcinoma. Cell 1994; 79:315–328.
15. Kurup A, Lin CW, Murry DJ, et al. Recombinant human angiostatin (rhAngiostatin) in combination with paclitaxel and carboplatin in patients with advanced non-small-cell lung cancer: a phase II study from Indiana University. Ann Oncol 2006; 17:97–103.
16. Ezekowitz RA, Mulliken JB, Folkman J. Interferon alfa-2a therapy for life-threatening hemangiomas of infancy. N Engl J Med 1992; 326:1456–1463.
17. Shepherd FA, Beaulieu R, Gelmon K, et al. Prospective randomized trial of two dose levels of interferon alfa with zidovudine for the treatment of Kaposi's sarcoma associated with human immunodeficiency virus infection: a Canadian HIV Clinical Trials Network study. J Clin Oncol 1998; 16:1736–1742.
18. Jett JR, Maksymiuk AW, Su JQ, et al. Phase III trial of recombinant interferon gamma in complete responders with small-cell lung cancer. J Clin Oncol 1994; 12:2321–2326.

19. Kelly K, Crowley JJ, Bunn PA Jr, et al. Role of recombinant interferon alfa-2a maintenance in patients with limited-stage small-cell lung cancer responding to concurrent chemoradiation: a Southwest Oncology Group study. J Clin Oncol 1995; 13:2924–2930.

20. Mattson K, Niiranen A, Pyrhonen S, et al. Natural interferon alfa as maintenance therapy for small cell lung cancer. Eur J Cancer 1992; 28A:1387–1391.

21. Lebeau B, Delsalmoniere P, Ozenne G, et al. Alpha Interferon as maintenance therapy for small cell lung cancer (SCLC). Proc ASCO 1999; 18:475a [abstr. 1832].

22. Holden SN, Morrow M, O'Bryant C, et al. Correlative biological assays used to guide dose escalation in a phase I study of the antiangiogenic aVB3 and a VB5 integrin antagonist EMD 121974 (EMD). Proc ASCO 2002; 21:28a [abstr. 110].

23. Teicher BA, Holden SA, Ara G, Korbut T, Menon K. Comparison of several antiangiogenic regimens alone and with cytotoxic therapies in the Lewis lung carcinoma. Cancer Chemother Pharmacol 1996; 38:169–177.

24. Teicher BA, Dupuis NP, Robinson MF, Emi Y, Goff DA. Antiangiogenic treatment (TNP-470/minocycline) increases tissue levels of anticancer drugs in mice bearing Lewis lung carcinoma. Oncol Res 1995; 7:237–243.

25. Herbst RS, Madden TL, Tran HT, et al. Safety and pharmacokinetic effects of TNP-470, an angiogenesis inhibitor, combined with paclitaxel in patients with solid tumors: evidence for activity in non-small-cell lung cancer. J Clin Oncol 2002; 20:4440–4447.

26. Kobayashi H, Eckhardt SG, Lockridge JA, et al. Safety and pharmacokinetic study of RPI.4610 (ANGIOZYME), an anti-VEGFR-1 ribozyme, in combination with carboplatin and paclitaxel in patients with advanced solid tumors. Cancer Chemother Pharmacol 2005; 56:329–336.

27. Irish JM, Kotecha N, Nolan GP. Mapping normal and cancer cell signalling networks: towards single-cell proteomics. Nat Rev Cancer 2006; 6:146–155.

28. Dy GK, Adjei AA. Angiogenesis inhibitors in lung cancer: a promise fulfilled. Clin Lung Cancer 2006; 7(suppl 4):S1; 45–149.

29. Hurwitz H, Dowlati A, Savage S, Fernando N, et al. Safety, tolerability and pharmacokinetics of oral administration of GW786034 in pts with solid tumors. J Clin Oncol 2005; ASCO Annual Meeting Proceedings. Vol. 23, No. 16S, Part I of II (suppl), 2005:3012.

30. GlaxoSmith Kline. Pazopanib (GW786034) Investigator's Brochure, Version 3, (December 2005). 2005.

31. Suttle A, Hurwitz H, Dowlati A, Fernando N, et al. Pharmacokinetics (PK) and tolerability of GW786034, a VEGFR tyrosine kinase inhibitor, after daily oral administration to patients with solid tumors. J Clin Oncol 2004; ASCO Annual Meeting Proceedings (Post-Meeting Edition). Vol. 22, No 14S (July 15 Supplement), 2004:3054.

32. Wedge SR, Kendrew J, Hennequin LF, et al. AZD2171: a highly potent, orally bioavailable, vascular endothelial growth factor receptor-2 tyrosine kinase inhibitor for the treatment of cancer. Cancer Res 2005; 65:4389–4400.

33. Drevs J, Medinger M, Mross K, et al. Phase I clinical evaluation of AZD2171, a highly potent VEGF receptor tyrosine kinase inhibitor, in patients with advanced tumors. J Clin Oncol 2005; ASCO Annual Meeting Proceedings. Vol. 23, No. 16S, Part I of II (June 1 Supplement), 2005:3002.

34. Wood JM, Bold G, Buchdunger E, et al. PTK787/ZK 222584, a novel and potent inhibitor of vascular endothelial growth factor receptor tyrosine kinases, impairs

vascular endothelial growth factor-induced responses and tumor growth after oral administration. Cancer Res 2000; 60:2178–2189.

35. Drevs J, Hofmann I, Hugenschmidt H, et al. Effects of PTK787/ZK 222584, a specific inhibitor of vascular endothelial growth factor receptor tyrosine kinases, on primary tumor, metastasis, vessel density, and blood flow in a murine renal cell carcinoma model. Cancer Res 2000; 60:4819–4824.

36. Morgan B, Thomas AL, Drevs J, et al. Dynamic contrast-enhanced magnetic resonance imaging as a biomarker for the pharmacological response of PTK787/ZK 222584, an inhibitor of the vascular endothelial growth factor receptor tyrosine kinases, in patients with advanced colorectal cancer and liver metastases: results from two phase I studies. J Clin Oncol 2003; 21:3955–3964.

37. Thomas AL, Morgan B, Horsfield MA, et al. Phase I study of the safety, tolerability, pharmacokinetics, and pharmacodynamics of PTK787/ZK 222584 administered twice daily in patients with advanced cancer. J Clin Oncol 2005; 23(18):4162–4171.

38. Hecht J, Trarbach T, Jaeger E, et al. A randomized, double-blind, placebo-controlled, phase III study in patients (pts) with metastatic adeno-carcinoma of the colon or rectum receiving first-line chemotherapy with oxaliplatin/5-fluorouracil/leucovorin and PTK787/ZK 222584 or placebo (CONFIRM-1). Proc Am Soc Clin Oncol 2005; 23: LBA3a.

39. Ruggeri B, Singh J, Gingrich D, et al. CEP-7055: a novel, orally active pan inhibitor of vascular endothelial growth factor receptor tyrosine kinases with potent antiangiogenic activity and antitumor efficacy in preclinical models. Cancer Res 2003; 63: 5978–5991.

40. Pili R, Carducci MA, Robertson P, Brown P, et al. A phase I study of the pan-VEGFR tyrosine kinase inhibitor, CEP-7055, in patients with advanced malignancy. Proc Am Soc Clin Oncol 2003; 22 [abstr. 831].

41. Rugo HS, Herbst RS, Liu G, et al. Phase I trial of the oral antiangiogenesis agent AG-013736 in patients with advanced solid tumors: pharmacokinetic and clinical results. J Clin Oncol 2005; 23:5474–5483.

42. Wickman G, Hallin M, Amundson K, et al. Further characterization of the potent VEGF/PDGF receptor tyrosine kinase inhibitor AG-013736 in preclinical tumor models for its angiogenesis and antitumor activity. Proc Am Assoc Cancer Res 2003; 44:752 [abstr. 3780].

43. Rini B, Rixe O, Bukowski R, et al. AG-013736, a multi-target tyrosine kinase receptor inhibitor, demonstrates anti-tumor activity in a phase 2 study of cytokine-refractory, metastatic renal cell cancer. J Clin Oncol 2005; ASCO Annual Meeting Proceedings. Vol. 23, No. 16S, Part I of II (June 1 Supplement), 2005:4509.

44. Nakamura K, Taguchi E, Miura T, et al. KRN951, a highly potent inhibitor of vascular endothelial growth factor receptor tyrosine kinases, has antitumor activities and affects functional vascular properties. Cancer Res 2006; 66:9134–9142.

45. Bruns CJ, Solorzano CC, Harbison MT, et al. Blockade of the epidermal growth factor receptor signaling by a novel tyrosine kinase inhibitor leads to apoptosis of endothelial cells and therapy of human pancreatic carcinoma. Cancer Res 2000; 60:2926–2935.

46. Kim SJ, Uehara H, Karashima T, et al. Blockade of epidermal growth factor receptor signaling in tumor cells and tumor-associated endothelial cells for therapy of androgen-independent human prostate cancer growing in the bone of nude mice. Clin Cancer Res 2003; 9:1200–1210.

47. Ciardiello F, Bianco R, Caputo R, et al. Antitumor activity of ZD6474, a small molecule VEGF receptor tyrosine kinase inhibitor, in human cancer cells with acquired resistance to EGF receptor-targeted drugs. Proc Am Soc Clin Oncol 2003; 22:205 [abstr. 820].

48. Hirata A, Ogawa S, Kometani T, et al. ZD1839 (Iressa) induces antiangiogenic effects through inhibition of epidermal growth factor receptor tyrosine kinase. Cancer Res 2002; 62:2554–2560.

49. Wedge SR, Ogilvie DJ, Dukes M, et al. ZD6474 inhibits vascular endothelial growth factor signaling, angiogenesis, and tumor growth following oral administration. Cancer Res 2002; 62:4645–4655.

50. Holden SN, Eckhardt SG, Basser R, et al. Clinical evaluation of ZD6474, an orally active inhibitor of VEGF and EGF receptor signaling, in patients with solid, malignant tumors. Ann Oncol 2005; 16:1391–1397.

51. Minami H, Ebi H, Tahara M, et al. A phase I study of an oral VEGF receptor tyrosine kinase inhibitor, ZD6474, in Japanese patients with solid tumors. Proc Am Soc Clin Oncol 2003; 22 [abstr. 778].

52. Natale R, Bodkin D, Govindan R, et al. ZD6474 versus gefitinib in patients with advanced NSCLC: final results from a two-part, double-blind, randomized phase II trial. J Clin Oncol 2006; 24 [abstr. 7000].

53. Miller KD, Trigo JM, Wheeler C, et al. A multicenter phase II trial of ZD6474, a vascular endothelial growth factor receptor-2 and epidermal growth factor receptor tyrosine kinase inhibitor, in patients with previously treated metastatic breast cancer. Clin Cancer Res 2005; 11:3369–3376.

54. Cunningham D, Humblet Y, Siena S, et al. Cetuximab monotherapy and cetuximab plus irinotecan in irinotecan-refractory metastatic colorectal cancer. N Engl J Med 2004; 351:337–345.

55. Moore MGL, Hamm J, et al. Erlotinib plus gemcitabine compared to gemcitabine alone in patients with advanced pancreatic cancer. A phase III trial of the National Cancer Institute of Canada Clinical Trials Group. J Clin Oncol 2005; 24 [abstr. 1].

56. Herbst RS, Giaccone G, Schiller JH, et al. Gefitinib in combination with paclitaxel and carboplatin in advanced non-small-cell lung cancer: a phase III trial—INTACT 2. J Clin Oncol 2004; 22:785–794.

57. Herbst RS, Prager D, Hermann R, et al. TRIBUTE: a phase III trial of erlotinib hydrochloride (OSI-774) combined with carboplatin and paclitaxel chemotherapy in advanced non-small-cell lung cancer. J Clin Oncol 2005; 23:5892–5899.

58. Sandler AB, Gray R, Brahmer J, et al. Randomized phase II/III Trial of paclitaxel (P) plus carboplatin (C) with or without bevacizumab (NSC # 704865) in patients with advanced non-squamous non-small cell lung cancer: an Eastern Cooperative Oncology Group (ECOG) Trial—E4599. J Clin Oncol 2005; 23 [abstr. 4].

59. Herbst R, Johnson B, Rowbottom J, et al. ZD6474 plus docetaxel in patients with previously-treated NSCLC: results of a randomized, placebo-controlled phase II trial. Lung Cancer 2005; 49:S35 [abstr. O-100].

60. Heymach JV, Johnson BE, Prager D, et al. A phase II trial of ZD6474 plus docetaxel in patients with previously treated NSCLC: follow-up results. J Clin Oncol 2006; 24 [abstr. 7016].

61. http://www.clinicaltrials.gov/ct/show/NCT00093392. Phase II randomized study of ZD6474, carboplatin, and paclitaxel in patients with previously untreated stage IIIB or IV or recurrent non-small cell lung cancer. Clinical Trials.gov [website].

62. http://www.clinicaltrials.gov/ct/show/NCT00312377. A phase III, randomized, double-blinded, multi-center, study to assess the efficacy of docetaxel (Taxotere™ in combination with ZD6474 (Zactima™) versus docetaxel (Taxotere™) with placebo in subjects with locally advanced or metastatic NSCLC. Clinical Trials.gov [website].

63. Baselga J, Rojo F, Dumez H, et al. Phase I study of AEE788, a novel multitargeted inhibitor of ErbB and VEGF receptor family tyrosine kinases: a pharmacokinetic-pharmacodynamic study to identify the optimal therapeutic dose regimen. J Clin Oncol 2005; ASCO Annual Meeting Proceedings. Vol. 23, No. 16S (June 1 supplement), 2005:3028.

64. Park YW, Younes MN, Jasser SA, et al. AEE788, a dual tyrosine kinase receptor inhibitor, induces endothelial cell apoptosis in human cutaneous squamous cell carcinoma xenografts in nude mice. Clin Cancer Res 2005; 11:1963–1973.

65. Wakelee H, Adjei AA, Halsey J, et al. A phase I dose-escalation and pharmacokinetic (PK) study of a novel spectrum selective kinase inhibitor, XL647, in patients with advanced solid malignancies (ASM). J Clin Oncol 2006; ASCO Annual Meeting Proceedings Part I. Vol. 24, No. 18S (June 20 supplement), 2006:3044.

66. O'Farrell AM, Abrams TJ, Yuen HA, et al. SU11248 is a novel FLT3 tyrosine kinase inhibitor with potent activity in vitro and in vivo. Blood 2003; 101:3597–3605.

67. Mendel DB, Laird AD, Xin X, et al. In vivo antitumor activity of SU11248, a novel tyrosine kinase inhibitor targeting vascular endothelial growth factor and platelet-derived growth factor receptors: determination of a pharmacokinetic/pharmacodynamic relationship. Clin Cancer Res 2003; 9:327–337.

68. Faivre S, Delbaldo C, Vera K, et al. Safety, pharmacokinetic, and antitumor activity of SU11248, a novel oral multitarget tyrosine kinase inhibitor, in patients with cancer. J Clin Oncol 2006; 24:25–35.

69. Socinski M, Novello S, Sanchez JM, et al. Efficacy and safety of sunitinib in previously treated, advanced non-small cell lung cancer: preliminary results of a multicenter phase II trial. J Clin Oncol 2006; ASCO Annual Meeting Proceedings Part I. Vol. 24, No. 18S (June 20 supplement), 2006:7001.

70. http://www.cancer.gov/search/ViewClinicalTrials.aspx?cdrid=462318&version=HealthProfessional&protocolsearchid=2500905.

71. Rosen L, Kurzrock R, Jackson E, et al. Phase I study of AMG 706 in patients with advanced solid tumors. ASCO Annual Meeting Proceedings, Vol. 23, No. 16S, Part I of II (June 1 supplement), 2005:3013.

72. Wilhelm SM, Carter C, Tang L, et al. BAY 43-9006 exhibits broad spectrum oral antitumor activity and targets the RAF/MEK/ERK pathway and receptor tyrosine kinases involved in tumor progression and angiogenesis. Cancer Res 2004; 64:7099–7109.

73. Wilhelm S, Chien DS. BAY 43-9006: preclinical data. Curr Pharm Des 2002; 8:2255–2257.

74. Moore M, Hirte HW, Siu L, et al. Phase I study to determine the safety and pharmacokinetics of the novel Raf kinase and VEGFR inhibitor BAY 43-9006, administered for 28 days on/7 days off in patients with advanced, refractory solid tumors. Ann Oncol 2005; 16:1688–1694.

75. Strumberg D, Richly H, Hilger RA, et al. Phase I clinical and pharmacokinetic study of the Novel Raf kinase and vascular endothelial growth factor receptor inhibitor BAY 43-9006 in patients with advanced refractory solid tumors. J Clin Oncol 2005; 23:965–972.

76. Ratain M, Eisen T, Stadler WM, et al. Final findings from a phase II, placebo-controlled, randomized discontinuation trial of sorafenib (BAY 43-9006) in patients with advanced renal cell carcinoma. Proc Am Soc Clin Oncol 2005; 23:4544a.

77. Escudier B, Szczylik C, Eisen T, et al. Randomized phase III trial of the Raf kinase and VEGFR inhibitor sorafenib (BAY 43-9006) in patients with advanced renal cell carcinoma. Proc Am Soc Clin Oncol 2005; 23:4510a.

78. Adjei A, Mandrekar S, Marks RS, et al. A phase I study of BAY 43-9006 and gefitinib in patients with refractory or recurrent non-small-cell lung cancer. J Clin Oncol 2005; ASCO Annual Meeting Proceedings. Vol. 23, No. 16S, Part I of II (June 1 supplement), 2005:3067.

79. Tolcher AW, Karp DD, O'Leary JJ, DeBono JS, et al. A phase I and biologic correlative study of an oral endothelial vascular growth factor receptor-2 (VEGFR-2) tyrosine kinase inhibitor, CP-547, 632 in patients with advanced solid tumors. Proc ASCO 2002; 21:84a [abstr. 334].

80. Roberts WG, Jani J, Beebe J, et al. Preclinical development of CP-547, 632, a novel VEGFR-2 inhibitor for cancer therapy. Proc ASCO 2002; 21:119a [abstr. 473].

81. Hoekstra R, de Vos FY, Eskens FA, et al. Phase I safety, pharmacokinetic, and pharmacodynamic study of the thrombospondin-1-mimetic angiogenesis inhibitor ABT-510 in patients with advanced cancer. J Clin Oncol 2005; 23:5188–5197.

82. Albert JM, Cao C, Geng L, Leavitt L, Hallahan DE, Lu B. Integrin alpha v beta 3 antagonist cilengitide enhances efficacy of radiotherapy in endothelial cell and non-small-cell lung cancer models. Int J Radiat Oncol Biol Phys 2006; 65:1536–1543.

83. Franks ME, Macpherson GR, Figg WD. Thalidomide. Lancet 2004; 363:1802–1811.

84. Riedel R, Crawford J, Dunphy F, et al. Phase II study of carboplatin, irinotecan, and thalidomide combination in patients with extensive stage small-cell lung cancer. Lung Cancer 2006; 54:431–432.

85. Baguley BC. Antivascular therapy of cancer: DMXAA. Lancet Oncol 2003; 4:141–148.

86. Vincent L, Kermani P, Young LM, et al. Combretastatin A4 phosphate induces rapid regression of tumor neovessels and growth through interference with vascular endothelial-cadherin signaling. J Clin Invest 2005; 115:2992–3006.

87. Rustin GJ, Price P, Stratford M, et al. Phase 1 study of weekly intravenous combretastatin A4 phophate: pharmacokinetics and toxicity. Proc Am Soc Clin Oncol 2001; 20 [abstr. 392].

88. Ciardiello F, Caputo R, Damiano V, et al. Antitumor effects of ZD6474, a small molecule vascular endothelial growth factor receptor tyrosine kinase inhibitor, with additional activity against epidermal growth factor receptor tyrosine kinase. Clin Cancer Res 2003; 9:1546–1556.

89. Jain RK. Normalization of tumor vasculature: an emerging concept in antiangiogenic therapy. Science 2005; 307:58–62.

4

Antiangiogenic Therapy for Lung Cancer: Antibodies and Other Novel Agents

Sarita Dubey

Division of Hematology/Oncology, University of California–San Francisco, San Francisco, California, U.S.A.

Ravi Salgia

Section of Hematology/Oncology, Department of Medicine, University of Chicago, Chicago, Illinois, U.S.A.

INTRODUCTION

Angiogenesis is a requirement for tumor growth (Fig. 1). Increased levels of angiogenesis are associated with poorer outcomes in several malignancies including lung cancer. Thus, inhibition of this process is a valid approach to treatment. Within the angiogenic pathway, there are multiple targets for intervention. Some of these targets have been successfully inhibited with agents that have shown preclinical or clinical efficacy. The preceding chapter describes the role of angiogenesis in malignancy and discusses the small molecule inhibitors currently under clinical investigations. This review discusses the role of antibodies and other novel agents in the treatment of lung cancer.

MEDIATORS OF ANGIOGENESIS

A brief review of angiogenesis is presented here (see Chapter 3).

Multiple mediators of angiogenesis have been identified—vascular endothelial growth factor (VEGF), platelet-derived growth factor, basic fibroblast growth factor (bFGF), transforming growth factor α (TGF α), interleukin (IL)-1, IL-6, integrins, urokinase plasminogen activator (uPA), and others (1). Among these factors, VEGF is the most potent. There are five isoforms of VEGF-(A–E) resulting from alternative splicing of VEGF gene, and three different types of VEGF tyrosine kinsase receptors (2). The VEGF receptors (VEGFR)1 fms-like tyrosine kinase (Flt1) and VEGFR2 kinease insert domain protein receptor (KDR) are located on endothelial cells, while VEGFR3 (Flt4) is located on lymph vessels. VEGF, through its key receptors VEGFR1 and KDR, stimulates endothelial cell survival and revascularization (3), and inhibition of VEGF in preclinical models decreases angiogenesis and suppresses tumor growth (4). In clinical series, approximately 50% or more of lung cancers have increased expression of VEGF and its receptor KDR (5–7). As one would expect, higher levels of VEGF expression are not only associated with increased nodal involvement but are also associated with decreased survival. Thus, the primary mediator of angiogenesis is not only responsible for tumor growth but is also a prognosticator of outcome.

INHIBITION OF ANGIOGENESIS

The strong evidence supporting the role of angiogenesis in tumor growth and prognosis led to the development of agents that can inhibit angiogenesis (Table 1). These inhibitors target various levels in the angiogenesis pathway and are in different levels of clinical development. Some of these inhibitors are discussed in this review, while a large class of these agents, the tyrosine kinase inhibitors, are discussed in the preceding chapter.

VEGF Inhibitors

Monoclonal Antibodies to VEGF

Bevacizumab (Avastin) is a recombinant humanized monoclonal antibody (Rhu-Mab) against VEGF-A. Its first approval for use in human cancers came after a randomized phase III trial in patients with chemo-naïve colorectal cancer (8). The addition

Table 1 Angiogenesis Inhibitors

Target	Mechanism of action	Drug
VEGF	Monoclonal antibody	Bevacizumab
VEGFR-2	Monoclonal antibody	IMC-1C11
VEGFR	Fusion protein of VEGFR 1 and 2	VEGF Trap/AVE-005
VEGFR	Tyrosine kinase inhibitors	PTK787, SU11248, AMG 706, GW786034, AZD2171, ZD6474, sorafenib
PDGFR	Tyrosine kinase inhibitors	PTK787, AZD2171, GW786034

Abbreviations: PDGFR, platelet-derived growth factor receptor; VEGF, vascular endothelial growth factor; VEGFR, vascular endothelial growth factor receptor.

of bevacizumab to chemotherapy produced a five months' improvement in overall survival ($P < 0.001$). In non–small-cell lung cancer (NSCLC), a phase II study included previously untreated subjects with advanced disease. Bevacizumab was used in combination with paclitaxel and carboplatin (9). Ninety-nine patients were randomized to carboplatin [area under the curve (AUC) = 6)] and paclitaxel (200 mg/m^2) every three weeks for six cycles or the same chemotherapy regimen plus a low (7.5 mg/kg) or high (15 mg/kg) dose of bevacizumab every three weeks. Objective response rates and median survival in the high-dose and low-dose bevacizumab arms and control arms were 32%/28%/19% and 18/12/15 months, respectively. Thus, the overall outcome was higher in the high-dose bevacizumab arm. Six life-threatening hemorrhages were seen in the bevacizumab arms and did not appear to be dose related. They were more commonly associated with squamous-cell carcinomas (31%) than adenocarcinoma, central tumors close to blood vessels, and cavitation as seen after radiation treatments. In the non–squamous-cell cohort, the risk of severe hemorrhage was low at 4%.

Based on the positive results of the phase II study and the increased hemorrhage seen in the squamous-cell cohort, a phase III study was designed with bevacizumab, carboplatin, and paclitaxel in previously untreated nonsquamous NSCLC patients (10). Eight hundred and seventy eight patients were randomized to receive carboplatin AUC 6 and paclitaxel 200 mg/m^2 on day 1 every 21 days or the same combination with bevacizumab 15 mg/kg on day 1 every 21 days. After completion of six treatment cycles, those on the bevacizumab arm continued to receive bevacizumab every three weeks until relapse or disease progression. Response rates and survivals were higher in the bevacizumab arm ($P = 0.003$) (Table 2). Both regimens were well tolerated with some differences. The toxicities that were higher with bevacizumab were grade 4 neutropenia (16.8% vs. 25%), grade 3 or 4 thromboembolism (3% vs. 3.8%), grade 3 or 4 hemorrhage (1% vs. 4.1%), and treatment-related deaths (2 patients vs. 15 patients). Of the fifteen treatment-related deaths with bevacizumab, five were attributed to pulmonary hemorrhage and five to febrile neutropenia. Pulmonary hemorrhage was seen in patients with tumors that were contiguous with major blood vessels, cavitation, or baseline history of hemoptysis. Thus, bevacizumab, a novel targeted agent, has demonstrated improved outcomes in addition to cytotoxic chemotherapy. The risk of hemorrhage can be decreased by patient selection. The results of this study led to

Table 2   Results of E4599

	Chemotherapy	Chemotherapy + bevacizumab	P value
Response rate %	15	35	<0.001
Progression-free survival (mo)	4.5	6.2	<0.001
Overall survival (mo)	10.3	12.3	0.003

Note: Phase III trial of chemotherapy with or without bevacizumab in non–small cell lung cancer.

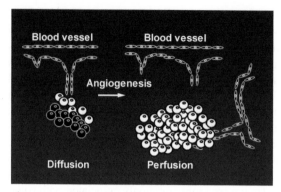

Figure 1   Malignant cells depend on diffusion of nutrients from blood vessels. Enlargement of tumors depends on successful perfusion of tumor by recruitment of new blood vessels.

the approval of this agent for its use in chemo-naïve NSCLC in combination with carboplatin and paclitaxel.

Combinations of angiogenesis inhibitors are not limited to chemotherapy alone. In patients with relapsed disease, bevacizumab was combined with EGFR inhibitor erlotinib in a phase I/II study (11). Of the 40 patients enrolled, 34 patients were treated at the phase II dose of erlotinib 150 mg orally daily and bevacizumab 15 mg/kg every three weeks intravenously. Twenty-two patients had two or more prior regimens. Disease control rate was 85%, with 20% partial response. Median overall survival and PFS were 12.6 months and 6.2 months, respectively. Based on the positive results of this study, a randomized phase III study of erlotinib with or without bevacizumab in patients with one prior chemotherapy treatment has been launched.

Inhibitors of VEGFR

Monoclonal Antibody to KDR

IMC-1C11 is a chimeric antibody to KDR and prevents ligand binding to the receptor. It thus inhibits VEGF-induced endothelial-cell activation and proliferation. A phase I study was conducted in patients with colorectal metastases (12). Stable disease was seen in four of the 14 patients, and significant decrease in tumor vascular perfusion was detected on dynamic enhanced magnetic resonance imaging (MRI) within four weeks of drug administration. Human antichimeric antibodies (HACA) were detected in seven of 14 patients. The drug was safe and tolerable. No grade 3 or 4 toxicities were seen. Grade 1 hemorrhage was seen in four patients.

VEGF Trap

VEGF trap is a fusion protein consisting of human VEGFR-1, VEGFR-2, and IgG constant domains. It has a high affinity for binding to VEGF and thus prevents binding of VEGF to VEGFR. A phase I study of this agent was conducted in patients with refractory solid tumors. The preliminary results indicate that drug-related grade 3 adverse events were uncommon and included fatigue, arthralgia, and voice disturbance (13). Dynamic contrast-enhanced, MRI-based evaluation is included in this study. No HACA antibodies were seen. One patient with renal-cell carcinoma developed stable disease for more than six months. Other ongoing phase I studies will evaluate the safety of this agent in combination with chemotherapy regimens.

Correlates of Antiangiogenic Activity

As discussed above, VEGF levels have an inverse correlation with outcome in NSCLC. Koukourakis et al. showed that the binding of VEGF to KDR causes conformal changes on the NH2 terminus, which is detected by specific antibodies (14). The VEGF/KDR complex is more representative of active angiogenesis than free VEGF alone. In 102 tumor samples from early NSCLC, the presence of this complex was a more powerful indicator and correlated with worse outcome than VEGF or standard microvessel density. In the randomized phase III study comparing chemotherapy against chemotherapy with bevacizumab, intercellular adhesion molecule (ICAM) levels were both prognostic as well as predictive of outcome to treatment. Baseline serum ICAM levels of below 260 ng/mL were associated with a one-year survival of 60% versus 25% in those with baseline levels above 260 ng/mL ($P = 0.00005$) (15). Higher levels of ICAM were also associated with poorer response (40% vs. 20%, $P = 0.02$) to treatment with chemotherapy and bevacizumab in comparison with lower levels. Similar effects of low ICAM levels were seen on PFS: 53% reduction in PFS ($P < 0.001$) when treated with chemotherapy in combination with bevacizumab. High baseline levels of VEGF were related to higher response rate to treatment with bevacizumab (33% vs. 7%, $P = 0.04$); however, this did not translate to improvement in overall survival. As is seen with many of these agents, stable disease may perhaps be a more common response than disease shrinkage and can be attributed to the noncytotoxic nature of these drugs. Decrease in tumor vascularity within four weeks of drug administration has been demonstrated with dynamic contrast enhanced MRI. Thus, this imaging modality is a potential surrogate for antitumor activity of this group of drugs.

CONCLUSION

Angiogenesis is vital for tumor growth. High levels of angiogenesis mediators inversely correlate with outcomes in lung cancer. Inhibition of angiogenesis is associated with suppression of tumor growth and increased delivery of chemotherapeutic drugs and hence with improved outcomes. The monoclonal antibody bevacizumab has been approved for its use in colorectal cancer and NSCLC in combination with chemotherapy. This new era of antitumor agents also presents new challenges. As would be expected with this class of drugs, major toxicities seen include pulmonary hemorrhage. Careful patient selection will reduce the likelihood of such events. As seen with other targeted agents, a patient enrichment strategy has the potential to increase response to treatment. Baseline levels of ICAM and VEGF appear to predict outcomes in response to bevacizumab. Confirmation of these associations in prospective studies may help to identify those who may benefit the most with antiangiogenic therapy. Dynamic contrast enhanced MRI is a promising new approach to detect drug activity in the absence of traditional responses or tumor shrinkage. Future studies will evaluate the role of several angiogenesis inhibitors as single agents and in combination with chemotherapy and other targeted agents.

ACKNOWLEDGMENT

This work is in part supported by an R01 (CA100750), American Cancer Society (RSG-02-244-04), and American Lung Association Discovery Award to Ravi Salgia.

REFERENCES

1. Herbst RS, Onn A, Sandler A. Angiogenesis and lung cancer: prognostic and therapeutic implications. J Clin Oncol 2005; 23(14):3243–3256.
2. Neufeld G, Cohen T, Gengrinovitch S, Poltorak Z. Vascular endothelial growth factor (VEGF) and its receptors. Faseb J 1999; 13(1):9–22.
3. Ferrara N, Gerber HP, LeCouter J. The biology of VEGF and its receptors. Nat Med 2003; 9(6):669–676.
4. Kim KJ, Li B, Winer J, Armanini M, Gillett N, Phillips HS, et al. Inhibition of vascular endothelial growth factor-induced angiogenesis suppresses tumour growth in vivo. Nature 1993; 362(6423):841–844.
5. O'Byrne KJ, Koukourakis MI, Giatromanolaki A, et al. Vascular endothelial growth factor, platelet-derived endothelial cell growth factor and angiogenesis in non–small-cell lung cancer. Br J Cancer 2000; 82(8):1427–1432.
6. Volm M, Koomagi R, Mattern J. Prognostic value of vascular endothelial growth factor and its receptor Flt-1 in squamous cell lung cancer. Int J Cancer 1997; 74(1): 64–68.
7. Ohta Y, Watanabe Y, Murakami S, et al. Vascular endothelial growth factor and lymph node metastasis in primary lung cancer. Br J Cancer 1997; 76(8):1041–1045.
8. Hurwitz H, Fehrenbacher L, Novotny W, et al. Bevacizumab plus irinotecan, fluorouracil, and leucovorin for metastatic colorectal cancer. N Engl J Med 2004; 350(23): 2335–2342.
9. Johnson DH, Fehrenbacher L, Novotny WF, et al. Randomized phase II trial comparing bevacizumab plus carboplatin and paclitaxel with carboplatin and paclitaxel alone in previously untreated locally advanced or metastatic non–small-cell lung cancer. J Clin Oncol 2004; 22(11):2184–2191.
10. Sandler A, Gray R, Perry MC, et al. Paclitaxel-carboplatin alone or with bevacizumab for non–small-cell lung cancer. N Engl J Med 2006; 355(24):2542–2550.

11. Herbst RS, Johnson DH, Mininberg E, et al. Phase I/II trial evaluating the anti-vascular endothelial growth factor monoclonal antibody bevacizumab in combination with the HER-1/epidermal growth factor receptor tyrosine kinase inhibitor erlotinib for patients with recurrent non–small-cell lung cancer. J Clin Oncol 2005; 23(11): 2544–2555.

12. Posey JA, Ng TC, Yang B, et al. A phase I study of anti-kinase insert domain-containing receptor antibody, IMC-1C11, in patients with liver metastases from colorectal carcinoma. Clin Cancer Res 2003; 9(4):1323–1332.

13. Dupont J, Rothenberg ML, Spriggs DR, et al. Safety and pharmacokinetics of intravenous VEGF Trap in a phase I clinical trial of patients with advanced solid tumors [abstr. 3029]. J Clin Oncol 2005; 23(16s):199s.

14. Koukourakis MI, Giatromanolaki A, Thorpe PE, et al. Vascular endothelial growth factor/KDR activated microvessel density versus CD31 standard microvessel density in non-small cell lung cancer. Cancer Res 2000; 60(11):3088–3095.

15. Dowlati A, Gray R, Johnson DH, Schiller JH, Brahmer J. Prospective correlative assessment of biomarkers in E4599 randomized phase II/III trial of carboplatin and paclitaxel ± bevacizumab in advanced non-small cell lung cancer (NSCLC) [abstr. 7027]. J Clin Oncol 2006; 24(18S):370s.

5

Epidermal Growth Factor Receptor Inhibition in Non–Small Cell Lung Cancer

Antonio Jimeno and Manuel Hidalgo

Sidney Kimmel Comprehensive Cancer Center at Johns Hopkins University School of Medicine, Baltimore, Maryland, U.S.A.

THE EPIDERMAL GROWTH FACTOR RECEPTOR

The epidermal growth–factor receptor (EGFR, HER1) is a member of the HER family of membrane receptors (HER1–4). The other members are HER2 (also termed ErbB2 or HER2/neu), HER3 (also termed ErbB3), and HER4 (also termed ErbB4). These receptors share the same molecular structure with an extracellular, cysteine-rich, ligand-binding domain, a single α-helix transmembrane domain, and an intracellular domain with tyrosine–kinase (TK) activity in the carboxy-terminal tail (excepting the HER3) (1). The TK domains of HER2 and HER4 show an 80% homology to that of the EGFR (2). Epidermal growth factor (EGF), transforming growth factor-α (TGF-α), and amphiregulin bind exclusively to the EGFR, whereas betacellulin and epiregulin bind both EGFR and HER4. Ligand binding induces EGFR homodimerization as well as heterodimerization with other types of HER proteins (3,4). HER2 does not bind to any known ligand, but it is the preferred heterodimerization partner for EGFR after ligand-induced activation (5). EGFR/EGFR homodimers are unstable, whereas EGFR/HER2 heterodimers are stable and recycle more rapidly to the cell surface (6).

EGFR dimerization induces TK-catalytic activity, which leads to the autophosphorilation in one or more of the five tyrosine residues in the carboxy-terminal tail, producing phosphotyrosine sites (Y992, Y1068, Y1086, Y1448, and Y1173) where adaptor and docking molecules ultimately bind (7). EGFR intracellular signaling is mainly mediated through two interrelated downstream pathways, the Ras-Raf-mitogen-activated protein kinases (MAPK, also known as extracytoplasmatic regulated kinases, ERK1 and ERK2) and the phosphatidylinositol 3-kinase/Akt pathways (8,9). ERKs regulate the transcription of molecules involved in cell proliferation, transformation, and metastasis development (10), whereas the Akt pathway is more relevant in cell-survival processes (11). An alternative route of EGFR-mediated transduction of extracellular signals is via the stress-activated protein kinase pathway that involves protein kinase C (PKC), although the basis of this regulation remains obscure. The finding that PKC has a role in EGFR transactivation and ERK regulation further complicates this regulatory mechanism (12). EGFR signaling ultimately causes increased proliferation (13), angiogenesis (14), metastasis (15), and decreased apoptosis (16). Under physiological conditions, ligand binding is required to activate EGFR; however, in tumor cells, there are additional mechanisms of EGFR activation. First, receptor overexpression leading to ligand-independent dimerization is commonly found in many different solid human tumors (17). Second, autocrine production of ligands (such as TGF-α) by tumor cells has been linked to receptor overexpression and may represent an efficient mechanism of EGFR-driven growth (18).

EGFR overexpression correlates with a worse clinical outcome in several cancers including non–small-cell lung cancer (NSCLC) and tumors of the prostate, breast, stomach, colon, ovary, and head and neck, further supporting their role in tumorigenesis (17,19,20). It is estimated that between 40% and 80% of NSCLC overexpress EGFR, and 20% to 30% overexpress HER2 (21–23). The pivotal role that the EGFR plays as a sensor of the extracellular environment and the maintenance of cellular homeostasis make it an a-priori ideal candidate for a cell in transformation to exploit in order to acquire advantageous features such as freedom of movement, nutrient independence, and immortality. The EGFR was proposed as a rational target for drug development more than 20 years ago (24,25). In this chapter, we will briefly discuss current and future approaches to the EGFR-targeted therapy focusing on NSCLC.

TARGETED THERAPY AGAINST THE EGFR

Numerous classes of drugs that target the EGFR are under development, and over the last few years, an increasing number of compounds directed against the EGFR have entered clinical development and are currently in clinical trials. Two strategies have been more extensively explored in clinical trials: the use of small molecules that compete with adenosine triphosphate (ATP) for binding to the receptor's kinase pocket, thus blocking receptor activation, also known as TK inhibitors (TKIs) and the use of monoclonal antibodies (MAbs) directed against the external domain of the receptor. In the next few paragraphs, we summarize the key clinical and translational research aspects in the development of these drugs.

TKIS AGAINST THE EGFR

TKIs compete with ATP for binding to the receptor's kinase pocket, thus blocking receptor activation. A large number of TKIs are currently being evaluated. They can be classified according to their selectivity (specific agents with HER1-selective activity, as opposed to nonspecific agents that target several members of the HER family or other receptors) and according to the reversibility of their interaction with their target (reversible or irreversible inhibitors) (Table 1). Two have received regulatory approval for use in NSCLC patients, gefitinib and erlotinib. A large number of other TKIs are currently being evaluated.

Gefitinib

Gefitinib (Iressa™, ZD1839, AstraZeneca, Wilmington, Delaware, U.S.A.) is an orally active, low molecular weight, synthetic quinazoline (26). Gefitinib reversibly and selectively targets the EGFR and blocks signal transduction processes implicated in the proliferation and survival of cancer cells with minimal activity against other TKs and serine/threonine kinases. Gefitinib prevents autophosphorilation of EGFR, resulting in the inhibition of downstream signaling pathways (27–29). Phase I clinical trials of gefitinib showed a favorable toxicity profile, mostly consisting in skin toxicity and diarrhea, and dose limiting toxicities (DLTs) were observed at doses well above that at which antitumor activity was seen (30–32). Two phase II studies have evaluated the clinical activity of gefitinib at two dose levels (250 and 500 mg) in patients with NSCLC that had failed at least one (210 patients) and at least two (216 patients) chemotherapy regimens for advanced disease, documenting response rates of 18.7% and 10.6%, respectively (33,34). In these studies, a higher dose did not improve response rate and caused an increased toxicity. Improvement in disease-related symptoms was significant in both trials. These results led to the limited or conditional approval of gefitinib 250 mg/day as monotherapy treatment for patients with locally advanced or metastatic NSCLC refractory to platinum-based and docetaxel chemotherapy in the United States and Japan, (among others) pending results from the placebo-controlled trial. However, the addition of gefitinib to standard chemotherapy has failed to induce an improvement in response or survival in chemo-naïve NSCLC

Table 1 Small Molecules Targeted at the EGFR Tyrosine Kinase

Drug	Type	EGFR IC$_{50}$ (μM)	HER-2 IC$_{50}$ (μM)	Phase of development
Gefitinib (Iressa™)	Selective, reversible	0.02	3.7	Approved
Erlotinib (Tarceva™)	Selective, reversible	0.02	3.5	Approved
Lapatinib (GW2016)	Bifunctional, reversible	0.01	0.009	III, II

Note: IC$_{50}$ values represent substrate phosphorylation assays.
Abbreviation: EGFR, epidermal growth factor receptor.

patients. Two placebo-controlled, double-blinded, phase III randomized trials evaluating chemotherapy (either gemcitabine-cisplatin or paclitaxel-cisplatin) plus either gefitinib (250–500 mg) or placebo have rendered negative results (Table 2) (35,36). A placebo-controlled phase III study investigated the effect on survival of gefitinib as second-line or third-line treatment in 1692 patients with locally advanced or metastatic NSCLC (39). The primary endpoint was survival in the overall population of patients and those with adenocarcinoma. Preplanned subgroup analyses showed longer survival in the gefitinib group than the placebo group for never-smokers [$n = 375$; 0.67 (0.49–0.92), $P = 0.012$; median survival 8.9 months vs. 6.1 months] and patients of Asian origin [$n = 342$; 0.66 (0.48–0.91), $P = 0.01$; median survival 9.5 months vs. 5.5 months], but treatment with gefitinib was not associated with significant improvement in survival in either coprimary endpoints. Based on these results, gefitinib was subsequently not granted full approval but was allowed to remain on the market for those patients who were still deriving benefit.

Erlotinib

Erlotinib (Tarceva™, OSI-774, OSI Pharmaceuticals, Uniondale, New York, USA) is a quinazoline derivative, which reversibly inhibits the kinase activity of EGFR. It has shown in vitro and in vivo activity in preclinical trials in multiple human cancer-cell lines, including ovarian, head and neck, and non–small-cell

Table 2 Results of Trials of Gefitinib and Erlotinib in Combination with Chemotherapy in the First-Line Treatment of Non–Small Cell Lung Cancer

Chemotherapy	Biologic agent	Response rate (%)	Median survival (mo)	One-year survival (%)	References
Gemcitabine and cisplatin	Placebo	44.8	11.1	45	(35)
	Gefitinib 250 mg	50.1	9.9	42	
	Gefitinib 500 mg	49.7	9.9	44	–
Paclitaxel and carboplatin	Placebo	33.6	9.9	42	(36)
	Gefitinib 250 mg	35.0	9.8	42	–
	Gefitinib 500 mg	32.1	8.7	38	–
Paclitaxel and carboplatin	Placebo	19.3	10.5	44	(37)
	Erlotinib 150 mg	21.5	10.6	47	–
			Median survival (days)		
Gemcitabine and cisplatin	Placebo	N/R	309	N/R	(38)
	Erlotinib 150 mg	–	301	–	

Abbreviation: N/R, not reported.

lung carcinoma (40,41). Erlotinib has been evaluated in several phase I studies using different doses and schedules, including weekly administration for three weeks every four weeks, and a continuous daily dosing (42,43). The schedule that was ultimately chosen for further evaluation consists on the daily administration of 150 mg orally, with higher doses resulting in dose-limiting diarrhea and cutaneous acneiform rash (42). The cutaneous toxicity was dose dependent, affected the face and upper trunk areas, appeared at the end of the first week of dosing, and progressively recovered even in patients who continued taking the same dose of erlotinib. Other toxicities were mild to moderate and consisted of nausea and vomiting, elevation in bilirubin, headaches, and mucositis. The preliminary results of several disease-directed studies have been presented. Erlotinib has demonstrated clinical activity as a single agent in patients with NSCLC, ovarian cancer, and head and neck cancer (44–46). A combined analysis of the data of these phase II studies has suggested that patients who develop rash of any grade had a statistically significant longer median survival (47). Erlotinib in combination with gemcitabine increased survival compared with gemcitabine alone as first-line therapy for advanced disease in a randomized trial in pancreatic cancer patients, and it recently received regulatory approval for this indication (48). Data from two phase III clinical trials in patients with NSCLC comparing standard chemotherapy regimens [cisplatin plus gemcitabine (38) and carboplatin plus paclitaxel (37)] with or without erlotinib showed that this approach failed to demonstrate a response or survival advantage. However, in a trial that randomized pretreated NSCLC patients to erlotinib:placebo in the ratio of 2:1, subjects receiving the study drug survived 6.7 months compared with 4.7 months of those taking placebo ($P < 0.001$), and this has been the first EGFR-targeted therapy to receive regulatory approval on the basis of prolongation of survival (49). In initial, small clinical trials, erlotinib has shown significant anti-tumor activity in the first-line treatment of advanced NSCLC (50). The discovery of activating mutations in the *EGFR* gene has prompted novel patient-selection strategies. Preliminary results from a clinical trial that sequenced the *EGFR* gene in chemo-naïve patients with NSCLC and treated those positive with erlotinib showed that 37 of 297 subjects were found to harbor a mutation, and 19 of 21 treated patients presented a response to therapy (51).

EKB-569

EKB-569 (Wyeth) is an oral, selective, and irreversible EGFR inhibitor. In an initial phase I study, EKB-569 has been reported to be safe both on an intermittent and on a continuous-dose schedule. The agent is well tolerated, with diarrhea and acneiform rash being the most common reported toxicities. Grade-3 diarrhea was the dose-limiting toxicity at doses of 100 mg/day, with 75 mg/day being the recommended dose for future studies (52). EKB-569 is currently being evaluated in NSCLC and in combination with chemotherapy for colo-rectal cancer.

Lapatinib

Lapatinib (GW572016, GlaxoSmithKline, Research Triangle Park, North Carolina, U.S.A.) is a 6-thiazolyquinazoline that reversibly inhibits the phosphorylation of both EGFR and HER2. This agent is currently undergoing clinical evaluation and in early clinical trials has shown a typical TKI-toxicity profile, with diarrhea and rash being the most relevant adverse events (53). It is in advanced phases of development in breast cancer. In a randomized phase II multicenter trial comparing two schedules and doses of lapatinib in patients with chemo-naive advanced or metastatic NSCLC, there were no significant drug-related toxicities. Efficacy results from this trial are pending (54).

ZD6474

ZD6474 (AstraZeneca, Wilmington, Delaware) is an oral, quinazoline derivative dual inhibitor of EGFR and the vascular endothelial growth–factor receptor. Phase I evaluation has shown ZD6474 to be well tolerated, with a pharmacokinetic profile appropriate for once-daily oral dosing and a half-life of above 120 hours (55). Phase II evaluation of ZD6474 has included two randomized studies of patients with NSCLC. In one of these trials, the efficacy of ZD6474 (300 mg) was compared with that of gefitinib in previously treated patients (56). The adverse event profile of ZD6474 was similar to that seen in previous trials and included rash, diarrhea, and asymptomatic QTc prolongation. A statistically significant improvement in time to progression was observed for ZD6474 compared with gefitinib (11.9 weeks vs. 8.1 weeks, $P = 0.011$). In a second trial, 127 patients with platinum-refractory NSCLC were treated with ZD6474 (100 or 300 mg) or placebo, in combination with docetaxel (75 mg/m^2 by IV infusion every 21 days) (57). Preliminary results show a nonsignificantly longer median time to progression for the combined arms versus docetaxel alone, and mature data are awaited. Based on these results, phase III trials are currently being planned.

HKI-272

HKI-272 (Wyeth) is an irreversible TKI with dual activity against EGFR and HER2. In vitro studies have shown activity of HKI-272 in NSCLC cell lines with acquired resistance to gefitinib (58). In preclinical xenograft studies, HKI-272 significantly reduced the growth of HER2- and EGFR-dependent tumors when given at doses between 10 and 40 mg/kg/day (59). Phase I trials to determine safety and tolerability and phase II studies in NSCLC are underway.

MONOCLONAL ANTIBODIES TARGETED AGAINST THE EGFR

Blocking altered biologic pathways with MAbs is one of the most successful therapeutic strategies currently under evaluation in cancer research, and the EGFR is one of the targets against which more MAbs are being developed (Table 3).

Table 3 Monoclonal Antibodies Targeting the EGFR

Monoclonal antibody	Properties	Trial status	Regimen	Tumor type
Cetuximab	Anti-EGFR	Approved	Combination with chemotherapy or radiation therapy	Colorectal and head and neck colon
Panitumumab (ABX-EGF)	Anti-EGFR	Approved	Monotherapy	Colorectal
Matuzumab (EMD72000)	Anti-EGFR	Phase I	Monotherapy	Head and neck, esophagus colon, cervix
MAb ICR62	Anti-EGFR	Phase I	Monotherapy	NSCLC, head and neck

Abbreviations: EGFR, epidermal growth factor receptor; NSCLC, non–small cell lung cancer; MAb, monoclonal antibody.

Cetuximab

Cetuximab (IMC-C225; Imclone Systems, New York, NY, USA) is a chimeric mouse-human MAb that binds the EGFR in its extracellular domain and blocks EGF-induced autophosphorilation of the EGFR cell lines in vitro (60), induces dimerization and downregulation of the EGFR (61), perturbs cell-cycle progression (62), and inhibits tumor-induced angiogenesis (63). In phase I studies, doses ranging from 5 to 400 mg/m^2 were explored without reaching a maximum tolerated dose. Pharmacokinetics analyses showed a nonlinear behavior, with saturation of drug clearance at doses over 200 mg/m^2, and therefore the dose regimen selected for phases II to III trials was a loading dose of 400 mg/m^2, followed by a weekly maintenance dose of 250 mg/m^2. Phase I trials revealed a favorable tolerability, with the most significant toxicity reported being an acneiform rash and folliculitis involving the face and upper chest that occurs in 80% of the patients (64–66). Hypersensitivity reactions have been reported, some of them occurring within minutes of the first infusion but are uncommon (<5%) and rarely life threatening. Other adverse effects include asthenia, fever, and alteration in liver-function tests.

Many have evaluated cetuximab alone or in combination with radiotherapy or chemotherapy in patients with squamous head and neck, renal, pancreatic, and colorectal cancer and NSCLC. Of special relevance are the results of a phase II trial that compared the objective-confirmed response rate of the combination of cetuximab plus irinotecan or of cetuximab as a single agent in patients with EGFR-positive, irinotecan-refractory colorectal cancer (67) that led to its initial regulatory approval.

Cetuximab monotherapy has shown modest activity in refractory NSCLC (68), and phase II trials of cetuximab combined with paclitaxel and carboplatin, and gemcitabine with carboplatin in patients with NSCLC have all shown it is possible to combine cetuximab safely with chemotherapy (69,70). In the two first-line trials, the 28.6% response rate in the gemcitabine study and the 29% response rate in the paclitaxel study do not appear to be higher than would be expected with chemotherapy alone. The addition of cetuximab to cisplatin plus vinorelbine versus chemotherapy alone as first-line treatment of patients with NSCLC showed response rates favoring the cetuximab group (53.3% vs. 32.2%), as did disease control rates (93.3% and 77.4%), although more mature reports are awaited (71).

Panitumumab

Panitumumab (ABX-EGF, Amgen, Thousand Oaks, California, USA) is a high-affinity, fully human MAb that binds the EGFR in its extracellular domain; blocks the binding of both EGF and TGF-α to various EGFR-expressing human carcinoma-cell lines; and inhibits EGFR tyrosine phosphorylation and cell proliferation (72). Full humanization prevents the development of antibodies against murine epitopes, a potential limitation of MAbs that could result in decreased efficacy. ABX-EGF has evidenced preclinical activity in vitro and in vivo, as single agent and in combination with cytotoxic agents in a wide range of human cancer-cell lines, including pancreatic, prostate, breast, head and neck, and renal human-cell lines (73). Based on these preclinical studies, a biomathematical model was developed to predict antitumor efficacy in patients, and maximum antitumor activity was calculated for maintenance doses between 1 and 3 mg/kg weekly. Initial clinical trials of ABX-EGF in heavily pretreated patients have reported encouraging results. A phase I trial was conducted with a weekly schedule with doses ranging from 0.01 to 2.5 mg/kg weekly for four consecutive weeks and every other week thereafter. In this study, treatment with ABX-EGF was well tolerated and no dose-limiting toxicities were reported (74). Biologic activity, evidenced by reversible acneiform skin rash, was observed at the 1.0 mg/kg dose level. A randomized phase II study is currently evaluating the activity of carboplatin/paclitaxel with or without the addition of panitumumab in patients with chemotherapy-naive advanced NSCLC.

Matuzumab

Matuzumab (EMD72000, Merck, Whitehouse Station, New Jersey, U.S.A.) is a humanized MAb directed at the EGFR, which has shown potent antitumor activity in preclinical studies (75,76). A significant difference with the above mentioned EGFR-targeted MAbs is a longer half-life, a feature that has prompted its evaluation every two and three weeks (77). Clinical activity was documented in subjects with colorectal and renal cancer. This study included pharmacodynamic assessment and correlative studies, evidencing that EMD72000 induced a complete inhibition of pEGFR and pMAPK with an increase in p27 in skin biopsies in all patients, whereas pAkt was only inhibited in responding patients. An expanded phase of the prior study has shown dose-dependent inhibition of downstream pathways in surrogate tissues, supporting an optimal biologic dose-seeking approach (78). A weekly schedule in patients with EGFR-expressing solid tumors has been recently reported, evidencing that headache and fever were dose limiting, and documenting a response rate of 23%, including patients with head and neck, color-ectal, and esophageal cancers (79). A phase II study of matuzumab in combination with pemetrexed in NSCLC is ongoing.

MAb ICR62

MAb ICR62 is a rat MAb that blocks binding of EGF and TGF-α to EGFR. In vitro, it inhibits growth of tumor cells that overexpress EGFR and in xenograft models eradicates EGFR-expressing tumors (80). In a phase I trial of 20 patients with squamous-cell cancers of lung and head and neck that expressed EGFR, no serious toxic effects were observed with doses up to 100 mg a day and biopsy samples taken from four patients who received doses of MAb ICR62 of 40 mg or greater showed localization of the antibody to cell membranes (81).

SUMMARY

The EGFR is a validated anticancer target whose successful exploitation has added novel agents to our current treatment protocols. Subsets of patients have shown to benefit the most from these therapies, and though these traits have yet to be completely defined, they are mostly of genetic nature. These are addressed elsewhere in this book. The discovery of *EGFR*-activating mutations, a potential predictor of efficacy for such a devastating disease as NSCLC, created a tremen-dous expectation from the oncology community and from the public. This break-through is an evident step toward individualized treatment for cancer, a global trend in Medicine that is particularly appealing in the management of advanced cancers where second therapeutic chances are not always an option. Despite the initial excitement that the discovery of activating *EGFR* mutations elicited, follow-up reports have shown that it may be over simplistic to extrapolate the gene-addiction paradigm to a disease with such complexities as NSCLC (where very few molecu-lar prognostic factors have been solidly validated). Although increases in the number of gene copies, protein expression, and *EGFR* mutations have been asso-ciated with TKI and MAb efficacy, objective responses to both gefitinib and erlotinib are also found in the absence of these features. This suggests that TKIs may affect, or be dependent for its activity on, additional genetic factors and/or signaling pathways and that may be essential for target expression, target rele-vance, and tumor-cell proliferation. It seems unlikely that we will be able to sim-plify decision-making schemas following a binary structure, and panels of selected molecular markers and genes will need to be evaluated to accurately classify lung-cancer patients according to their genotype in order to make therapeutic decisions.

REFERENCES

1. Wells A. EGF receptor. Int J Biochem Cell Biol 1999; 31:637–643.
2. Arteaga CL. The epidermal growth factor receptor: from mutant oncogene in nonhuman cancers to therapeutic target in human neoplasia. J Clin Oncol 2001; 19: 32S–40S.

3. Pinkas-Kramarski R, Soussan L, Waterman H, et al. Diversification of neu differentiation factor and epidermal growth factor signaling by combinatorial receptor interactions. Embo J 1996; 15:2452–2467.
4. Yarden Y, Sliwkowski MX. Untangling the ErbB signalling network. Nat Rev Mol Cell Biol 2001; 2:127–137.
5. Graus-Porta D, Beerli RR, Daly JM, Hynes NE. ErbB-2, the preferred heterodimerization partner of all ErbB receptors, is a mediator of lateral signaling. Embo J 1997; 16:1647–1655.
6. Worthylake R, Opresko LK, Wiley HS. ErbB-2 amplification inhibits down-regulation and induces constitutive activation of both ErbB-2 and epidermal growth factor receptors. J Biol Chem 1999; 274:8865–8874.
7. Schlessinger J. Cell signaling by receptor tyrosine kinases. Cell 2000; 103:211–225.
8. Blenis J. Signal transduction via the MAP kinases: proceed at your own RSK. Proc Natl Acad Sci USA 1993; 90:5889–5892.
9. Burgering BM, Coffer PJ. Protein kinase B (c-Akt) in phosphatidylinositol-3-OH kinase signal transduction. Nature 1995; 376:599–602.
10. Lewis TS, Shapiro PS, Ahn NG. Signal transduction through MAP kinase cascades. Adv Cancer Res 1998; 74:49–139.
11. Cantley LC. The phosphoinositide 3-kinase pathway. Science 2002; 296: 1655–1657.
12. Tebar F, Llado A, Enrich C. Role of calmodulin in the modulation of the MAPK signalling pathway and the transactivation of epidermal growth factor receptor mediated by PKC. FEBS Lett 2002; 517:206–210.
13. Giordano A, Rustum YM, Wenner CE. Cell cycle: molecular targets for diagnosis and therapy: tumor suppressor genes and cell cycle progression in cancer. J Cell Biochem 1998; 70:1–7.
14. de Jong JS, van Diest PJ, van der Valk P, Baak JP. Expression of growth factors, growth-inhibiting factors, and their receptors in invasive breast cancer. II. Correlations with proliferation and angiogenesis. J Pathol 1998; 184:53–57.
15. Wells A. Tumor invasion: role of growth factor-induced cell motility. Adv Cancer Res 2000; 78:31–101.
16. Gibson EM, Henson ES, Haney N, Villanueva J, Gibson SB. Epidermal growth factor protects epithelial-derived cells from tumor necrosis factor-related apoptosis-inducing ligand-induced apoptosis by inhibiting cytochrome c release. Cancer Res 2002; 62: 488–496.
17. Salomon DS, Brandt R, Ciardiello F, Normanno N. Epidermal growth factor-related peptides and their receptors in human malignancies. Crit Rev Oncol Hematol 1995; 19:183–232.
18. Grandis JR, Melhem MF, Gooding WE, et al. Levels of TGF-alpha and EGFR protein in head and neck squamous cell carcinoma and patient survival. J Natl Cancer Inst 1998; 90:824–832.
19. Woodburn JR. The epidermal growth factor receptor and its inhibition in cancer therapy. Pharmacol Ther 1999; 82:241–250.
20. Nicholson RI, Gee JM, Harper ME. EGFR and cancer prognosis. Eur J Cancer 2001; 37(suppl 4):S9–S15.
21. Rusch V, Klimstra D, Venkatraman E, Pisters PW, Langenfeld J, Dmitrovsky E. Overexpression of the epidermal growth factor receptor and its ligand transforming growth factor alpha is frequent in resectable non-small cell lung cancer but does not predict tumor progression. Clin Cancer Res 1997; 3:515–522.

22. Fontanini G, De Laurentiis M, Vignati S, et al. Evaluation of epidermal growth factor-related growth factors and receptors and of neoangiogenesis in completely resected stage I–IIIA non-small-cell lung cancer: amphiregulin and microvessel count are independent prognostic indicators of survival. Clin Cancer Res 1998; 4:241–249.

23. Shi D, He G, Cao S, et al. Overexpression of the c-erbB-2/neu-encoded p185 protein in primary lung cancer. Mol Carcinog 1992; 5:213–218.

24. Masui H, Kawamoto T, Sato JD, Wolf B, Sato G, Mendelsohn J. Growth inhibition of human tumor cells in athymic mice by anti-epidermal growth factor receptor monoclonal antibodies. Cancer Res 1984; 44:1002–1007.

25. Sato JD, Kawamoto T, Le AD, Mendelsohn J, Polikoff J, Sato GH. Biological effects in vitro of monoclonal antibodies to human epidermal growth factor receptors. Mol Biol Med 1983; 1:511–529.

26. Barker AJ, Grundy W, et al. Studies leading to the identification of ZD 1839 (IRESSA): an orally active, selective epidermal growth factor receptor tyrosine kinase inhibitor targeted to the treatment of cancer. Bioorg Med Chem 2001; 11:1911–1914.

27. Barker AJ, Gibson KH, Grundy W, et al. Studies leading to the identification of ZD1839 (IRESSA): an orally active, selective epidermal growth factor receptor tyrosine kinase inhibitor targeted to the treatment of cancer. Bioorg Med Chem Lett 2001; 11:1911–1914.

28. Anderson NG, Ahmad T, Chan K, Dobson R, Bundred NJ. ZD1839 (Iressa), a novel epidermal growth factor receptor (EGFR) tyrosine kinase inhibitor, potently inhibits the growth of EGFR-positive cancer cell lines with or without erbB2 overexpression. Int J Cancer 2001; 94:774–782.

29. Ciardiello F, Caputo R, Bianco R, et al. Inhibition of growth factor production and angiogenesis in human cancer cells by ZD1839 (Iressa), a selective epidermal growth factor receptor tyrosine kinase inhibitor. Clin Cancer Res 2001; 7:1459–1465.

30. Baselga J, Rischin D, Ranson M, et al. Phase I safety, pharmacokinetic, and pharmacodynamic trial of ZD1839, a selective oral epidermal growth factor receptor tyrosine kinase inhibitor, in patients with five selected solid tumor types. J Clin Oncol 2002; 20:4292–4302.

31. Herbst RS, Maddox AM, Rothenberg ML, et al. Selective oral epidermal growth factor receptor tyrosine kinase inhibitor ZD1839 is generally well-tolerated and has activity in non-small-cell lung cancer and other solid tumors: results of a phase I trial. J Clin Oncol 2002; 20:3815–3825.

32. Ranson M, Hammond LA, Ferry D, et al. ZD1839, a selective oral epidermal growth factor receptor-tyrosine kinase inhibitor, is well tolerated and active in patients with solid, malignant tumors: results of a phase I trial. J Clin Oncol 2002; 20:2240–2250.

33. Fukuoka M, Yano S, Giaccone G, et al. Multi-institutional randomized phase II trial of gefitinib for previously treated patients with advanced non-small-cell lung cancer. J Clin Oncol 2003; 21:2237–2246.

34. Kris MG, Natale RB, Herbst RS, et al. Efficacy of gefitinib, an inhibitor of the epidermal growth factor receptor tyrosine kinase, in symptomatic patients with non-small cell lung cancer: a randomized trial. JAMA 2003; 290:2149–2158.

35. Giaccone G, Herbst RS, Manegold C, et al. Gefitinib in combination with gemcitabine and cisplatin in advanced non-small-cell lung cancer: a phase III trial—INTACT 1. J Clin Oncol 2004; 22:777–784.

36. Herbst RS, Giaccone G, Schiller JH, et al. Gefitinib in combination with paclitaxel and carboplatin in advanced non-small-cell lung cancer: a phase III trial—INTACT 2. J Clin Oncol 2004; 22:785–794.

37. Herbst RS, Prager D, Hermann R, et al. TRIBUTE: a phase III trial of erlotinib hydro-chloride (OSI-774) combined with carboplatin and paclitaxel chemotherapy in advanced non-small-cell lung cancer. J Clin Oncol 2005; 23:5892–5899.

38. Gatzemeier U, Pluzanska A, Szczesna A, et al. Results of a phase III trial of erlotinib (OSI-774) combined with cisplatin and gemcitabine (GC) chemotherapy in advanced non-small cell lung cancer (NSCLC) [abstr. 7010]. Proc Am Soc Clin Oncol 2004; J Clin Oncol 22:14S.

39. Thatcher N, Chang A, Parikh P, et al. Gefitinib plus best supportive care in previously treated patients with refractory advanced non-small-cell lung cancer: results from a randomised, placebo-controlled, multicentre study (Iressa Survival Evaluation in Lung Cancer). Lancet 2005; 366:1527–1537.

40. Pollack VA, Savage DM, Baker DA, et al. Inhibition of epidermal growth factor recep-tor-associated tyrosine phosphorylation in human carcinomas with CP-358,774: dynamics of receptor inhibition in situ and antitumor effects in athymic mice. J Pharmacol Exp Ther 1999; 291:739–748.

41. Moyer JD, Barbacci EG, Iwata KK, et al. Induction of apoptosis and cell cycle arrest by CP-358,774, an inhibitor of epidermal growth factor receptor tyrosine kinase. Cancer Res 1997; 57:4838–4848.

42. Hidalgo M, Siu LL, Nemunaitis J, et al. Phase I and pharmacologic study of OSI-774, an epidermal growth factor receptor tyrosine kinase inhibitor, in patients with advanced solid malignancies. J Clin Oncol 2001; 19:3267–3279.

43. Karp D FD, Tensfeldt TG, et al. A phase I dose escalation study of epidermal growth factor receptor (EGFR) tyrosine kinase (TK) inhibitor CP-358,774 in patients (pts) with advanced solid tumors. Lung Cancer 2000; 29:72.

44. Perez-Soler R, Chachoua A, Huberman M, et al. A phase II trial of the epidermal growth factor receptor (EGFR) tyrosine kinase inhibitor OSI-774, following platinum-based chemotherapy, in patients (pts) with advanced, EGFR-expressing, non-small cell lung cancer (NSCLC) [abstr. 1235]. Proc Am Soc Clin Oncol 2001; 20:310.

45. Finkler N, Gordon A, Crozier M, et al. Phase II evaluation of OSI-774, a potent oral antagonist of the EGFR-TK in patients with advanced ovarian carcinoma [abstr. 831]. Proc Am Soc Clin Oncol 2001; 20:208.

46. Soulieres D, Senzer NN, Vokes EE, Hidalgo M, Agarwala SS, Siu LL. Multicenter phase II study of erlotinib, an oral epidermal growth factor receptor tyrosine kinase inhibitor, in patients with recurrent or metastatic squamous cell cancer of the head and neck. J Clin Oncol 2004; 22:77–85.

47. Clark G, Pérez-Soler R, Siu LA, Gordon A, Santabárbara P. Rash severity is predictive of increased survival with erlotinib HCl [abstr. 786]. Proc Am Soc Clin Oncol 2003:196.

48. Immervoll H, Hoem D, Kugarajh K, Steine SJ, Molven A. Molecular analysis of the EGFR-RAS-RAF pathway in pancreatic ductal adenocarcinomas: lack of muta-tions in the BRAF and EGFR genes. Virchows Arch 2006; 448(6):788–796. EPub. 2006, Apr. 6.

49. Shepherd FA, Rodrigues Pereira J, Ciuleanu T, et al. Erlotinib in previously treated non-small-cell lung cancer. N Engl J Med 2005; 353:123–132.

50. Giaccone G, Gallegos Ruiz M, Le Chevalier T, et al. Erlotinib for frontline treatment of advanced non-small cell lung cancer: a phase II study. Clin Cancer Res 2006; 12:6049–6055.

51. Paz-Ares L, Sanchez J, García-Velasco A, et al. A prospective phase II trial of erlotinib in advanced non-small cell lung cancer (NSCLC) patients (p) with mutations in the

tyrosine kinase (TK) domain of the epidermal growth factor receptor (EGFR). J Clin Oncol 2006; ASCO Annual Meeting Proceedings Part I 2006; 24:18S:7020.

52. Hidalgo M, Erlichman C, Rowinsky E, et al. Phase 1 trial of EKB-569, an irreversible inhibitor of the epidermal growth factor receptor (EGFR), in patients with advanced solid tumors [abstr. 65]. Proc Am Soc Clin Oncol 2002; 21:25.

53. Burris HA 3rd, Hurwitz HI, Dees EC, et al. Phase I safety, pharmacokinetics, and clinical activity study of lapatinib (GW572016), a reversible dual inhibitor of epidermal growth factor receptor tyrosine kinases, in heavily pretreated patients with metastatic carcinomas. J Clin Oncol 2005; 23:5305–5313.

54. Ross H, Blumenschein G, Dowlati A, et al. Preliminary safety results of a phase II trial comparing two schedules of lapatinib (GW572016) as first line therapy for advanced or metastatic non-small cell lung cancer. J Clin Oncol 2005; ASCO Annual Meeting Proceedings Vol. 23:16S, Part I of II (June 1 Supplement), 2005:7099.

55. Holden SN, Eckhardt SG, Basser R, et al. Clinical evaluation of ZD6474, an orally active inhibitor of VEGF and EGF receptor signaling, in patients with solid, malignant tumors. Ann Oncol 2005; 16:1391–1397.

56. Natale R, Bodkin D, Govindan R, et al. ZD6474 versus gefitinib in patients with advanced NSCLC: final results from a two-part, double-blind, randomized phase II trial. J Clin Oncol 2006; ASCO Annual Meeting Proceedings Part I. Vol 24, No. 18S (June 20 Supplement), 2006:7000.

57. Heymach J, Johnson B, Prager D, et al. A phase II trial of ZD6474 plus docetaxel in patients with previously treated NSCLC: follow-up results. J Clin Oncol 2006; ASCO Annual Meeting Proceedings Part I. Vol. 24, No. 18S (June 20 Supplement), 2006:7016.

58. Kwak EL, Sordella R, Bell DW, et al. Irreversible inhibitors of the EGF receptor may circumvent acquired resistance to gefitinib. Proc Natl Acad Sci USA 2005; 102: 7665–7670.

59. Rabindran SK, Discafani CM, Rosfjord EC, et al. Antitumor activity of HKI-272, an orally active, irreversible inhibitor of the HER-2 tyrosine kinase. Cancer Res 2004; 64:3958–3965.

60. Goldstein NI, Prewett M, Zuklys K, Rockwell P, Mendelsohn J. Biological efficacy of a chimeric antibody to the epidermal growth factor receptor in a human tumor xenograft model. Clin Cancer Res 1995; 1:1311–1318.

61. Fan Z, Lu Y, Wu X, Mendelsohn J. Antibody-induced epidermal growth factor receptor dimerization mediates inhibition of autocrine proliferation of A431 squamous carcinoma cells. J Biol Chem 1994; 269:27595–27602.

62. Wu X, Rubin M, Fan Z, et al. Involvement of p27KIP1 in G1 arrest mediated by an anti-epidermal growth factor receptor monoclonal antibody. Oncogene 1996; 12:1397–1403.

63. Ciardiello F, Bianco R, Damiano V, et al. Antiangiogenic and antitumor activity of anti-epidermal growth factor receptor C225 monoclonal antibody in combination with vascular endothelial growth factor antisense oligonucleotide in human GEO colon cancer cells. Clin Cancer Res 2000; 6:3739–3747.

64. Robert F, Ezekiel MP, Spencer SA, et al. Phase I study of anti-epidermal growth factor receptor antibody cetuximab in combination with radiation therapy in patients with advanced head and neck cancer. J Clin Oncol 2001; 19:3234–3243.

65. Baselga J, Pfister D, Cooper MR, et al. Phase I studies of anti-epidermal growth factor receptor chimeric antibody C225 alone and in combination with cisplatin. J Clin Oncol 2000; 18:904–914.

66. Shin DM, Donato NJ, Perez-Soler R, et al. Epidermal growth factor receptor-targeted therapy with C225 and cisplatin in patients with head and neck cancer. Clin Cancer Res 2001; 7:1204–1213.

67. Cunningham D, Humblet Y, Siena S, et al. Cetuximab monotherapy and cetuximab plus irinotecan in irinotecan-refractory metastatic colorectal cancer. N Engl J Med 2004; 351:337–45.

68. Lynch T, Lilenbaum R, Bonomi P, et al. A phase II trial of cetuximab as therapy for recurrent non-small cell lung cancer (NSCLC) [abstr. 7084]. Proc Am Soc Clin Oncol 2004; 23:634.

69. Thienelt CD, Bunn PA Jr, Hanna N, et al. Multicenter phase I/II study of cetuximab with paclitaxel and carboplatin in untreated patients with stage IV non-small-cell lung cancer. J Clin Oncol 2005; 23:8786–8793.

70. Robert F, Blumenschein G, Herbst RS, et al. Phase I/IIa study of cetuximab with gemcitabine plus carboplatin in patients with chemotherapy-naive advanced non-small-cell lung cancer. J Clin Oncol 2005; 23:9089–9096.

71. Rosell R, Daniel C, Ramlau R, et al. Randomized phase II study of cetuximab in combination with cisplatin (C) and vinorelbine (V) vs. CV alone in the first-line treatment of patients (pts) with epidermal growth factor receptor (EGFR)-expressing advanced non-small-cell lung cancer (NSCLC) [abstr. 7012]. Proc Am Soc Clin Oncol 2004; 23:618.

72. Yang XD, Jia XC, Corvalan JR, Wang P, Davis CG. Development of ABX-EGF, a fully human anti-EGF receptor monoclonal antibody, for cancer therapy. Crit Rev Oncol Hematol 2001; 38:17–23.

73. Lynch DH, Yang XD. Therapeutic potential of ABX-EGF: a fully human anti-epidermal growth factor receptor monoclonal antibody for cancer treatment. Semin Oncol 2002; 29:47–50.

74. Figlin R, Belldegrun A, Crawford J, et al. ABX-EGF, a fully human anti-epidermal growth factor receptor (EGFR) monoclonal antibody (mAb) in patients with advanced cancer: phase 1 clinical results [abstr. 35]. Proc Am Soc Clin Oncol 2002; 21:10.

75. Hambek M, Solbach C, Schnuerch HG, et al. Tumor necrosis factor alpha sensitizes low epidermal growth factor receptor (EGFR)-expressing carcinomas for anti-EGFR therapy. Cancer Res 2001; 61:1045–1049.

76. Knecht R, Peters S, Adunka O, Strebhardt K, Gstoettner W, Hambek M. Carcinomas unresponsive to either cisplatinum or anti-EGFR therapy can be growth inhibited by combination therapy of both agents. Anticancer Res 2003; 23:2577–2583.

77. Tabernero J, Rojo F, Jimenez E, et al. A phase I PK and serial tumor and skin pharmacodynamic (PD) study of weekly (q1w), every 2-week (q2w) or every 3-week (q3w) 1-hour (h) infusion EMD72000, a humanized monoclonal anti-epidermal growth factor receptor (EGFR) antibody, in patients (pt) with advanced tumors [abstr. 770]. Proc Am Soc Clin Oncol 2003; 22:192.

78. Salazar R, Tabernero J, Rojo F, et al. Dose-dependent inhibition of the EGFR and signalling pathways with the anti-EGFR monoclonal antibody (MAb) EMD 72000 administered every three weeks (q3w). A phase I pharmacokinetic/pharmacodynamic (PK/PD) study to define the optimal biological dose (OBD) [abstr. 2002]. Proc Am Soc Clin Oncol 2004; 23:127.

79. Vanhoefer U, Tewes M, Rojo F, et al. Phase I study of the humanized antiepidermal growth factor receptor monoclonal antibody EMD72000 in patients with advanced

solid tumors that express the epidermal growth factor receptor. J Clin Oncol 2004; 22:175–184.

80. Hoffmann T, Hafner D, Ballo H, Haas I, Bier H. Antitumor activity of anti-epidermal growth factor receptor monoclonal antibodies and cisplatin in ten human head and neck squamous cell carcinoma lines. Anticancer Res 1997; 17:4419–4425.

81. Modjtahedi H, Hickish T, Nicolson M, et al. Phase I trial and tumour localisation of the anti-EGFR monoclonal antibody ICR62 in head and neck or lung cancer. Br J Cancer 1996; 73:228–235.

6

Epidermal Growth Factor Receptor Targeted Therapy—Markers of Sensitivity and Response

Rafal Dziadziuszko

Division of Medical Oncology, Department of Medicine, University of Colorado Health Sciences and Cancer Center, Aurora, Colorado, U.S.A., and Department of Oncology and Radiotherapy, Medical University of Gdańsk, Gdańsk, Poland

Barbara Szostakiewicz

Department of Oncology and Radiotherapy, Medical University of Gdańsk, Gdańsk, Poland

Fred R. Hirsch

Division of Medical Oncology, Department of Medicine, University of Colorado Health Sciences and Cancer Center, Aurora, Colorado, U.S.A.

INTRODUCTION

Recent advances in molecular biology and translational research of lung cancer have resulted in the incorporation of novel agents into the treatment of this disease. Importance of epidermal growth factor receptor (EGFR) pathway for the development and progression of non–small cell lung cancer (NSCLC) was recognized in the last decade (1), and clinical development of new agents targeting this pathway was initiated. Two classes of compounds interfering with EGFR are currently in use for the treatment of solid malignancies, including small, orally available

EGFR tyrosine kinase inhibitors (EGFR TKIs), gefitinib (Iressa™), and erlotinib (Tarceva™), and monoclonal antibodies—cetuximab (C225, Erbitux™). Many other new agents targeting EGFR pathway are in development, including a dual inhibitor of EGFR and HER2 tyrosine kinases, lapatinib (GW572016) and inhibitor of EGFR, HER2, and HER3 tyrosine kinases, canertinib (CI-1033) (2); irreversible EGFR TKIs (EKB-569, HKI-272, and HKI-357) (3,4), several monoclonal antibodies—ABX-EGF (panitumumab) (5), EMD 72000 (matuzumab) (6), and 2C4 (pertuzumab)—an anti-HER2 monoclonal antibody that prevents receptor heterodimerization with other EGFR family members (7).

After initial reports of promising efficacy of EGFR TKIs, gefitinib and erlotinib, in NSCLC, it was realized that these agents are active only in a proportion of patients, with some 10% to 15% of Western NSCLC populations eliciting response and another 20% to 30% of patients experiencing stable disease and symptomatic benefit (8–10). Thus, the disease control will be achieved in approximately 40% of NSCLC patients who previously failed on chemotherapy. In the last three years, large efforts were undertaken on how to select the populations of patients who are most likely to benefit from EGFR TKIs, based on identified clinical and molecular markers of sensitivity or resistance. Much less is known on predictive markers for treatment benefit with monoclonal antibodies, although some biomarkers of sensitivity may also pertain to this class of agents. The present review will discuss the predictive role of clinical and molecular markers for response and survival benefit to EGFR-targeted therapies in NSCLC.

Several important points need to be addressed prior to discussion of specific biomarkers of sensitivity or resistance. Predictive biomarkers define a population of patients who achieve treatment benefit (increased response and/or prolonged survival) when treated with active drug as compared to placebo. Prognostic biomarkers identify the population of patients with better or worse prognosis regardless of treatment; that is, indicate more indolent or more aggressive course of the disease. The best estimation of predictive role of biomarker is through its analysis in placebo-controlled trials, in which treatment benefit can be compared to placebo in subsets of patients with positive and negative biomarker test. In single arm or retrospective studies, predictive role of the biomarker should be interpreted with caution because it may be obscured by its prognostic significance.

The clinical definition of sensitivity includes both increased response rate and prolonged survival. It should be noted that populations of patients who respond to targeted therapies may be considerably different than populations of patients who benefit from prolonged survival, for which disease stabilization may contribute to the success of therapy, as indicated in a recent trial of renal cancer (11). Hence, markers of response benefit may not always be the same as markers of survival benefit.

Finally, the largest amount of information on markers of increased sensitivity to EGFR-targeted therapies comes from clinical trials with EGFR TKIs, gefitinib and erlotinib. The questions asked in these studies vary extensively (i.e., monotherapy vs. combination studies, drugs and doses used, phase of the study, and patient populations) and therefore the conclusions regarding biomarker analyses should be interpreted in the context of these particular studies.

CLINICAL FEATURES

Several clinical features have been associated with the benefit to EGFR TKI therapy. Of these, never-smoking history is probably the strongest predictor of increased response and prolonged survival after the treatment with gefitinib and erlotinib. In the United States, never-smokers represent approximately 10% to 15% of newly diagnosed lung cancer patients (12), whereas in the Far East, this proportion may be as high as 30% (13). In phase-I and phase-II studies with EGFR TKIs, this clinical feature was infrequently reported. In the retrospective analysis of 139 patients treated with single-agent gefitinib, response rate in never-smokers was 36% versus 8% in ever-smokers (14). In two prospective, placebo-controlled randomized trials with EGFR TKIs as second- or third-line therapy, the BR.21 and ISEL, the response rates in never-smokers were 25% and 18% versus 4% and 5% in ever-smokers, respectively (Table 1) (15,16).

Most importantly, both studies showed a significant survival advantage in the subsets of never smokers treated with erlotinib or gefitinib, respectively. In the analysis of the BR.21 study with erlotinib, hazard ratio (HR, a coefficient indicating the relative reduction of the risk of death) in never-smokers was 0.42 as compared to 0.87 in ever-smokers (19). In this study, particular treatment benefit was observed in never-smoking patients with positive EGFR immunostaining (HR = 0.28). Based on these data, several clinical studies are assessing the role of EGFR TKIs as the first-line treatment of advanced NSCLC never-smoking patients.

Early in the clinical development of EGFR TKIs, it was realized that these drugs produce increased responses in patients of Asian origin. In IDEAL 1 (Iressa™ Dose Evaluation in Advanced Lung cancer) phase-II study assessing two doses of single-agent gefitinib in chemotherapy-pretreated NSCLC, response rates were 27.5% in Japanese patients as compared to 10.4% in non-Japanese patients (8). Increased response rates to erlotinib in Asians were also observed in the BR.21 study (18.9% vs. 7.5% in non-Asians) (17) and to gefitinib in the ISEL trial (12.4% vs. 6.8% in non-Asians) (16). In both studies, the use of EGFR TKIs in subgroups of patients of Asian descent was associated with significant survival benefit as compared to placebo (Table 1).

Although all four phase-III studies exploring combination of chemotherapy and EGFR TKIs in the first-line treatment of NSCLC were negative (18,20–22), significant association between benefit from erlotinib and never-smoking history was found in the TRIBUTE study, in which the median survival of never-smoking patients receiving paclitaxel, carboplatin, and erlotinib was 22.5 months versus 10.1 months in never-smokers who received chemotherapy and placebo (18). Smoking history was not addressed in the reports of the remaining phase-III clinical trials addressing the role of concomitant chemotherapy and EGFR TKIs. Based on this finding, combination of erlotinib and chemotherapy in the first-line treatment of NSCLC in never-smokers warrants further investigation.

Table 1 Clinical Markers of Sensitivity to Epidermal Growth Factor Receptor Tyrosine Kinase Inhibitors in Selected Large Studies

Clinical marker	Study (Ref.)	Number of patients	Drug (dose)	Proportion positive	Response rates: positive vs. negative	Survival hazard ratio (95% CI)
Never-smoking history	Shepherd et al.—BR.21 (17)	731	Erlotinib (150 mg)	20%	24.7% vs. 3.9%	0.4 (0.3–0.6)
Never-smoking history	Thatcher et al.—ISEL (16)	1692	Gefitinib (250 mg)	22%	18.1% vs. 5.3%	0.67 (0.49–0.92)
Never-smoking history	Miller et al.—retrospective (14)	139	Gefitinib (250 mg, 90%) (500 mg, 10%)	26%	36.1% vs. 7.6%	NR
Never-smoking history	Herbst et al.—TRIBUTE (18)	1079	Erlotinib (150 mg)	10.7%	30% vs. 11%[a]	0.49 (0.28–0.85)[a]
Asian origin	Shepherd et al.—BR.21 (17)	731	Erlotinib (150 mg)	12.7%	18.9% vs. 7.5%	0.6 (0.4–1.0)
Asian origin	Thatcher et al.—ISEL (16)	1692	Gefitinib (250 mg)	20.2%	12.4% vs. 6.8%	0.66 (0.48–0.91)
Asian origin	Fukuoka et al.—IDEAL 1 (8)	210	Gefitinib (250 mg, 50%) (500 mg, 50%)	48.8%	27.5% vs. 10.4%	NR
Adenocarcinoma histology	Shepherd et al.—BR.21 (17)	731	Erlotinib (150 mg)	49.9%	13.9% vs. 4.1%	0.7 (0.6–0.9)
Adenocarcinoma histology	Thatcher et al.—ISEL (16)	1692	Gefitinib (250 mg)	45%	11.9% vs. 4.8%	0.84 (0.70–1.02)
Adenocarcinoma with BAC features	Miller et al.—retrospective (14)	139	Gefitinib (250 mg, 90%) (500 mg, 10%)	17%	38% vs. 10%	NR
Female gender	Shepherd et al.—BR.21 (17)	731	Erlotinib (150 mg)	21.3%	14.4% vs. 6%	0.8 (0.6–1.1)
Female gender	Thatcher et al.—ISEL (16)	1692	Gefitinib (250 mg)	33%	14.7% vs. 5.1%	0.8 (0.6–1.0)[b]
Female gender	Miller et al.—retrospective (14)	139	Gefitinib (250 mg, 90%) (500 mg, 10%)	65%	18.7% vs. 8.3%	NR

[a]Comparison of erlotinib, paclitaxel, and carboplatin vs. placebo, paclitaxel, and carboplatin in never-smoking patients; all other comparisons are for epidermal growth factor receptor tyrosine kinase inhibitor vs. placebo in subsets of patients with positive clinical marker.
[b]Data extracted from graph (Fig. 1).
Abbreviations: BAC, bronchioloalveolar carcinoma; CI, confidence interval; NR, not reported.

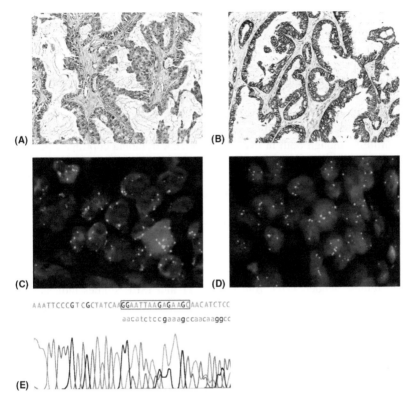

Figure 1 (*See color insert*.) Example biomarker analysis of a lung tumor with bronchi-oloalveolar histology (**A**) ×200, with strong EGFR protein expression (**B**) DAKO Pharm Dx staining kit, ×200, *EGFR* gene amplification (**C**) Hybridization with the LSI EGFR SpectrumOrange/CEP SpectrumGreen probe, Vysis, Abbott Molecular, high *HER2* gene copy number (**D**) Hybridization with the Path Vysion HER-2 DNA Probe Kit, Vysis, Abbott Molecular and *EGFR* exon 19 E746 A750 deletion (**E**) Sequencing analyzed in Genetic Analyzer ABI PRISM 310. *Source*: From Ref. 103.

Adenocarcinoma histology was associated with higher response rates to EGFR TKIs in numerous retrospective and prospective studies (Table 1). The response rates to gefitinib or erlotinib in patients with adenocarcinoma histology enrolled in prospective monotherapy studies remain in the order of 12% to 14%, as compared to 4% to 5% in patients with other histological types of NSCLC. In the subset of adenocarcinomas, bronchioloalveolar carcinoma (BAC) features are particularly predictive of response to EGFR TKIs. In the retrospective study of 139 patients treated with gefitinib, response rate in patients with BAC features was 38% versus 14% in patients with non-BAC adenocarcinomas (14). After adjustment for other clinical markers of sensitivity in the multivariate analysis, odds ratio of response for tumors with BAC features was 13.5 as compared to nonadenocarcinomas in this study. Kris et al. reported 25% response rate and 58%

one-year survival probability with erlotinib in patients with tumors classified as BAC (23). In the Southwest Oncology Group (SWOG) 0126 study, a phase-II clinical trial that specifically addressed the role of gefitinib 500 mg daily in patients with BAC, response rates were 17% among previously untreated patients and 9% in patients who failed chemotherapy (24). It should be noted however that despite increased response rate in adenocarcinoma patients who participated in BR.21 study, survival benefit in favor of erlotinib was also observed in nonadeno-carcinoma subsets of patients (17). Similar tendency was noted in the ISEL trial with gefitinib, although both in overall and adenocarcinoma coprimary popula-tions the survival benefit from gefitinib was not significant (16).

The probability of response to EGFR TKIs also depends on gender. Female NSCLC patients have 14% to 25% response rates to EGFR TKIs as compared to 3% to 8% in male NSCLC patients (Table 1). In the BR.21 and ISEL trials, survival benefit was however not limited to females treated with erlotinib, as indi-cated by similar HRs for both genders (16,17).

In summary, four clinical features are associated with increased responsive-ness to EGFR TKIs: never-smoking history, Asian origin, adenocarcinoma histol-ogy, and female gender. Data from the BR.21 and ISEL studies indicate that survival benefit is observed also in other subsets of patients, although certainly the magnitude of this benefit is greatest in never-smokers and Asians. Clinical mark-ers of sensitivity to EGFR TKIs may be used to guide physicians on whom to treat with EGFR TKIs, although such selection would select only a small proportion of patients who could otherwise derive survival benefit from EGFR TKIs. Clearly, more robust markers are needed for appropriate selection of patients to EGFR TKI therapy, and significant scientific efforts have been made to identify molecular predictors of treatment benefit.

EGFR IMMUNOHISTOCHEMISTRY

It was anticipated that the presence of molecular target is the most important and straightforward marker of sensitivity to molecular-targeted therapies. EGFR immunohistochemical staining is the most widely available and the most commonly used method to evaluate the presence and the degree of EGFR protein expression. Several clinical studies have addressed the associations of treatment benefit and EGFR immunohistochemistry (IHC). The results of these studies are conflicting due to different methodologies—use of different antibodies, different scoring systems, but also different populations of patients investigated clinically. These studies are summarized in Table 2 and discussed below. Example of posi-tive EGFR immunostaining is shown in Figure 1B.

Early clinical data indicated that EGFR immunostaining was not predictive of the treatment benefit from EGFR TKIs. Bailey et al. performed EGFR immu-nostaining in tumor samples from 157 patients participating in phase-II gefitinib studies using DAKO Cytomation EGFR pharmDx assay (Dako Corp. Glostrup, Denmark). Authors used quantitative scoring system taking into account percent-age of positive cells and the intensity of staining. Using objective response and

Table 2 EGFR Protein Expression as a Marker of Sensitivity to EGFR Tyrosine Kinase Inhibitors[a]

Study (Ref.)	Number of patients	Drug (dose)	Antibody	Scoring system (cut point)	Proportion positive	Response rates: positive vs. negative	Survival hazard ratio (95% CI)
Tsao et al.— BR.21 (15)	325	Erlotinib (150 mg)	Dako PharmD× Staining Kit	Percent of positive cells (10%)	57%	11% vs. 4%	0.68[b] (0.49–0.95)
Hirsch et al.— ISEL (25)	379	Gefitinib (250 mg)	Dako PharmD× Staining Kit	Percent of positive cells (10%)	69.7%	8.2% vs. 1.5%	0.77[b] (0.56–1.08)
Cappuzzo et al.— retrospective (26)	98	Gefitinib (250 mg)	Zymed	Percent of positive cells × staining intensity (200)	59%	21% vs. 5%	0.60[c] (0.36–1.01)
Parra et al. retrospective (27)	50	Gefitinib (250 mg)	EGFR Ab-10	Four-point (2+/3+)	46%	17.3% vs. 3.7%	NR[d]

[a]Two negative studies of Bailey et al. (28,29) presented as abstracts only are not included.
[b]Hazard ratio comparing erlotinib or gefitinib to placebo in immunohistochemistry-positive group of patients.
[c]Hazard ratio comparing EGFR immunohistochemistry-negative and positive patients treated with gefitinib.
[d]Hazard ratio was not reported; worse survival in gefitinib-treated patients with high *EGFR* expression was found.
Abbreviations: CI, confidence interval; EGFR, epidermal growth factor receptor.

symptom improvement as end points, no cutoff of EGFR IHC could be identified to associate with treatment outcome (28). The same group reported no predictive value of EGFR immunostaining for response or survival benefit in the subsequent EGFR IHC study based on tumor samples from 516 patients accrued in two gefitinib phase-III clinical trials, INTACT 1 and 2 (Iressa NSCLC Trials Assessing Combination Treatment) (29). Cappuzzo et al. analyzed EGFR (Zymed Laboratories, San Francisco, California, U.S.) and HER2 (DAKO Herceptest, Copenhagen, Denmark) immunostaining in 63 gefitinib-treated, locally advanced, or metastatic NSCLC patients. Combination of both biomarkers did not associate with response or survival (30). The same antibody from Zymed was used in the retrospective study of 102 relapsed patients treated with gefitinib, but with different scoring system, based on the percentage of positive cells and staining intensity (26). In this study, staining intensity was graded on zero to four scale and multiplied by percent of positive cells, resulting in IHC score ranging from 0 to 400. Cut-off point of 200 defined tumors with moderate or strong staining as IHC-positive (59% of patients) and no or weak staining as IHC-negative (41% of patients). This study also evaluated associations of *EGFR* gene copy number, *EGFR* mutations, and phosphorylated Akt (p-Akt) expression with treatment outcome. Positive EGFR immunostaining was linked to significantly better response rate (21% vs. 5%), superior progression-free (median 5.2 vs. 2.3 months), and overall survival (median 11.5 vs. 5.0 months).

Biomarker analysis of the BR.21 study showed that EGFR IHC, evaluated by DAKO Cytomation EGFR pharmDx assay, appears predictive of treatment outcome (15). EGFR immunostaining with DAKO antibody was positive in 57% of patients using cut-off point of 10% cells with membranous staining of at least weak intensity. EGFR positivity was associated with slightly higher response rate (11% vs. 4% in EGFR-negative patients) and with increased survival (HR = 0.68 vs. 0.93, respectively). Interaction test with treatment (indicating comparison of HRs for erlotinib between positive and negative subsets) was not significant ($P = 0.25$). Biomarker analysis of the ISEL trial, using the same antibody and cut point, also indicated a higher response in EGFR-positive as compared to EGFR-negative patients (8.2% vs. 1.5%) (25). Although treatment benefit was only slightly and nonsignificantly better in the subset of EGFR-positive patients (HR = 0.77) than in overall population (HR = 0.89), approximately 30% EGFR-negative patients did not derive any benefit from gefitinib (HR = 1.57). The interaction test with treatment was statistically significant ($P = 0.049$), indicating that EGFR immunostaining does predict different outcome in gefitinib-treated advanced NSCLC patients. In conclusion, some data suggest improved outcome in EGFR IHC-positive patients, although controversies exist on different methodologies used across the studies. More importantly, EGFR IHC-negative patients are unlikely to benefit from EGFR TKIs, and it may be considered as a negative predictive factor indicating who should not be treated with these drugs.

Several important issues regarding the routine use of EGFR IHC remain to be considered. DAKO Cytomation EGFR pharmDx assay is most often used in the clinical studies assessing the association with the efficacy of EGFR inhibitors.

In a study of 230 tumor samples from colorectal cancer patients, three different commercially available antibodies for EGFR IHC from DAKO, Zymed, and Ventana (Tucson, Arizona, U.S.) were compared (31). The use of antibodies from Ventana and Zymed resulted in higher number of positive samples as compared to DAKO, regardless of cut-off points defining positivity. Another study addressed the influence of different fixatives and storage time to assess EGFR staining results with DAKO Cytomation EGFR PharmDx assay in colorectal, lung, and head and neck carcinomas. Use of different fixatives resulted in slightly different results, and positive EGFR IHC inversely correlated with storage time across all fixatives (32). These data suggest that choice of fixative, antibody, and length of sample storage may all affect the results of IHC testing. There is also no universal agreement on the optimal cut-off point to define IHC positivity (33). The analysis of different cut-off points of IHC in the BR.21 erlotinib study showed that higher cut-off points than the one predefined in the trial (i.e., 10% of positive cells of any staining intensity) do not lead to better prediction of survival benefit (34). Automated assessment becomes more popular for certain immunohistochemical applications (35) with aims to improve interobserver variability and to provide a high throughput platform. The comparisons of EGFR IHC by automated and manual scoring to predict sensitivity to EGFR inhibitors have not been performed.

EGFR GENE COPY NUMBER

In breast cancer patients, amplification of the *HER2* gene detected by fluorescence in situ hybridization (FISH) is a powerful predictive factor for treatment benefit from anti-HER2 monoclonal antibody, trastuzumab, recommended for use in clinical practice (36). It may be speculated that genomic gain of *EGFR* is a factor contributing to growth advantage of NSCLC cells and may be an important biomarker of sensitivity to EGFR TKIs. Investigators from the University of Colorado Cancer Center developed an original scoring system for *EGFR* gene copy number assessed by FISH in which tumors were classified into six categories, based on ascending number of gene copies per cell (26). FISH-negative samples were classified as those with no or low genomic gain (≥4 copies of the gene per cell in <40% of cells), and FISH-positive samples were defined as tumors with high gene copy number (≥4 copies of the gene per cell in ≥40% of cells) or amplification (tight gene clusters and a ratio of gene/chromosome per cell ≥2, or ≥15 gene copies per cell in ≥10% of the cells). To date, four major studies have addressed the association between *EGFR* gene copy number by FISH and treatment outcome to EGFR TKIs. All four studies demonstrated clinically important treatment benefit in patients with high *EGFR* gene copy number (Table 3), and this test is now being validated in prospective clinical studies in enriched population of NSCLC patients. Examples of *EGFR* and *HER2* gene copy number assessments by FISH are shown in Figure 1C and 1D.

Cappuzzo et al. analyzed 102 gefitinib-treated patients according to EGFR protein expression, p-Akt expression, *EGFR* gene copy number by FISH, and *EGFR* mutations (26). Patients who were FISH-positive had significantly better

Table 3 Epidermal Growth Factor Receptor Gene Copy Number as a Marker of Sensitivity to Epidermal Growth Factor Receptor Tyrosine Kinase Inhibitors

Study (Ref.)	Number of patients	Drug (dose)	Method of gene copy number evaluation (cut point)	Proportion positive	Response rates: positive vs. negative	Survival hazard ratio (95% CI)
Cappuzzo et al.—retrospective (26)	102	Gefitinib (250 mg)	FISH (high polysomy and gene amplification)	32.3%	36% vs. 3%	0.44[a] (0.23–0.82)
Hirsch et al.—SWOG 0126 (37)	81	Gefitinib (500 mg)	FISH (high polysomy and gene amplification)	32.0%	26% vs. 11%	0.50[a,b] (0.25–0.97)
Tsao et al.—BR.21 (15)	125	Erlotinib (150 mg)	FISH (high polysomy and gene amplification)	45%	20% vs. 2%	0.44[c] (0.23–0.82)
Hirsch et al.—ISEL (25)	370	Gefitinib (250 mg)	FISH (high polysomy and gene amplification)	30.8%	16.4% vs. 3%	0.61[c] (0.36–1.04)
Bell et al. (38)—IDEAL	90	Gefitinib (250 mg and 500 mg)	Quantitative PCR (>4)	8%	29% vs. 15%	NR
INTACT	453			7%	56% vs. 53%[d]	2.03[c] (0.67–6.13)
Dziadziuszko et al.—retrospective (39)	82	Gefitinib (250 mg)	Quantitative PCR (>median)	51%	12% vs. 10%	1.04[a] (0.61–1.76)
Takano et al.—retrospective (40)	66	Gefitinib (250 mg)	Quantitative PCR (≥3)	44%	72% vs. 38%	0.80[a] (0.42–1.50)

[a]Comparison of patients with high versus low *EGFR* gene copy number.
[b]Hazard ratio was recalculated from original publication for consistency in the table.
[c]Comparison within high *EGFR* gene copy number subset of patients receiving EGFR inhibitor vs. placebo.
[d]Indicates response rates to chemotherapy and EGFR inhibitor versus chemotherapy and placebo.
Abbreviations: CI, confidence interval; EGFR, epidermal growth factor receptor; PCR, polymerase chain reaction.

response rate (36% vs. 3% in FISH-negative patients), median time-to-progression (9.0 months vs. 2.5 months, respectively), and median overall survival (18.7 months vs. 7.0 months, respectively). The association of FISH positivity and superior survival was confirmed in multivariate survival analysis. Evaluation of *EGFR* gene copy number by FISH was also performed in tumor samples from 81 participants of SWOG 0126 study, assessing the role of gefitinib in BAC and adenocarcinoma with bronchioloalveolar features. In this study, FISH-positive patients had about 50% reduction in the risk of death as compared to FISH-negative patients (37). Data from the ISEL trial are based on the subset of 370 patients, represent the largest evaluation of this biomarker in the study of EGFR TKIs in advanced NSCLC, and favor *EGFR* gene copy number assessment by FISH as a clinically useful predictor of treatment benefit from gefitinib (25). The response rate in FISH-positive patients was 16% as compared to 3% in FISH-negative patients, and the median survival was almost doubled (8.3 months in gefitinib-treated FISH-positive patients vs. 4.5 months in FISH-positive patients treated with placebo, corresponding to HR of 0.61). Patients with high *EGFR* copy number treated with placebo had slightly inferior survival when compared to patients with low *EGFR* gene copy number (4.5 months vs. 6.2 months, respectively), indicating that increased *EGFR* gene copy number by FISH is purely predictive for the benefit from EGFR TKI and not a prognostic indicator. The lack of prognostic value of EGFR FISH is also supported by the results of *EGFR* gene copy number assessment from surgically treated NSCLC patients (41) and in NSCLC patients treated with chemotherapy alone (42). Molecular analysis of tumor samples from the BR.21 trial was performed using FISH according to the same criteria, although at a different institution. Although FISH result could be obtained only in 125 out of 221 samples (57%), the subset of FISH-positive patients achieved significant treatment benefit from erlotinib (20% response rate and a HR of 0.44), whereas this benefit was modest in FISH-negative patients (2% response rate and a HR of 0.85) (15).

EGFR gene copy number may be heterogeneous within different areas of the same tumor and between the primary and metastatic site, influencing the result of the FISH analysis (43). Clinical significance of tumor heterogeneity with regard to sensitivity to EGFR TKIs is presently unknown. Other techniques of gene copy number assessment include quantitative polymerase chain reaction (qPCR) and chromogenic in situ hybridization (CISH). In the former method, copy number of the gene of interest is compared to that of the housekeeping gene, and expressed as a relative ratio. Direct comparison of *EGFR* gene copy number assessment by FISH and qPCR in 82 advanced NSCLC patients showed no significant association between FISH positivity and qPCR results (39). In this study, *EGFR* gene copy number by qPCR was not associated with outcome of gefitinib-treated patients (Table 3). Molecular analysis of IDEAL (phase-II) and INTACT (phase-III studies comparing chemotherapy and gefitinib vs. chemotherapy and placebo) demonstrated no predictive value of *EGFR* gene amplification by qPCR for treatment outcome (38). In a study from Japan on 66 gefitinib-treated patients, increased *EGFR* gene copy number by qPCR was linked to higher response rate and increased time-to-progression, but not overall survival (40). At present, we need more definitive data to explain why the results of *EGFR* gene copy number quantification by FISH and qPCR are different with respect to its predictive value for EGFR TKI treatment benefit. Quantification of gene copy number by FISH is possible in individual tumor cells, whereas qPCR techniques assess gene copy number in a pool of cells, which may also contain inflammatory and stromal components. Tumor microdissection may help to ensure that the assessment is carried out in areas abundant in tumor cells, but this procedure significantly increases the assay cost. In qPCR technique, quantification of the reference gene copy number presents additional challenge due to the possibility of its deletion or amplification in tumor cells. CISH technique implements an enzymatic reaction to detect the DNA probe hybridized to the gene of interest. The main advantage of this technology is the use of light instead of fluorescent microscope enabling the reader to score the signals in histological sections. Data on CISH gene copy number evaluation and sensitivity to EGFR TKIs are sparse. In a group of 44 NSCLC patients treated with gefitinib or erlotinib, *EGFR* gene copy number by CISH did not associate with response rate (44). A comparison study between CISH and FISH is currently ongoing.

In summary, EGFR TKIs produce significant survival benefit in pretreated populations of patients with high *EGFR* gene copy number evaluated by FISH, as demonstrated by four studies involving almost 700 patients. Several phase-II prospective clinical studies with patient selection based on FISH or combination of FISH and other biomarkers are currently underway in the adjuvant, first- and second-line setting. There is no data to support the equivalence of *EGFR* gene copy number testing by FISH, qPCR, or CISH for the purpose of patient selection to EGFR-targeted therapies.

EGFR MUTATIONS

Mutations in the region coding tyrosine kinase domain of the *EGFR* gene occur in approximately 10% to 20% of North American or European surgically treated NSCLC patients (45–47) and approximately 30% to 50% of operable NSCLC patients from Far East (46,48). These mutations were discovered by two investigator groups from Boston in 2004, and linked to increased responsiveness to EGFR TKIs (49,50). Three different types of *EGFR* mutations have been identified, including in-frame deletions in exon 19, single nucleotide substitutions in exons 18, 20, and 21, and in-frame duplications/insertions in exon 20. The most common mutations include E746-A750 exon 19 deletion and missense mutation in exon 21, leading to the substitution of arginine for leucine at position 858 of the protein (L858R) (46,47). In two large cohorts of surgically treated patients from various geographical regions, exon 19 deletions were detected in 46% and exon 21 point mutations were detected in 39% of patients harboring mutations (46,47). All identified mutations are located close to the adenosine triphosphate-binding pocket of the kinase domain, resulting in deregulation of the kinase activity. The majority of the mutations identified are heterozygous, suggesting that they are likely dominant.

Rare exon 20 T790M point mutation was linked to acquired or de novo resistance to EGFR TKIs (51,52). A recent study documented that these mutations may be present in a small subset of tumor cells prior to the start of EGFR-targeted therapy and these cells subsequently give rise to the relapse through a clonal selection process (53). Numerous studies documented an association between *EGFR* mutations and clinical features predicting increased response to EGFR TKIs— that is, Asian origin, never-smoking history, female gender, and adenocarcinoma histology, suggesting mutations as underlying cause of increased sensitivity to EGFR TKIs (46,54).

In vitro studies confirm higher sensitivity of lung cancer cell lines harboring *EGFR* mutations to EGFR TKIs. Investigators identified several NSCLC cell lines with mutations of *EGFR* that are sensitive to treatment with gefitinib and erlotinib (55–57). H3255 cell line harboring L858R point mutation was found to be the most sensitive to gefitinib (57). There is growing body of evidence suggesting that tumors with *EGFR* mutations have different biologic features compared to tumors with wild-type receptors. The gefitinib-sensitive cell lines with *EGFR* mutations have the potential to transduce signals that are qualitatively distinct from those mediated by wild-type *EGFR*. Cells harboring *EGFR* mutations are more sensitive to pharmacological inhibition of proteins involved in the control of apoptosis, Akt or signal transduction and activation of transcription (STAT), whereas cells expressing wild-type *EGFR* signal mainly through ras pathway controlling cell proliferation (56). Survival of *EGFR* mutant cell lines is dependent on the signaling through pathways controlling apoptosis, and treatment with gefitinib or erlotinib causes rapid and massive programmed cell death. This effect is also consistent with rapid responses to EGFR TKIs observed in NSCLC patients. Data from cell line studies (55) but also from NSCLC tumor samples indicate that the occurrence of mutations is associated with high *EGFR* gene copy number (26,40,58), and mutated *EGFR* allele is preferentially amplified (40).

The most common method to detect mutations is bidirectional sequencing after amplification of the regions most likely to contain mutations (exons 18–21) (15,25,49,50) (Fig. 1E). Other techniques used for this purpose include single strand conformation polymorphism analysis of PCR products (45), mutation-specific PCR (59), or allele-specific PCR (25)—these techniques are designed to detect most common mutation types and do not allow for detection of novel or rare mutations. Allele-specific PCR and its product digestion by SURVEYOR (a commercially available CEL I endonuclease) with subsequent analysis by high performance liquid chromatography was reported to be a highly sensitive method of mutation detection, particularly suitable for mutation screening (60). Other currently developed highly sensitive techniques include high-resolution melting analysis (61) and peptide nucleic acid-locked nucleic acid PCR clamp (62). The clinical significance of higher mutation detection rate through increased sensitivity of these tests is presently unknown. Due to possible artifacts of mutation analysis, especially from paraffin-embedded tumor samples (63), it is generally recommended to confirm the presence of mutations by an alternative technique.

Detection of *EGFR* mutations is now possible in the serum samples allowing for serial testing at various time points during treatment (64).

Increased responsiveness to gefitinib and erlotinib in patients whose tumors harbor *EGFR* mutations was observed in large number of studies, with response rates ranging from 16% to 89% (Table 4).

Lower response rates in prospective trials (16% in the BR.21 and 37.5% in the ISEL) as compared to retrospective studies (54–89%) indicate possible patient selection bias in the latter studies. An association of *EGFR* mutations and increased survival of patients treated with gefitinib or erlotinib was reported mainly in cohorts of patients from the Far East (40,58,66,69–70) (Table 4). This association was however not confirmed in prospective, placebo-controlled trials. In the BR.21, HRs comparing erlotinib to placebo were almost the same in patients with and without *EGFR* mutations, indicating more indolent course of the disease and lack of predictive value of mutation testing (15). The molecular analysis of this study was criticized for unexpectedly high rate of uncommon mutations that could represent false-positive findings (63), but updated analysis confined to patients with exon 19 and 21 "classical" mutations did not change the study conclusions (71). In the ISEL trial, there were too few events for meaningful survival comparisons (25). In the INTACT and the TRIBUTE trials, testing the addition of gefitinib or erlotinib to the first-line chemotherapy in NSCLC, patients with mutations had favorable survival irrespective whether they received active drug or placebo, supporting the notion that *EGFR* mutations represent more indolent biology of NSCLC and have prognostic implication (38,65). More recent data indicate that the subsets of EGFR TKI-treated patients with exon 19 deletions survive longer as compared to those with exon 21 point mutations (72–74). The precise role of *EGFR* mutations to select patients for treatment with EGFR TKIs remains to be established. A prospective phase-II study with gefitinib was conducted in 16 *EGFR* mutation-positive NSCLC patients who fulfilled the enrollment criteria and were selected from 99 chemo-naïve patients subjected to mutation screening (75). The response rate to gefitinib (250 mg daily) was 75% and median progression-free survival was almost 10 months with no significant toxicity. A preliminary report from the Spanish Lung Cancer Study Group showed 90% response to erlotinib (150 mg daily) in *EGFR* mutant patients who constituted 12.5% of screened chemotherapy-naïve NSCLC population. These results are very encouraging; however, they also indicate that the population of NSCLC patients identified by mutation testing is relatively small even in the Far East.

OTHER BIOMARKERS

Downstream Signaling Proteins

Activation of EGFR pathways controlling cell proliferation or apoptosis depends upon phosphorylation of kinases involved in intracellular signaling (PI3K/Akt and ras/Raf/MAPK pathways, respectively). In vitro data support the observation

Table 4 Epidermal Growth Factor Receptor Mutations as a Marker of Sensitivity to Epidermal Growth Factor Receptor Tyrosine Kinase Inhibitors in Selected Large Studies

Study (Ref.)	Number of patients	Drug (dose)	Methods of *EGFR* mutation analysis	Proportion positive	Response rates: positive vs. negative	Survival hazard ratio (95% CI)
Tsao et al.—BR.21 (15)	197	Erlotinib (150 mg)	Sequencing	22.6%	16% vs. 7%	0.77 (0.40–1.50)[a]
Hirsch et al.—ISEL (25)	215	Gefitinib (250 mg)	Sequencing + amplificati on refractory mutation system	12.1%	37.5% vs. 2.6%	NR[a]
Bell et al. (38)—IDEAL	79	Gefitinib (250 mg and 500 mg)	Sequencing	18%	46% vs. 10%	NR[a]
INTACT	312			10%	72% vs. 55%[b]	1.77 (0.50–6.23)[b]
Eberhard et al.—TRIBUTE (65)	228	Erlotinib (150 mg)	Sequencing (repeated for confirmation)	12.7%	53% vs. 18%[b]	NR (NS)[a]
Mitsudomi et al.—retrospective (66)	59	Gefitinib (250 mg)	Sequencing	56%	83% vs. 10%	0.342 (0.117–0.998)[c]
Takano et al.—retrospective (40)	66	Gefitinib (250 mg)	Sequencing + pyrosequencing	59%	82% vs. 11%	0.27 (0.13–0.53)[c]
Cappuzzo et al.—retrospective (26)	89	Gefitinib (250 mg)	Sequencing	17%	54% vs. 5%	NR (NS)[c]
Cortes-Funes et al. (67)	83	Gefitinib (250 mg)	Sequencing	12%	60% vs. 8.8%	0.32 (0.12–0.91)[c,d]
Han et al. (68)	90	Gefitinib (250 mg)	Sequencing	18.9%	64.7% vs. 13.7%	0.16 (0.046–0.52)[c]

[a]Comparison within high *EGFR* gene copy number mutant subset of patients receiving EGFR inhibitor versus placebo.
[b]Comparison of chemotherapy and EGFR inhibitor versus chemotherapy and placebo.
[c]Comparison of patients with versus without *EGFR* mutations.
[d]Hazard ratio was recalculated from original publication for consistency in the table.
Abbreviations: EGFR, epidermal growth factor receptor; NR, not reported; NR (NS), exact hazard ratio not reported, difference in survival was not significant.

of selective activation of antiapoptotic Akt and STAT pathways in cell lines transfected with mutant *EGFR* and link these findings to increased sensitivity of cell lines to gefitinib (56). High level of phosphorylated kinases located in apoptotic pathway could thus indicate sensitivity to EGFR-targeted therapies. Phosphorylated Akt and phosphorylated MAPK were evaluated by IHC in a cohort of 103 patients treated with gefitinib (76). High levels of p-Akt were associated with female gender, never-smoking history, and bronchioloalveolar histology. Patients with tumors positive for p-Akt had significantly higher response rate and superior time-to-progression, but not overall survival. MAPK activation was not associated with treatment outcome and subsequent study reported similar results (26). The predictive significance of p-Akt immunostaining was not confirmed in molecular analysis of samples from patients enrolled in the ISEL study (25). Phosphorylated Erk kinase (p-Erk) is a marker of activation of ras/Raf/MAPK pathway. In a study of 87 patients from Korea, Han et al. found that high expression of p-Erk is linked to lower response rate and time-to-progression of patients treated with gefitinib (68). The limitation of the studies on phosphorylated proteins in tumor samples is related to their short half-life—the assay result may be affected by the time and method of tissue sample fixation.

Mutations in *K-ras* oncogene occur in approximately 5% to 40% of tumors from NSCLC patients (25,46,48,65,77), predominantly in adenocarcinomas. These mutations are associated with smoking history and male gender (48) and are almost always mutually exclusive with *EGFR* mutations (46,48,65,78), suggesting different molecular genetic pathways underlying the development of lung cancer in smokers versus never-smokers (48). The role of *K-ras* mutations as a prognostic marker in NSCLC remains controversial, with several studies showing its negative prognostic value but also a number of studies showing no prognostic significance (reviewed by Aviel-Ronen et al.) (79). In vitro and clinical data suggest that *K-ras* mutations may be associated with resistance to EGFR TKIs (80–82). In molecular analysis of the TRIBUTE study that compared chemotherapy and erlotinib to chemotherapy and placebo, *K-ras* mutations were detected in 21% patients (65). The response rate in *K-ras* mutant patients treated with chemotherapy and erlotinib was nonsignificantly inferior to response rate of patients receiving chemotherapy and placebo (8% vs. 23%). *K-ras* mutant patients had significantly inferior survival when treated with chemotherapy and erlotinib versus chemotherapy and placebo (HR = 2.1, 95% CI: 1.1–3.8). Molecular analysis of the ISEL trial found *K-ras* mutations in codons 12 and 13 in only 8% of patients and none of them responded to gefitinib (25). Limited number of patients with *K-ras* mutations prevented meaningful survival comparisons. A retrospective study of Endoh et al. found that patients harboring *K-ras* mutations have significantly inferior response and survival as compared to wild-type patients (83). In conclusion, activation of ras/Raf/MAPK pathway seems to associate with resistance to EGFR TKIs in vitro and in vivo, whereas activation of PI3K/Akt pathway seems to associate with sensitivity. Clinical importance of these predictive features, including *K-ras* mutation testing, needs to be further studied before their use in making treatment decisions in patients.

Other Members of EGFR/HER Family of Receptors

EGF receptor heterodimerization, particularly with HER2, is more potent signal trigger than homodimerization in response to ligand stimulation (84). Higher expression of other members of EGFR/HER family of receptors may thus indicate sensitivity to agents blocking EGFR pathway. In vitro data show that transfection of HER2 cDNA into *EGFR* wild-type cell lines with low HER2 levels significantly increases their sensitivity to gefitinib (85). In a group of 63 gefitinib-treated patients, Cappuzzo et al. could not find any correlation between HER2 expression determined by IHC and treatment outcome (30). However, in another cohort of patients treated with gefitinib, high *HER2* gene copy number was found to associate with response rate, time-to-progression, and a trend toward improved survival (86).

Downregulation of HER3 expression in gefitinib-sensitive cell lines is associated with decreased sensitivity to gefitinib, indicating its possible role to predict sensitivity (87). There are no published studies addressing the value of HER3 IHC in tumor samples of patients treated with EGFR TKIs. Gefitinib-treated patients with tumors containing high *HER3* gene copy numbers were reported to achieve higher response rate, time-to-progression, but not overall survival, compared to patients with low *HER3* copy numbers (88).

Markers of Epithelial–Mesenchymal Transition

Epithelial-mesenchymal transition (EMT) is a complex process by which epithelial cells are converted to cells with migration propensities. This process is highly important during embryonic development, but also constitutes an important mechanism of tumor progression in many tumors of epithelial origin (89). E-cadherin is involved in forming cell–cell junctions and linking them to cytoplasmic actin microfilaments through α-catenin and β-catenin. Loss of E-cadherin is a hallmark of EMT and indicates worse prognosis in many tumor types, including lung cancer (90). Thompson et al. showed that low levels of E-cadherin and high levels of fibronectin and vimentin are indicative of lack of sensitivity of the lung cancer cell lines and tumor xenographs to erlotinib (91). Through gene array study, Yauch et al. demonstrated that erlotinib-insensitive cell lines have multigene signature indicative of EMT. Erlotinib-sensitive cell lines were characterized by high expression of epithelial-related genes such as *E-cadherin, plakophilin-3*, and *stratifin1*, whereas insensitive lines had high expression of genes indicative of mesenchymal phenotype such as *vimentin, ZEB-1*, and *epimorphin*. The same study reported a trend toward better progression-free and overall survival in patients with E-cadherin–positive tumors who received chemotherapy and erlotinib as compared to chemotherapy and placebo in the TRIBUTE study, although the small patient number with available biopsies precludes any meaningful conclusions. Witta et al. demonstrated marked increase in sensitivity of resistant lung cancer cell lines transfected with *E-cadherin* gene (92). Modulation of *E-cadherin* expression through addition of histone deacetylase inhibitor, MS-275, leads to a significant increase of sensitivity to gefitinib in vitro (92). The strategy of combined histone deacetylase and EGFR inhibition is currently tested in phase-II clinical studies.

Serum Proteomics

All the candidate-predictive markers described so far have been tissue-based. The tissue-based assays share the same limitations of the material availability, tumor heterogeneity, and invasiveness of the procedure. Development of serum or plasma-based predictive assays has the potential to overcome these limitations. Preliminary encouraging report on proteomic profiling of serum from gefitinib-treated patients was presented by Solomon et al. at 2006 American Society of Clinical Oncology Annual Meeting (93). The proteomic signature indicative of significantly longer progression-free and overall survival was identified in the training set of Italian gefitinib-treated patients and successfully validated in the independent cohort of Japanese patients. The proteomic signature did not have prognostic significance in advanced-NSCLC patients treated with chemotherapy or in early stage surgical series. These promising data warrant further testing in placebo-controlled clinical studies.

Combination of Biomarkers

In a study combining the data from two cohorts of patients treated with gefitinib (26,37), Hirsch et al. analyzed outcome of patients according to *EGFR* gene copy number by FISH and according to IHC (94). Both studies used Zymed antibody for immunostaining and used a cut point of 200 on a scale from 0 to 400. Patients with both positive markers (23%) had impressive 41% response rate and median survival of 21 months. Moderate benefit was observed in patients (47%) who had one test positive—10% response rate and median survival of 10 months, whereas patients with double negative test (30%) appeared not to benefit from this treatment—they had 2% response rate and median survival of six months. This study suggested that population of patients with both negative tests does not achieve any benefit from gefitinib and should not be offered this treatment. Data on multiple biomarkers from large phase-III clinical studies are relatively sparse. In the ISEL study, patients with high *EGFR* gene copy number and positive EGFR immunostaining had survival advantage that was similar to the whole group of patients with high *EGFR* gene copy number (HR of 0.55 and 0.61, respectively, comparing gefitinib to placebo) (25). Multivariate analysis of biomarkers in the BR.21 study is not informative due to small number of patients within the subsets (15). Clearly, more data are needed from large prospective clinical trials or trials in enriched patient populations in order to establish a paradigm for the proper selection of patients to EGFR-targeted therapies using multiple markers.

CETUXIMAB AND OTHER DRUGS

The clinical value of cetuximab in the treatment of NSCLC is not established and much less is known about molecular markers that could predict sensitivity to this and other antibodies against EGFR. In vitro data suggest that cetuximab is a less potent cell growth inhibitor than erlotinib in NSCLC cell lines harboring *EGFR* mutations, but has similar potency as erlotinib in cell lines with wild-type *EGFR* (95). Three phase-II clinical trials exploring combination of cetuximab and chemotherapy have been reported, indicating the possibility of outcome improvement as compared to chemotherapy alone (96–98). All these studies were performed in patients selected by positive IHC, which was observed in approximately 80% to 90% of screened patients. Based on results of these trials, large randomized phase-III study is ongoing in Europe. Radiation Therapy Oncology Group sponsored study (RTOG-0324) exploring the role of cetuximab in combination with radiochemotherapy in stage-III NSCLC patients has completed patient accrual and biomarker analysis is planned in this study. Limiting patient enrollment in cetuximab trials to EGFR IHC-positive subsets does not allow for determination of IHC as a predictive marker of treatment benefit. It should be noted however that EGFR IHC-negative colorectal cancer patients appear to have a reasonable chance of response to cetuximab (99), and the intensity of EGFR IHC staining does not correlate with outcome of cetuximab-treated relapsed colorectal cancer patients (100). Data from another colorectal cancer trial (101) indicate that some of the markers discussed in this chapter, as *EGFR* gene copy number detected by FISH, could also be relevant for cetuximab benefit in NSCLC, but this awaits confirmation.

FUTURE DIRECTIONS

Despite initial enthusiasm for targeted therapies in the treatment of lung cancer, the outcomes of large phase-III clinical studies performed in unselected patients have been disappointing. While the optimal sequencing of EGFR TKIs with chemotherapy continues to be investigated, we have learned that early identification of markers associated with treatment benefit is essential for the successful implementation of the novel agents into the clinical practice. In Western NSCLC patients, *EGFR* gene copy number evaluated by FISH is associated with a significant and clinically meaningful survival benefit in randomized trials exploring the value of EGFR TKIs in the second- or third-line setting. Predictive role of *EGFR* mutations to select patients to treatment with EGFR TKIs remains to be established, particularly in Western NSCLC patients, as none of the prospective studies could demonstrate their predictive role for survival benefit. The current challenge is how to find the optimal strategy to select patients for the first-line treatment and adjuvant treatment after surgery, and a number of clinical studies are ongoing to answer these questions. A phase-II clinical study with single-agent erlotinib or chemotherapy and erlotinib given on days 2 to 16 of each chemotherapy cycle is currently ongoing in chemo-naïve advanced-stage NSCLC patients with positive EGFR FISH or IHC test. A large phase-III clinical study [randomized double blind trial in adjuvant NSCLC with tarceva (RADIANT)] exploring the efficacy of erlotinib as adjuvant treatment in surgically treated NSCLC patients with EGFR-positive tumors is open to accrual in several countries with *EGFR* gene copy number used as a stratification factor. Another currently ongoing phase-II trial tests induction gefitinib in early stage lung carcinomas with limited smoking history and/or bronchioloalveolar features (102). Patients who respond to induction treatment or harbor *EGFR* mutations are also treated postoperatively. These and other clinical studies should define the role of predictive biomarkers for EGFR inhibitors in the first-line and adjuvant settings. For the new agents explored in lung cancer, it is essential to collect the biomarker information early in their development.

REFERENCES

1. Hirsch FR, Scagliotti GV, Langer CJ, et al. Epidermal growth factor family of receptors in preneoplasia and lung cancer: perspectives for targeted therapies. Lung Cancer 2003; 41(suppl 1):S29–S42.
2. Heymach JV, Nilsson M, Blumenschein G, et al. Epidermal growth factor receptor inhibitors in development for the treatment of non-small cell lung cancer. Clin Cancer Res 2006; 12:4441s-4445s.
3. Kwak EL, Sordella R, Bell DW, et al. Irreversible inhibitors of the EGF receptor may circumvent acquired resistance to gefitinib. Proc Natl Acad Sci USA 2005; 102:7665–7670.
4. Sequist LV, Dziadziuszko R. Update on epidermal growth factor receptor inhibitor development in lung cancer. J Thorac Oncol 2006; 1:740–743.
5. Crawford J, Swanson P, Prager D, et al. Panitumumab, a fully human antibody, combined with paclitaxel and carboplatin versus paclitaxel and carboplatin alone for first line treatment of advanced non-small cell lung cancer (NSCLC): a primary analysis. Paper presented at the European Cancer Conference, 2005, Paris, France, 2005.
6. Kollmannsberger C, Schittenhelm M, Honecker F, et al. A phase I study of the humanized monoclonal anti-epidermal growth factor receptor (EGFR) antibody EMD 72000 (matuzumab) in combination with paclitaxel in patients with EGFR-positive advanced non-small-cell lung cancer (NSCLC). Ann Oncol 2006; 17: 1007–1013.
7. Adams CW, Allison DE, Flagella K, et al. Humanization of a recombinant monoclonal antibody to produce a therapeutic HER dimerization inhibitor, pertuzumab. Cancer Immunol Immunother 2006; 55:717–727.
8. Fukuoka M, Yano S, Giaccone G, et al. Multi-institutional randomized phase II trial of gefitinib for previously treated patients with advanced non-small-cell lung cancer (The IDEAL 1 Trial). J Clin Oncol 2003; 21:2237–2246.
9. Kris MG, Natale RB, Herbst RS, et al. Efficacy of gefitinib, an inhibitor of the epidermal growth factor receptor tyrosine kinase, in symptomatic patients with non-small cell lung cancer: a randomized trial. JAMA 2003; 290:2149–2158.
10. Perez-Soler R. Phase II clinical trial data with the epidermal growth factor receptor tyrosine kinase inhibitor erlotinib (OSI-774) in non-small-cell lung cancer. Clin Lung Cancer 2004; 6(suppl 1):S20–S23.
11. Ratain MJ, Eisen T, Stadler WM, et al. Phase II placebo-controlled randomized discontinuation trial of sorafenib in patients with metastatic renal cell carcinoma. J Clin Oncol 2006; 24:2505–2512.
12. Annual smoking-attributable mortality, years of potential life lost, and productivity losses—United States, 1997–2001. MMWR Morb Mortal Wkly Rep 2005; 54: 625–628.

13. Toh CK, Gao F, Lim WT, et al. Never-smokers with lung cancer: epidemiologic evidence of a distinct disease entity. J Clin Oncol 2006; 24:2245–2251.

14. Miller VA, Kris MG, Shah N, et al. Bronchioloalveolar pathologic subtype and smoking history predict sensitivity to gefitinib in advanced non-small-cell lung cancer. J Clin Oncol 2004; 22:1103–1109.

15. Tsao MS, Sakurada A, Cutz JC, et al. Erlotinib in lung cancer—molecular and clinical predictors of outcome. N Engl J Med 2005; 353:133–144.

16. Thatcher N, Chang A, Parikh P, et al. Gefitinib plus best supportive care in previously treated patients with refractory advanced non-small-cell lung cancer: results from a randomised, placebo-controlled, multicentre study (Iressa Survival Evaluation in Lung Cancer). Lancet 2005; 366:1527–1537.

17. Shepherd FA, Rodrigues PJ, Ciuleanu T, et al. Erlotinib in previously treated non-small-cell lung cancer. N Engl J Med 2005; 353:123–132.

18. Herbst RS, Prager D, Hermann R, et al. TRIBUTE: a phase III trial of erlotinib hydrochloride (OSI-774) combined with carboplatin and paclitaxel chemotherapy in advanced non-small-cell lung cancer. J Clin Oncol 2005; 23:5892–5899.

19. Clark GM, Zborowski DM, Santabarbara P, et al. Smoking history and epidermal growth factor receptor expression as predictors of survival benefit from erlotinib for patients with non-small-cell lung cancer in the National Cancer Institute of Canada Clinical Trials Group Study BR.21. Clin Lung Cancer 2006; 7:389–394.

20. Gatzemeier U, Pluzanska A, Szczesna A, et al. Results of a phase III trial of erlotinib (OSI-774) combined with cisplatin and gemcitabine (GC) chemotherapy in advanced non-small cell lung cancer (NSCLC). Proc Am Soc Clin Oncol 2004; 22(suppl 14S):7010.

21. Giaccone G, Herbst RS, Manegold C, et al. Gefitinib in combination with gemcitabine and cisplatin in advanced non-small-cell lung cancer: a phase III trial—INTACT 1. J Clin Oncol 2004; 22:777–784.

22. Herbst RS, Giaccone G, Schiller JH, et al. Gefitinib in combination with paclitaxel and carboplatin in advanced non-small-cell lung cancer: a phase III trial—INTACT 2. J Clin Oncol 2004; 22:785–794.

23. Kris MG, Sandler A, Miller V, et al. Cigarette smoking history predicts sensitivity to erlotinib: results of a phase II trial in patients with bronchioloalveolar carcinoma (BAC). Proc Am Soc Clin Oncol 2004; 22(suppl 14S):7062.

24. West HL, Franklin WA, McCoy J, et al. Gefitinib therapy in advanced bronchioloalveolar carcinoma: Southwest Oncology Group Study S0126. J Clin Oncol 2006; 24:1807–1813.

25. Hirsch FR, Varella-Garcia M, Bunn PA Jr, et al. Molecular predictors of outcome with gefitinib in a phase III placebo-controlled study in advanced non-small-cell lung cancer. J Clin Oncol 2006; 24:5034–5042.

26. Cappuzzo F, Hirsch FR, Rossi E, et al. Epidermal growth factor receptor gene and protein and gefitinib sensitivity in non-small-cell lung cancer. J Natl Cancer Inst 2005; 97:643–655.

27. Parra HS, Cavina R, Latteri F, et al. Analysis of epidermal growth factor receptor expression as a predictive factor for response to gefitinib ('Iressa', ZD1839) in non-small-cell lung cancer. Br J Cancer 2004; 91:208–212.

28. Bailey LR, Kris MG, Wolf M, et al. Tumor EGFR membrane staining is not clinically relevant for predicting response in patients receiving gefitinib ('Iressa', ZD1939) monotherapy for pretreated advanced non-small-cell lung cancer: IDEAL1 and 2. Proc Am Assoc Cancer Res 2003:44(Abstr. LB-212).

29. Bailey LR, Janas MSK, Bindlsev N, et al. Evaluation of epidermal growth factor receptor (EGFR) as a predictive marker in patients with non-small-cell lung cancer (NSCLC) receiving first-line gefitinib combined with platinum-based chemotherapy. Proc Am Soc Clin Oncol 2004; 22(suppl 14S):7013.

30. Cappuzzo F, Gregorc V, Rossi E, et al. Gefitinib in pretreated non-small-cell lung cancer (NSCLC): analysis of efficacy and correlation with HER2 and epidermal growth factor receptor expression in locally advanced or metastatic NSCLC. J Clin Oncol 2003; 21:2658–2663.

31. Penault-Llorca F, Cayre A, Arnould L, et al. Is there an immunohistochemical technique definitively valid in epidermal growth factor receptor assessment? Oncol Rep 2006; 16:1173–1179.

32. Atkins D, Reiffen KA, Tegtmeier CL, et al. Immunohistochemical detection of EGFR in paraffin-embedded tumor tissues: variation in staining intensity due to choice of fixative and storage time of tissue sections. J Histochem Cytochem 2004; 52:893–901.

33. Dei Tos AP, Ellis I. Assessing epidermal growth factor receptor expression in tumours: what is the value of current test methods? Eur J Cancer 2005; 41: 1383–1392.

34. Clark GM, Zborowski DM, Culbertson JL, et al. Clinical utility of epidermal growth factor receptor expression for selecting patients with advanced non-small cell lung cancer for treatment with erlotinib. J Thorac Oncol 2006; 1:837–846.

35. Bankfalvi A, Boecker W, Reiner A. Comparison of automated and manual determination of HER2 status in breast cancer for diagnostic use: a comparative methodological study using the Ventana BenchMark automated staining system and manual tests. Int J Oncol 2004; 25:929–935.

36. Bast RC Jr, Ravdin P, Hayes DF, et al. 2000 update of recommendations for the use of tumor markers in breast and colorectal cancer: clinical practice guidelines of the American Society of Clinical Oncology. J Clin Oncol 2001; 19:1865–1878.

37. Hirsch FR, Varella-Garcia M, McCoy J, et al. Increased epidermal growth factor receptor gene copy number detected by fluorescence in situ hybridization associates with increased sensitivity to gefitinib in patients with bronchioloalveolar carcinoma subtypes: a Southwest Oncology Group Study. J Clin Oncol 2005; 23: 6838–6845.

38. Bell DW, Lynch TJ, Haserlat SM, et al. Epidermal growth factor receptor mutations and gene amplification in non-small-cell lung cancer: molecular analysis of the IDEAL/INTACT gefitinib trials. J Clin Oncol 2005; 23:8081–8092.

39. Dziadziuszko R, Witta SE, Cappuzzo F, et al. Epidermal growth factor receptor messenger RNA expression, gene dosage, and gefitinib sensitivity in non-small cell lung cancer. Clin Cancer Res 2006; 12:3078–3084.

40. Takano T, Ohe Y, Sakamoto H, et al. Epidermal growth factor receptor gene mutations and increased copy numbers predict gefitinib sensitivity in patients with recurrent non-small-cell lung cancer. J Clin Oncol 2005; 23:6829–6837.

41. Hirsch FR, Varella-Garcia M, Bunn PA Jr, et al. Epidermal growth factor receptor in non-small-cell lung carcinomas: correlation between gene copy number and protein expression and impact on prognosis. J Clin Oncol 2003; 21:3798–3807.

42. Dziadziuszko R, Holm B, Skov BG, et al. Epidermal growth factor receptor gene copy number and protein level are not associated with outcome of non-small-cell lung cancer patients treated with chemotherapy. Ann Oncol 2007; 18:447–452.

43. Italiano A, Vandenbos FB, Otto J, et al. Comparison of the epidermal growth factor receptor gene and protein in primary non-small-cell-lung cancer and metastatic sites: implications for treatment with EGFR-inhibitors. Ann Oncol 2006; 17:981–985.

44. Miller VA, Zakowski M, Riely GJ, et al. EGFR mutation, immunohistochemistry (IHC) and chromogenic in situ hybridization (CISH) as predictors of sensitivity to erlotinib and gefitinib in patients (pts) with NSCLC. Proc Am Soc Clin Oncol 2005; 23(suppl 16S):7031.

45. Marchetti A, Martella C, Felicioni L, et al. EGFR mutations in non-small-cell lung cancer: analysis of a large series of cases and development of a rapid and sensitive method for diagnostic screening with potential implications on pharmacologic treatment. J Clin Oncol 2005; 23:857–865.

46. Shigematsu H, Lin L, Takahashi T, et al. Clinical and biological features associated with epidermal growth factor receptor gene mutations in lung cancers. J Natl Cancer Inst 2005; 97:339–346.

47. Yang SH, Mechanic LE, Yang P, et al. Mutations in the tyrosine kinase domain of the epidermal growth factor receptor in non-small cell lung cancer. Clin Cancer Res 2005; 11:2106–2110.

48. Tam IY, Chung LP, Suen WS, et al. Distinct epidermal growth factor receptor and KRAS mutation patterns in non-small cell lung cancer patients with different tobacco exposure and clinicopathologic features. Clin Cancer Res 2006; 12: 1647–1653.

49. Lynch TJ, Bell DW, Sordella R, et al. Activating mutations in the epidermal growth factor receptor underlying responsiveness of non-small-cell lung cancer to gefitinib. N Engl J Med 2004; 350:2129–2139.

50. Paez JG, Janne PA, Lee JC, et al. EGFR mutations in lung cancer: correlation with clinical response to gefitinib therapy. Science 2004; 304:1497–1500.

51. Kobayashi S, Boggon TJ, Dayaram T, et al. EGFR mutation and resistance of non-small-cell lung cancer to gefitinib. N Engl J Med 2005; 352:786–792.

52. Pao W, Miller VA, Politi KA, et al. Acquired resistance of lung adenocarcinomas to gefitinib or erlotinib is associated with a second mutation in the EGFR kinase domain. PLoS Med 2005; 2:e73.

53. Inukai M, Toyooka S, Ito S, et al. Presence of epidermal growth factor receptor gene T790M Mutation as a minor clone in non-small cell lung cancer. Cancer Res 2006; 66:7854–7858.

54. Kosaka T, Yatabe Y, Endoh H, et al. Mutations of the epidermal growth factor receptor gene in lung cancer: biological and clinical implications. Cancer Res 2004; 64:8919–8923.

55. Amann J, Kalyankrishna S, Massion PP, et al. Aberrant epidermal growth factor receptor signaling and enhanced sensitivity to EGFR inhibitors in lung cancer. Cancer Res 2005; 65:226–235.

56. Sordella R, Bell DW, Haber DA, et al. Gefitinib-sensitizing EGFR mutations in lung cancer activate anti-apoptotic pathways. Science 2004; 305:1163–1167.

57. Tracy S, Mukohara T, Hansen M, et al. Gefitinib induces apoptosis in the EGFR L858R non-small-cell lung cancer cell line H3255. Cancer Res 2004; 64:7241–7244.

58. Taron M, Ichinose Y, Rosell R, et al. Activating mutations in the tyrosine kinase domain of the epidermal growth factor receptor are associated with improved survival in gefitinib-treated chemorefractory lung adenocarcinomas. Clin Cancer Res 2005; 11:5878–5885.

59. Endo K, Konishi A, Sasaki H, et al. Epidermal growth factor receptor gene mutation in non-small cell lung cancer using highly sensitive and fast TaqMan PCR assay. Lung Cancer 2005; 50:375–384.

60. Janne PA, Borras AM, Kuang Y, et al. A rapid and sensitive enzymatic method for epidermal growth factor receptor mutation screening. Clin Cancer Res 2006; 12:751–758.

61. Takano T, Ohe Y, Furuta K, et al. EGFR mutations detected by high resolution melting analysis (HRMA) as a predictor of response and survival in non-small cell lung cancer (NSCLC) patients treated with gefitinib. Proc Am Soc Clin Oncol 2006; 24(suppl 18S):7075.

62. Nagai Y, Miyazawa H, Huqun, et al. Genetic heterogeneity of the epidermal growth factor receptor in non-small cell lung cancer cell lines revealed by a rapid and sensitive detection system, the peptide nucleic acid-locked nucleic acid PCR clamp. Cancer Res 2005; 65:7276–7282.

63. Marchetti A, Felicioni L, Buttitta F. Assessing EGFR mutations. N Engl J Med 2006; 354:526–528.

64. Kimura H, Kazahara K, Shibata K, et al. EGFR mutation of tumor and serum in gefitinib-treated patients with chemotherapy-naive non-small cell lung cancer. J Thorac Oncol 2006; 1:260–267.

65. Eberhard DA, Johnson BE, Amler LC, et al. Mutations in the epidermal growth factor receptor and in KRAS are predictive and prognostic indicators in patients with non-small-cell lung cancer treated with chemotherapy alone and in combination with erlotinib. J Clin Oncol 2005; 23:5900–5909.

66. Mitsudomi T, Kosaka T, Endoh H, et al. Mutations of the epidermal growth factor receptor gene predict prolonged survival after gefitinib treatment in patients with non-small-cell lung cancer with postoperative recurrence. J Clin Oncol 2005; 23:2513–2520.

67. Cortes-Funes H, Gomez C, Rosell R, et al. Epidermal growth factor receptor activating mutations in Spanish gefitinib-treated non-small-cell lung cancer patients. Ann Oncol 2005; 16:1081–1086.

68. Han SW, Kim TY, Hwang PG, et al. Predictive and prognostic impact of epidermal growth factor receptor mutation in non-small-cell lung cancer patients treated with gefitinib. J Clin Oncol 2005; 23:2493–2501.

69. Chou TY, Chiu CH, Li LH, et al. Mutation in the tyrosine kinase domain of epidermal growth factor receptor is a predictive and prognostic factor for gefitinib treatment in patients with non-small cell lung cancer. Clin Cancer Res 2005; 11:3750–3757.

70. Zhang XT, Li LY, Mu XL, et al. The EGFR mutation and its correlation with response of gefitinib in previously treated Chinese patients with advanced non-small-cell lung cancer. Ann Oncol 2005; 16:1334–1342.

71. Shepherd F. BR.21 biomarker update. Paper presented at Targeted Therapies for the Treatment of Lung Cancer Meeting, Santa Monica, CA, USA, Jan 26–28, 2006.

72. Hirsch FR, Franklin WA, McCoy J, et al. Predicting clinical benefit from EGFR TKIs: not all EGFR mutations are equal. Proc Am Soc Clin Oncol 2006; 24(suppl 18S):7072.

73. Jackman DM, Yeap BY, Sequist LV, et al. Exon 19 deletion mutations of epidermal growth factor receptor are associated with prolonged survival in non-small cell lung cancer patients treated with gefitinib or erlotinib. Clin Cancer Res 2006; 12: 3908–3914.

74. Riely GJ, Pao W, Pham D, et al. Clinical course of patients with non-small cell lung cancer and epidermal growth factor receptor exon 19 and exon 21 mutations treated with gefitinib or erlotinib. Clin Cancer Res 2006; 12:839–844.
75. Inoue A, Suzuki T, Fukuhara T, et al. Prospective phase II study of gefitinib for chemotherapy-naive patients with advanced non-small-cell lung cancer with epidermal growth factor receptor gene mutations. J Clin Oncol 2006; 24:3340–3346.
76. Cappuzzo F, Magrini E, Ceresoli GL, et al. Akt phosphorylation and gefitinib efficacy in patients with advanced non-small-cell lung cancer. J Natl Cancer Inst 2004:1133–1141.
77. Jassem J, Jassem E, Jakobkiewicz-Banecka J, et al. P53 and K-ras mutations are frequent events in microscopically negative surgical margins from patients with nonsmall cell lung carcinoma. Cancer 2004; 100:1951–1960.
78. Soung YH, Lee JW, Kim SY, et al. Mutational analysis of EGFR and K-RAS genes in lung adenocarcinomas. Virchows Arch 2005; 446:483–488.
79. Aviel-Ronen S, Blackhall FH, Shepherd FA, et al. K-ras mutations in non-small-cell lung carcinoma: a review. Clin Lung Cancer 2006; 8:30–38.
80. Gumerlock P, Holland WS, Chen H, et al. Mutational analysis of K-ras and EGFR implicates K-ras as a resistance marker in the Southwest Oncology Group (SWOG) trial S0126 of bronchioalveolar carcinoma patients. Proc Am Soc Clin Oncol 2005; 23(suppl 16S):7008.
81. Janmaat ML, Rodriguez JA, Gallegos-Ruiz M, et al. Enhanced cytotoxicity induced by gefitinib and specific inhibitors of the Ras or phosphatidyl inositol-3 kinase pathways in non-small cell lung cancer cells. Int J Cancer 2006; 118:209–214.
82. Pao W, Wang TY, Riely GJ, et al. KRAS mutations and primary resistance of lung adenocarcinomas to gefitinib or erlotinib. PLoS Med 2005; 2:e17.
83. Endoh H, Yatabe Y, Kosaka T, et al. PTEN and PIK3CA expression is associated with prolonged survival after gefitinib treatment in EGFR-mutated lung cancer patients. J Thorac Oncol 2006; 1:629–634.
84. Mosesson Y, Yarden Y. Oncogenic growth factor receptors: implications for signal transduction therapy. Semin Cancer Biol 2004; 14:262–270.
85. Hirata A, Hosoi F, Miyagawa M, et al. HER2 overexpression increases sensitivity to gefitinib, an epidermal growth factor receptor tyrosine kinase inhibitor, through inhibition of HER2/HER3 heterodimer formation in lung cancer cells. Cancer Res 2005; 65:4253–4260.
86. Cappuzzo F, Varella-Garcia M, Shigematsu H, et al. Increased HER2 gene copy number is associated with response to gefitinib therapy in epidermal growth factor receptor-positive non-small-cell lung cancer patients. J Clin Oncol 2005; 23: 5007–5018.
87. Engelman JA, Janne PA, Mermel C, et al. ErbB-3 mediates phosphoinositide 3-kinase activity in gefitinib-sensitive non-small cell lung cancer cell lines. Proc Natl Acad Sci USA 2005; 102:3788–3793.
88. Cappuzzo F, Toschi L, Domenichini I, et al. HER3 genomic gain and sensitivity to gefitinib in advanced non-small-cell lung cancer patients. Br J Cancer 2005; 93:1334–1340.
89. Thiery JP. Epithelial-mesenchymal transitions in tumour progression. Nat Rev Cancer 2002; 2:442–454.
90. Bremnes RM, Veve R, Gabrielson E, et al. High-throughput tissue microarray analysis used to evaluate biology and prognostic significance of the E-cadherin pathway in non-small-cell lung cancer. J Clin Oncol 2002; 20:2417–2428.

91. Thomson S, Buck E, Petti F, et al. Epithelial to mesenchymal transition is a determinant of sensitivity of non-small-cell lung carcinoma cell lines and xenografts to epidermal growth factor receptor inhibition. Cancer Res 2005; 65:9455–9462.

92. Witta SE, Gemmill RM, Hirsch FR, et al. Restoring E-cadherin expression increases sensitivity to epidermal growth factor receptor inhibitors in lung cancer cell lines. Cancer Res 2006; 66:944–950.

93. Solomon B, Gregorc V, Taguchi F, et al. Prediction of clinical outcome in non-small cell lung cancer (NSCLC) patients treated with gefitinib using Matrix-Assisted Laser Desorption/Ionization-Time of Flight Mass Spectrometry (MALDI-TOF MS) of serum. Proc Am Soc Clin Oncol 2006; 24(suppl 18S):7004.

94. Hirsch FR, Varella-Garcia M, Cappuzzo F, et al. Combination of EGFR gene copy number and protein expression predicts outcome for advanced non-small cell lung cancer patients treated with gefitinib. Ann Oncol 2007 advanced access online doi: 1093/annonc/mdm003.

95. Mukohara T, Engelman JA, Hanna NH, et al. Differential effects of gefitinib and cetuximab on non-small-cell lung cancers bearing epidermal growth factor receptor mutations. J Natl Cancer Inst 2005; 97:1185–1194.

96. Robert F, Blumenschein G, Herbst RS, et al. Phase I/IIa study of cetuximab with gemcitabine plus carboplatin in patients with chemotherapy-naive advanced non-small-cell lung cancer. J Clin Oncol 2005; 23:9089–9096.

97. Rosell R, Daniel C, Ramlau R, et al. Randomized phase II study of cetuximab in combination with cisplatin (C) and vinorelbine (V) vs. CV alone in the first-line treatment of patients (pts) with epidermal growth factor receptor (EGFR)-expressing advanced non-small-cell lung cancer (NSCLC). Proc Am Soc Clin Oncol 2004; 22(suppl 14S):7012.

98. Thienelt CD, Bunn PA Jr, Hanna N, et al. Multicenter phase I/II study of cetuximab with paclitaxel and carboplatin in untreated patients with stage IV non-small-cell lung cancer. J Clin Oncol 2005; 23:8786–8793.

99. Chung KY, Shia J, Kemeny NE, et al. Cetuximab shows activity in colorectal cancer patients with tumors that do not express the epidermal growth factor receptor by immunohistochemistry. J Clin Oncol 2005; 23:1803–1810.

100. Cunningham D, Humblet Y, Siena S, et al. Cetuximab monotherapy and cetuximab plus irinotecan in irinotecan-refractory metastatic colorectal cancer. N Engl J Med 2004; 351:337–345.

101. Moroni M, Veronese S, Benvenuti S, et al. Gene copy number for epidermal growth factor receptor (EGFR) and clinical response to anti-EGFR treatment in colorectal cancer: a cohort study. Lancet Oncol 2005; 6:279–286.

102. Kris MG, Pao W, Zakowski M, et al. Prospective trial with preoperative gefitinib to correlate lung cancer response with EGFR exon 19 and 21 mutations and to select patients for adjuvant therapy. Proc Am Soc Clin Oncol 2006; 24(suppl 18S):7021.

103. Dziadziuszko R, Siemiatkowska A, Limon J, et al. Unusual chemosensitivity of advanced bronchioalveolar carcinoma after gefitinib response and progression: a case report. J Thorac Oncol 2007; 2:91–92.

7

Other Novel Targeted Therapies in Lung Cancer

Kyriakos P. Papadopoulos and Anthony W. Tolcher
South Texas Accelerated Research Therapeutics, Division of Medical Oncology, University of Texas Health Science Center at San Antonio, San Antonio, Texas, U.S.A.

INTRODUCTION

Although incremental advances have been made in the treatment of lung cancer, even the incorporation of currently available targeted agents into the therapeutic armamentarium has failed to improve the outcome of the majority of patients. Several randomized phase-III clinical trials have confirmed that first-line treatment of stage IIIB to IV non–small cell lung cancer (NSCLC) with platinum-based chemotherapy regimens increases response and survival (1). While none of the platinum doublets incorporating third-generation cytotoxic agents such as the taxanes or gemcitabine appears to be superior, each has a particular toxicity profile and the choice of therapy is often dictated by physician or patient preference and cost (2). Overall response rates range from 17% to 30%, with one- and two-year survival rates of 31% to 36% and 10% to 13%, respectively. Triplet cytotoxic chemotherapy may increase response but rarely proves more effective (3,4). The concurrent addition of erlotinib and gefitinib, small molecule tyrosine kinase inhibitors targeting the epidermal growth factor receptor (EGFR), to conventional cytotoxic doublets also fails to improve outcome except in a small subgroup of nonsmokers (5–8). More encouraging is a phase-III study in a select group of chemotherapy-naïve stage IIIb to IV nonsquamous NSCLC patients, where paclitaxel and carboplatin with the antivascular endothelial growth factor antibody bevacizumab shows significant improvement over chemotherapy alone, with response rate of 27.2%, progression free survival (PFS) of 6.4 months, and median survival of 12.5 months one- and two-year survival of 51.9% and 22.1%, respectively (9). Although the response rate with salvage therapy is low, cytotoxic agents such as docetaxel and pemetrexed afford a survival benefit to patients who have failed first-line treatment (10,11). In patients unselected for EGFR mutations and failing first- and second-line cytotoxic therapy, erlotinib but not gefitinib improves response and survival (12,13). Combination of erlotinib with bevacizumab may increase efficacy in these patients (14).

In patients with small cell lung cancer (SCLC), little progress has been made in improving outcome in patients with extensive stage disease beyond that achieved with cisplatin and etoposide, with median survival still only 8 to 10 months. Confirmation of improved outcome from irinotecan- and cisplatin-based regimens is awaited (15,16).

Since only a minority of patients with lung cancer respond to therapy and many are elderly with significant comorbidity, there is a need to identify agents that individually or in combination with existing cytotoxic or biologic drugs can improve outcome without a significant negative impact on quality of life.

Impaired apoptosis is a hallmark of malignant transformation and lung cancer is no exception. Technologic advances and an increasing understanding of the mechanisms of apoptosis have made possible several strategies of targeted anticancer therapy directed at proteins within the intrinsic, extrinsic, and common apoptotic pathways that are reviewed in this chapter. The ultimate goal of any such therapy is to achieve tumor death, either alone or by increasing sensitivity and decreasing resistance to standard chemotherapy and radiation therapy.

TARGETING THE BCL-2 FAMILY—BCL-2, BCL-XL, AND MCL-1

The Bcl-2 family of proteins plays a central role in apoptosis by regulating the mitochondrial membrane permeability that mediates the intrinsic pathway of caspase activation (17). The important function played in malignancy by the antiapoptotic members of the Bcl-2 family has made them a logical and attractive target for anticancer drug development in lung cancer.

Characteristic of the Bcl-2 family are four conserved amphipathic α-helical regions termed Bcl-2 homology (BH)1 to 4 domains. All members share one or more of these conserved BH domains but have a distinct structure and function. These domains allow for Bcl-2 family members to be classified into three subclasses (Table 1). The antiapoptotic multidomain members Bcl-2, Bcl-xL, Bcl-w, Bfl-1, and Mcl-1 share BH1 to 4 domains; the proapoptotic multidomain proteins Bax and Bak contain BH1 to 3 domains, and finally the proapoptotic "BH3-only" family members, which as their name indicates, have only a single BH3 domain and appear to play specific activating or sensitizing roles in controlling apoptosis (18,19). Interaction between the Bcl-2 family members, mediated by the amphipathic α-helical BH3 unit, is an important regulatory mechanism of apoptosis. The BH3 α-helix of one protein associates

Table 1 Bcl-2 Family Members

Bcl-2 homology domains	Function		Members
BH1–4	Antiapoptotic		Bcl-2, Bcl-xL, Bfl-1, Bcl-w, Mcl-1
BH1–3	Proapoptotic	Effectors	Bak, Bax
BH3 only	Proapoptotic	Activators	Bid, Bim
	Proapoptotic	Sensitizers	Bad, Bik, Bmf, Hrk, Noxa, Puma

with a large hydrophobic pocket of the multidomain binding partner and either activates or inhibits its function. An understanding of the structure and interaction of the various members of the Bcl-2 family, and of other proteins outside of this protein family, has fortified a current model of control of mitochondrial membrane-mediated apoptosis that emphasizes the pivotal role of Bax and Bak and their activation by specific BH3 domains (20,21).

Death stimuli that promote programmed cell death, including DNA damage or microtubule disruption by cytotoxic chemotherapy or radiation, appear to trigger activation of BH3-only proteins by a number of mechanisms including phosphorylation, ubiquitination, and proteolytic cleavage (Fig. 1) (22). BH3-only proteins such as Puma and Noxa are transcriptionally induced by p53 (23,24),

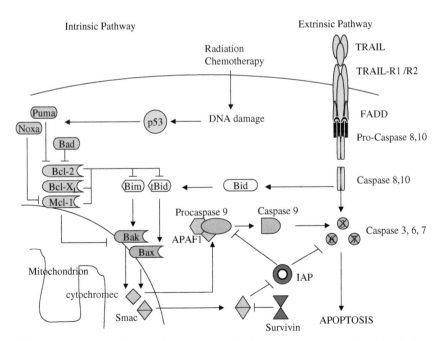

Figure 1 Intrinsic and extrinsic pathways mediating apoptotic cell death. *Abbreviations*: FADD, fas-associated death domain; IAP, inhibitor of apoptosis proteins; TRAIL, tumor necrosis factor–related apoptosis-inducing ligand.

while phosphorylation may play an important role in the activation and control of Bim and Bad (25). Bid is activated by caspase-8 and plays a unique role in connecting the extrinsic death receptor pathway to the intrinsic apoptosis pathway (26).

"Activator" BH3-only proteins (such as Bid and Bim) may initiate apoptosis by interacting with and inducing Bax and Bak oligomerization (18). The multidomain antiapoptotic proteins Bcl-2 and Bcl-xL are integral membrane proteins and can sequestrate these activating BH3-only proteins and abrogate the activation of apoptosis. Antiapoptotic proteins can also directly interact with and inhibit Bax and Bak oligomerization. "Sensitizer" BH3-only proteins (such as Bad, Bik, Bmf, Hrk, Noxa, and Puma) may apply their proapoptotic effect by competitively binding antiapoptotic Bcl-2 family members, preventing them from sequestering the activator BH3-only proteins (18). These sensitizer BH3-only proteins display selectivity for the antiapoptotic proteins they bind. For example, Noxa is highly specific for Mcl-1 and Bfl-1, while Bad is more selective for Bcl-2 and Bcl-xL (18,27,28).

Inactive Bax monomers are loosely attached to the mitochondrial outer membrane (MOM) or in the cytosol, while Bak monomers are in the mitochondrial membrane. Once Bax and Bak are activated by activator BH3-only proteins, they homo-oligomerize in the MOM. A number of non–Bcl-2 family proteins have been identified that can interact with and modulate Bax/Bak function (29–31). The MOM becomes permeable following Bak and Bax oligomerization and subsequently proteins in the mitochondrial intermembrane space, in particular cytochrome c and second mitochondria-derived activator of caspase (Smac), escape into the cytoplasm. The released cytochrome c interacts with apoptotic protease-activating factor 1 that binds procaspase-9 forming the apoptosome, which activates caspase-9. Activated caspase-9 is then able to activate the effector protease caspase-3, leading to cleavage of target proteins, DNA fragmentation, and cell death.

Both NSCLC and SCLC can overexpress Bcl-2 (32,33). Although its prognostic significance remains uncertain, Bcl-2 may contribute to chemotherapy and radiotherapy resistance (32–36). Overexpression of other antiapoptotic proteins, particularly Mcl-1 and Bcl-xL, has also been demonstrated in lung cancer and are associated with resistance to therapy or poor prognosis (37,38). Attempts at inhibition of antiapoptotic Bcl-2 family proteins have encompassed interruption of mRNA function by antisense oligonucleotides (ASOs) and the development of small molecule antagonists targeting the antiapoptotic proteins.

BCL-2, BCL-XL, AND MCL-1 ANTISENSE OLIGONUCLEOTIDES

ASO are short synthetic sequences of single-strand DNA that can bind to complimentary target mRNA, resulting in inhibition of mRNA translation and degradation of the bound target mRNA by RNase H, a ubiquitous endonuclease (39). Phosphorothioate analogues of the natural phosphodiester backbone of oligonucleotides are more resistant to degradation and employed in the manufacture of ASOs intended for clinical use (40). In addition to their inhibition of mRNA, there is evidence that some ASO have off-target nonantisense effects, particularly immune stimulation via their CpG repeats.

Downregulation of Bcl-2 and Bcl-xL by antisense is sufficient in some models to induce apoptotic cell death. Not surprisingly, in light of the extensive body of work highlighting its critical role in abrogating cell death, Bcl-2 has been the early focus of ASO targeting (41). The anti Bcl-2 mRNA agent furthest advanced in clinical testing is oblimersen (G3139, Genasense™, Genta, Berkely Heights, New Jersey, U.S.A.). Oblimersen is an 18-base antisense phosphorothioate oligonucleotide targeting the first six codons of the human Bcl-2 mRNA open reading frame. Preclinical in vitro and lung cancer xenograft models have demonstrated the activity of oblimersen in decreasing Bcl-2 mRNA and protein levels, inhibiting tumor growth and increasing survival (42). In tumors where diminished apoptosis may not be critical to cell survival but is only one component of chemoresistance, oblimersen may function to enhance sensitivity of tumors to chemotherapy. Following from this, several combination studies have been conducted with oblimersen and a variety of chemotherapeutic agents including docetaxel (43,44). In lung cancer in particular, oblimersen was combined with carboplatin and etoposide in a phase-I trial of 16 patients with untreated extensive stage SCLC (45). The regimen appeared to be well tolerated and of 14 evaluable patients, 86% had a partial response (PR). Notably no evidence of Bcl-2 suppression in peripheral blood mononuclear cells was observed. A second phase-I trial of oblimersen and paclitaxel in chemorefractory SCLC patients found the regimen to be tolerable but no responses were observed in 12 patients treated (46). A randomized phase-II study of docetaxel with or without oblimersen has been undertaken in previously treated NSCLC patients but no results from this trial are available. Three phase-III randomized trials, respectively, in myeloma, melanoma, and chronic lymphocytic leukemia (CLL) addressing whether oblimersen improves the efficacy of standard chemotherapy have yielded positive results only for CLL and its role, if any, in the treatment of lung cancer remains to be defined (47–49). Next generation ASO with locked nucleic acid modifications that have higher target affinity and stability are under clinical development (50,51). Second-generation antisense Bcl-xL oligonucleotide has been shown to effectively induce apoptosis in lung adenocarcinoma cell lines (52), and bispecific oligonucleotides targeting the mRNA homology region of both Bcl-2 and Bcl-xL have shown preclinical efficacy in inducing apoptosis in vitro in NSCLC and SCLC cells (53).

Of more recent interest as a target for ASO has been Mcl-1. Mcl-1 protein is widely expressed in a number of hematologic and solid tumors including lung cancer and there is increasing evidence for its oncogenic nature (37,54–56). Mcl-1 mRNA and protein undergo rapid turnover and has a short half-life (one to two hours) making it more amenable to reduction by ASO than Bcl-2 and Bcl-xL (56). A combination of Mcl-1 ASOs with chemotherapy may be a promising strategy to overcome chemoresistance in lung cancer (57). Interestingly, recent data from work with the multikinase inhibitor sorafenib showing that at least part of this drugs activity may be mediated by inhibition of Mcl-1 add credence to Mcl-1 as a promising target for antitumor drug development (58). The potential of ASO therapy targeting the Bcl-2 family has not yet been realized. Next generation ASO, with increased affinity and stability and potentially less toxicity, may fulfill this promise.

SMALL MOLECULE INHIBITORS OF BCL-2, BCL-XL, AND MCL-1

Elucidation of the structure and function of specific BH3-only proteins in inhibiting antiapoptotic Bcl-2–like proteins has prompted efforts to identify small molecule inhibitors that might be of clinical utility. Several of these molecules, some showing preclinical activity in lung cancer cells, are now entering phase-I clinical trials (Table 1) (59–61). One such agent is gossypol and its more active enantiomer (–)-gossypol, a polyphenolic component of cottonseed oil, which binds to antiapoptotic Bcl-2 members and have antitumor activity in a variety of tumor cell lines (62–64). Preliminary data from a phase-I trial of an orally available (–)-gossypol preparation AT-101, shown to inhibit Bcl-2, Bcl-xL and Mcl-1, report three of four NSCLC patients receiving 20 to 40 mg/day of drug having stable disease for 2.5 to 4 months (61).

For SCLC, most promising of the small molecules still in preclinical development is ABT737 (65). ABT737 is an inhibitor of the antiapoptotic proteins Bcl-2, Bcl-xL, and Bcl-w, which was discovered using nuclear magnetic resonance-based screening and structure-based design (65). Two chemical compounds binding to sites at the hydrophobic pocket on Bcl-xL were identified and then chemically joined. The resultant molecule was modified to improve affinity for the binding site and decrease nonspecific binding to human albumin. ABT737 displays a two- to threefold order of magnitude greater binding affinity (Ki < 1 nM) than previously described Bcl-2–binding molecules. Similar to Bad, ABT737 binds and inhibits antiapoptotic Bcl-2 family proteins but does not directly activate the proapoptotic proteins, Bax and Bak (65). ABT737 alone caused complete regression of established SCLC tumor xenografts and shows synergy with chemotherapy and radiation in various tumor cell lines including NSCLC. The drug was well tolerated with minor hematologic toxicity. These preclinical data suggest that ABT737 may be effective for the treatment of SCLC and may enhance the efficacy of chemotherapy and radiation in NSCLC.

TARGETING THE TRAIL RECEPTORS—TRAIL-R1 AND TRAIL-R2

Induction of apoptosis via the extrinsic pathway of caspase activation is mediated by the cell surface death receptors of the tumor necrosis factor (TNF) receptor superfamily (66,67). Binding of ligand to these death receptors activates the cytoplasmic death domain, which in turn recruits the adaptor molecule Fas-associated death domain (FADD) and caspase-8, forming the death-inducing signal complex

Table 2 Drugs Targeting Antiapoptotic Bcl-2 Family Members

Agent	Target	Strategy	Development stage
Oblimersen	Bcl-2	Antisense oligonucleotides	Phase III
Anti-Bcl-xL	Bcl-xL	Antisense oligonucleotides	Preclinical
Bispecific Bcl-2 and Bcl-xL	Bcl-2 and Bcl-xL	Antisense oligonucleotides	Preclinical
Anti-Mcl-1	Mcl-1	Antisense oligonucleotides	Preclinical
Gossypol	Bcl-2 (Bcl-xL, Bcl-b and Bfl-1)	Small molecule inhibitor	Phase II
GX15-070	Bcl-2 (? other)	Small molecule inhibitor	Phase I
AT-101	Bcl-2, Bcl-xL, Mcl-1	Small molecule inhibitor	Phase I
ABT737	Bcl-2, Bcl-xL, Bcl-w	Small molecule inhibitor	Preclinical

(Fig. 1) (68). Once dimerized, the initiator caspase-8 is cleaved and depending on cell type (69) can activate both Bid in the intrinsic pathway and executioner caspases 3, 6, and 7 to achieve cell death. Of the eight death receptors identified, most clinically relevant for lung cancer are TNF-related apoptosis-inducing ligand (TRAIL) receptor 1 (TRAIL-R1, DR4) and TRAIL receptor 2 (TRAIL-R2, DR5) and their associated ligand TRAIL (70). TRAIL-R1 and TRAIL-R2 are abundantly expressed on lung and other cancer cells but not normal tissue (71,72). Two decoy TRAIL-binding receptors TRAIL-R3 (DcR1) and TRAIL-R4 (DcR2) having absent or truncated death domains are also expressed on tumor cells. These decoy receptors do not signal apoptosis and may mediate resistance to TRAIL (73). Identification of these death receptors and their ligand has presented an opportunity for selective tumor killing via the extrinsic apoptotic pathway (Tables 2 and 3).

TRAIL AND TOLL RECEPTOR-9 AGONISTS

Although recombinant soluble TRAIL demonstrates significant preclinical antitumor activity and can be safely administered to nonhuman primates (74), concerns of potential hepatotoxicity have hampered clinical development of this agent and a phase-I trial of recombinant Apo2L/TRAIL has only recently been completed (75). Preliminary results in 58 patients with a variety of tumors show that Apo2L/TRAIL therapy, which activates both TRAIL-R1 and TRAIL-R2, appears to be safe and well tolerated with evidence of antitumor activity. There were few grades-3 to 4 toxicities and no drug-related dose-limiting toxicities at a dose of 15 mg/kg. One patient with chondrosarcoma demonstrated a PR. Further studies in combination with chemotherapy and other targeted therapies are planned.

Functional TRAIL protein expression is restricted to immune cells including T-cells, natural killer (NK)-cells, monocytes, and dendritic cells. Interferon

Table 3   Drugs Targeting Members of the Extrinsic and Postmitochondrial
Apoptosis Pathways

Agent	Target	Strategy	Development stage
Recombinant Apo2L/TRAIL	TRAIL-R1 and R2	TRAIL agonist	Phase I
PF3512676	TLR9 agonist	CpG oligodeoxynucleotide: indirectly upregulates TRAIL	Phase III
IMO-2055 (HYB2055)	TLR9 agonist	CpG oligodeoxynucleotide immunomer	Phase I
Mapatumumab	TRAIL-R1	Agonist antibody	Phase II
Lexatumumab	TRAIL-R2	Agonist antibody	Phase I
AEG35156	XIAP	Antisense oligonucleotide	Phase I
YM155	Survivin	Small molecule inhibitor	Phase II
EM-1421	Survivin and Cdc2	Small molecule inhibitor	Phase I
Survivin peptides	Survivin	MHC class-I cellular immunity	Phase I

Abbreviations: TRAIL, tumor necrosis factor–related apoptosis-inducing ligand; TRAIL-R1, TRAIL receptor; TLR, toll-like receptor; XIAP, X-linked inhibitor of apoptosis protein.

(IFN) can induce TRAIL expression in these immune cells and may contribute to the antitumor effect seen in patients treated with IFN (76–78). Unmethylated CpG motifs binding to transmembrane Toll-like receptors (TLR), of which at least 10 have been identified, can also function to stimulate both innate and adaptive antitumor immunity (79). There is evidence that at least in part, some of this stimulatory effect might be mediated by TRAIL (80,81). Development of TLR9 agonists, which are small (8–30 bases long), nonantisense synthetic oligodeoxynucleotides (ODNs) mimicking the CpG motif, able to activate TLR9s on plasmacytoid dendritic and B-cells have entered into clinical testing (82,83). Based on sequence variations, there are three classes of first-generation CpG ODNs, namely A-, B-, and C-class with distinct immunostimulatory activity (84). C-class CpG ODNs can induce a Th1-immune activating response in dendritic cells. The resultant cytokine-mediated stimulation of tumor-antigen–specific cytotoxic T-lymphocytes (CTLs) and NK-cells with upregulation of TRAIL/Apo-2L may enhance cell-mediated antitumor immunity against lung cancer cells (85). Interestingly, there is evidence for functionally active TLR9 expression on NSCLC cells and tissue (86). Stimulation of lung tumor cells with CpG ODNs induces production of monocyte chemoattractant protein 1, shown to mediate NK-cell suppression of xenograft lung adenocarcinoma metastases (87). How the interaction between the immune system and lung cancer cells and the microenvironment mediates tumor killing remains to be elucidated.

CpG ODNs have potential for immune stimulation when used as a single agent, as a vaccine adjuvant, and in combination with chemo- and radiation therapy. PF-3512676 CPG 7909 (Promune), a phosphorothioate oligonucleotide with repeat chains of deoxycytosine-deoxyguanosine, is the first in this new class of targeted agents to be tested clinically. In a small 2:1 randomized phase-II trial of first-line therapy for NSCLC, weekly subcutaneous administration of 0.2 mg/kg PF-3512676 in combination with doublet taxane/platinum chemotherapy showed a nonstatistically significant survival advantage over chemotherapy alone (median 12.7 months vs. 6.8 months, one-year survival 50% vs. 36% hazard ratio = 0.71, and $P = 0.16$) (88). Seventy-five patients received the combination therapy and were treated until disease progression or four to six cycles. The physician-determined response rates were 37% and 19%, respectively ($P = 0.048$). Independent radiologic review of 91 available films reported response rates of 22% and 11%. Notably, the independently confirmed response rate of 11% in the chemotherapy-alone arm is less than expected with this regimen. Treatment was well tolerated with minor injection-site reactions and flu-like symptoms. Grade-4 neutropenia occurred more frequently in the combined than the chemotherapy-only group (49% vs. 22%). Other grades 3 to 4 adverse events included thrombocytopenia (15% vs. 3%) and dehydration (45% vs. 14%). A phase-III trial in lung cancer is currently planned in Europe and the United States.

Based on the results of structure-activity studies, a new second generation of CpG ODNs containing 3'-3'-attached novel structures termed immunomers has been developed (89). A phase-I trial of one such TLR9 agonist, IMO-2005 (HYB2055), has been reported in solid tumors (90). Weekly subcutaneous injections of IMO-2055 induced immunologic activity with increases in cytokines including IL-12, a cytokine with both immunostimulatory and antiangiogenic effects. Adverse events were local injection reactions and flu-like symptoms. Further clinical studies are planned to confirm the role of these agents in the treatment of lung cancer.

TRAIL RECEPTOR ANTIBODIES

As noted previously, recombinant soluble TRAIL has only recently completed phase-I testing. More advanced in development is the promising strategy focusing on developing antibody agonists specific to the functional TRAIL receptors. Mapatumumab [HGS-ETR1 (TRM-1), Human Genome Sciences, Rockville, Maryland, U.S.A.] and lexatumumab (HGS-ETR2) are fully humanized monoclonal antibody agonists to TRAIL-R1 and TRAIL-R2, respectively. Preclinical in vitro and human tumor xenograft data demonstrate single-agent induction of apoptosis, growth inhibition, and cytotoxicity by these antibodies in NSCLC (91). Enhanced cytotoxicity and tumor growth inhibition of lung cancer tumors have also been shown when mapatumumab and lexatumumab are combined with cisplatin chemotherapy (91,92). These data collectively support further study of these antibodies in NSCLC patients. Interestingly, receptor expression is not a reliable indicator of sensitivity to the TRAIL receptor antibodies (91). Both mapatumumab and lexatumumab have undergone phase-I evaluation, with doses of

10 mg/kg for both drugs showing good tolerance and stable disease as best response (93,94). A subsequent multicenter phase-II trial evaluating the efficacy and safety of mapatumumab in 32 heavily pretreated patients with relapsed or recurrent NSCLC has been completed (95). Mapatumumab at 10 mg/kg every three weeks for up to four cycles was administered and patients with stable or responding disease could continue on treatment. With the exception of lymphopenia, no grade-3 toxicity exceeded 7% and no treatment-related severe adverse events occurred. Median PFS was 1.2 months and 29% of patients had stable disease (SD) of 2.3 months median duration. Plans to evaluate mapatumumab in combination with chemotherapy in patients with NSCLC are ongoing. To date, mapatumumab at doses of 10 or 20 mg/kg has been safely combined with paclitaxel (200 mg/m^2) and carboplatin [area under the curve (AUC) 6] every 21 days in a phase-I trial involving 28 patients (96). There were no unexpected toxicities, no evidence of drug–drug interactions, and evidence of PR in three patients with NSCLC.

TARGETING THE IAP FAMILY—XIAP

Caspase activation and execution in the common postmitochondrial apoptotic pathway is under regulatory control by inhibitor of apoptosis proteins (IAP), providing a further potential opportunity for intervention with targeted anticancer therapy (97). The IAP family members XIAP, cIAP1, and cIAP2 have characteristic baculovirus IAP repeat (BIR) and RING finger domains (98,99). The BIR domains of IAP interfere with processing and activation of caspase-9 and directly bind and inhibit activated terminal effector caspase-3 and -7. The RING domain mediates selective ubiquitination and degradation of IAP-caspase complexes, further abrogating apoptosis. Smac released from mitochondria with cytochrome c can bind and sequestrate IAP, allowing caspases to escape regulation and accomplish apoptosis. Overexpression of IAP is associated with resistance to chemotherapy and apoptosis; inhibiting IAP thus promotes caspase activation and tumor cell death.

XIAP ANTISENSE OLIGONUCLEOTIDES

XIAP is the best studied of the IAP and its prominent role in inhibiting both the initiation and the execution of caspase activity makes it a promising target for therapeutic intervention (100,101). Contrary to most instances where high expression of XIAP is associated with poor outcome, patients with resected NSCLC that overexpresses XIAP have better survival than patients with low XIAP expression (102). No such prognostic utility was detected in advanced stage disease (103). These data may reflect the complex interaction between apoptosis-associated proteins or limitations of the current studies, and require further confirmation.

Structurally XIAP has three BIR domains, with evidence suggesting that the BIR3 domain binds and inhibits caspase-9 and the BIR2 domain and its *N*-terminal linker inhibits caspase-3 and -7 (104). Binding sites on these BIR domains are potential targets for small molecule inhibitors, of which several are in preclinical development (105–107). The use of ASO to target the XIAP protein is furthest advanced and in clinical testing. ASO to XIAP can induce apoptosis in H460 lung cancer cells and sensitize cells to chemotherapy (108). In lung cancer xenograft models, XIAP ASOs decrease XIAP protein by 85%, inhibit tumor growth, and are synergistic with docetaxel and vinorelbine chemotherapy (108,109). Preliminary results of a phase-I study of AEG35156, a 19 base second-generation ASO to XIAP, have been reported (110). With 17 patients treated with AEG35156, as a seven-day continuous infusion every three weeks, one patient with breast cancer had an unconfirmed PR at the maximum tolerated dose (MTD) of 125 mg/m^2, with preliminary evidence of XIAP mRNA reduction. Thrombocytopenia and transaminitis were dose limiting. A phase-I trial of AEG35156 and docetaxel has been initiated, the outcome of which may have relevance for patients with lung cancer.

TARGETING THE IAP FAMILY—SURVIVIN

Survivin is a member of the IAP family, characterized by having a single BIR domain but lacking the RING finger motif (97). Instead, it has an extended C-terminal α-helical coiled-coil domain and forms a bow tie-shaped homodimer in solution (111). Survivin can interact with caspases, but may play a more important role in selectively binding and sequestrating Smac, thus preventing its interaction with other IAP proteins and consequently inhibiting apoptosis (112). Survivin also plays a role in preserving cell viability and regulating mitosis in tumor cells (113). It assists with cytokinesis by binding to microtubules and forming a complex with Aurora B (114). A number of splicing variants of survivin have been identified, including survivin-2B, -3B, 2α, and ΔEx3, the exact function of which has not been defined (115–119). With few exceptions, survivin is not expressed in differentiated normal tissue (120). The preferential expression of survivin in tumors, its ability to block apoptosis and regulate cancer cell proliferation, and its correlation with poor clinical outcome make survivin a novel target for therapy. Expression of survivin in lung cancer has been demonstrated (121), with high levels of expression predictive of poor outcome suggesting a potential role for anti-survivin therapy in this cancer (122,123). In preclinical models, strategies to inhibit survivin have included hammerhead ribozymes, siRNAs, and ASOs (124–126). The small molecule inhibitors YM155 and EM-1421 and vaccines directed against survivin have entered clinical testing.

SMALL MOLECULE INHIBITORS OF SURVIVIN

YM155 is a small molecule inhibitor of survivin that selectively suppresses survivin expression without affecting other IAP or Bcl-2 family proteins (127). Preclinical data show significant in vitro antiproliferative activity and antitumor activity in lung cancer xenograft mouse models, without concomitant significant weight loss or hematologic toxicity. Combination with taxanes and platinum drugs increases efficacy without an increase in toxicity. A phase-I study of YM155 in solid malignancies has been completed (128). YM155 was administered to 41 patients as a continuous infusion over seven days every three weeks. The MTD was determined as 4.8 mg/m^2/day. At this dose, stomatitis, arthralgia, and fever were the predominant toxicities, but none was severe. There were no grades 3 to 4 hematologic toxicities. Three of five refractory non-Hodgkin's lymphoma (NHL) patients demonstrated a PR and one of three NSCLC patients had a minor response. A phase-II study in NSCLC is currently recruiting patients.

EM-1421 (tetra-*O*-methyl nordihydroguaiaretic acid, formerly named M4N) is another small molecule showing potential as an inhibitor of survivin (129). EM-1421 induces apoptosis by suppressing survivin gene expression and causes arrest at the G2-M phase of the cell cycle by inhibiting Cdc2 mRNA transcription and protein expression (130). EM-1421 appears to interfere with the binding of the Sp1 transcription factor to the Sp1-dependent promoter sites of Cdc2 and survivin. Decrease in levels of Cdc2 and hence Cdc2 kinase may further destabilize survivin, since phosphorylation of survivin by Cdc2 kinase increases its stability (131). Dual suppression of Cdc2 and survivin thus may be cumulative in promoting apoptosis. Xenograft tumor models confirm decreased protein expression and tumor growth inhibition by EM-1421 (132), and EM-1421 is currently in phase-I testing.

ANTISURVIVIN IMMUNOTHERAPY

The overexpression of survivin in lung and other tumors but minimally in normal tissue has made it an attractive target for immunotherapy. The immunogenicity of survivin has been confirmed by the detection of spontaneous survivin antigen-specific CTLs and anti-survivin antibodies in patients with lung cancer (133–135). A number of survivin-derived epitopes binding a range of major-histocompatibility complex (MHC) class-I alleles have been identified (136) and initial clinical phase-I trials incorporating survivin peptides have confirmed the ability to generate survivin-specific CTLs (137–140). Further exploration of this immunotherapeutic approach in lung patients at various stages of disease seems warranted.

TARGETING THE PROTEASOME

Controlled protein degradation to maintain cell homeostasis is mediated by the ubiquitin-proteasome pathway (Fig. 2) (141). The ubiquitin-conjugating system targets proteins for degradation by attaching the activated ubiquitin polypeptide in a posttranslational modification known as ubiquitylation (142). Polyubiquinated proteins serve as the substrate for proteolysis by the proteasome core, a 20S multisubunit structure of four stacked rings with a catalytic inner chamber. Among

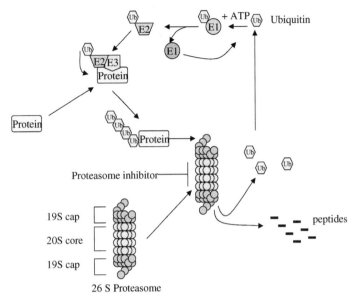

Figure 2 The ubiquitin-proteasome pathway. *Abbreviations*: E1, ubiquitin-activating enzyme; E2, ubiquitin-conjugating enzyme; E3, ubiquitin ligase enzyme; Protein, proteins relevant to lung cancer undergoing degradation include IkB, p21, p27, and p53.

proteins degraded by the ubiquitin-proteasome pathway are those involved in apoptosis, cell cycle progression, and transcription (143). Exposure to IFN-γ results in exchange of low-molecular-weight protease subunits for constitutive beta subunits, modifies the cleavage specificities of the proteasome, and yields an immunoproteasome that is key to generating peptides for eventually bind to MHC class-I molecules (144). Ubiquination can also function as a signal for kinase activation and protein trafficking.

Inhibition of the ubiquitin-proteasomal pathway can lead to growth inhibition, cell cycle disruption, and apoptosis. Malignant cells are selectively sensitive to proteasome inhibition and activity appears to be independent of p53 status. Although an important mechanism of action of proteasome inhibition in both SCLC and NSCLC cells is the inhibition of NF-kB activation as a result of decreased degradation of I-kB, a number of other mechanisms likely play a role, including several intersecting with the apoptosis pathways (143). The activity of proteasome inhibitors may be mediated in part by sustained activation of the JNK pathway, which promotes proapoptotic Bax activity through phosphorylation of 14-3-3 proteins (145). Levels of proapoptotic Bim and Bik also increase due to inhibition of proteasome-mediated degradation. Increase in Bax, increased phosphorylation, and inactivation of Bcl-2 may also contribute to increased apoptosis.

FIRST-GENERATION PROTEASOME INHIBITOR

The proteasome inhibitor bortezomib is a boronic acid dipeptide that reversibly interferes with the chymotryptic-like activity of the 20S proteasome and immunoproteasome (146). Bortezomib can induce growth inhibition and apoptosis in a number of lung cancer cell lines. In NSCLC H460 cells treated with bortezomib, there is an increase in bcl-2 phosphorylation and cleavage, with G2-M phase arrest, followed by apoptosis (147). The combination of bortezomib with a number of chemotherapy agents has also been investigated. Some in vivo studies suggest the sequence of administration to be important; gemcitabine and carboplatin chemotherapy with or followed by bortezomib is synergistic while bortezomib followed by chemotherapy is antagonistic in a mouse xenograft model of lung cancer (148). The preclinical sequence-dependent cytotoxicity data for bortezomib and docetaxel suggest antagonism when both agents are given together, but no difference in efficacy whether docetaxel is added before or after tumor exposure to bortezomib (149).

Bortezomib is the first inhibitor of the ubiquitin-proteasomal pathway to be approved for clinical use. In a phase-I study in patients with solid tumors (150) in which eight patients with NSCLC were entered, one patient with bronchoalveolar carcinoma had a PR of three months duration. Dose-limiting toxicity included sensory neuropathy, diarrhea, and fatigue. In another disease-specific phase-I trial of bortezomib incorporating pharmacodynamic correlates, 23 previously treated NSCLC patients received bortezomib 1.3/1.5 mg/m^2 on day 1, 4, 8, and 11 every 21 days. There was a PR in a patient with adenocarcinoma and nine patients had SD, five for more than four cycles (151). A number of phase-II studies are exploring the role of bortezomib in bronchoalveolar carcinoma and in patients with adenocarcinoma who have failed EGFR inhibitor therapy. Single-agent activity in NSCLC was also demonstrated in a randomized phase-II study of bortezomib or bortezomib and docetaxel in 155 previously treated NSCLC patients. The response rates were 8% versus 9%, time to progression 1.5 months versus 4 months, and median survival time 7.4 months versus 7.8 months for bortezomib and bortezomib/docetaxel, respectively. Treatment-related severe adverse events were similar (49% vs. 51%) (152). The sequence specificity of bortezomib and docetaxel is being evaluated in a phase-II study in patients failing first-line therapy.

Additional combination phase-I trials have been conducted, including those with gemcitabine and paclitaxel/carboplatin. In the bortezomib and gemcitabine study, nine of the patients had lung cancer (153). The MTD was determined as bortezomib 1 mg/m^2 on day 1, 4, 8, and 11 and gemcitabine 1000 mg/m^2 on day 1 and 8 every 21 days with the most common grades 3 to 4 toxicities being neutropenia (29%) and thrombocytopenia (19%). One patient with NSCLC who had previously progressed on gemcitabine had a PR and three other lung cancer patients had SD. A phase-I study of bortezomib and paclitaxel/carboplatin explored the sequence dependence of these drugs (154). A total of 53 patients with advanced solid tumors received either paclitaxel/carboplatin followed by bortezomib on day 2, 5, and 8 or bortezomib on day 1, 4, and 8 with paclitaxel/carboplatin on day 2 every 21 days. Neutropenia and fatigue were more common with the first regimen, which also showed poorer response rate (PR 4% vs. 21.4%), suggesting that sequence may be important for toxicity and efficacy. Recently reported is a phase-II Southwest Oncology Group trial (S0339) in chemo-naïve patients with late-stage disease tested a regimen of gemcitabine 1000 mg/m^2 on day 1 and 8, and carboplatin AUC 5 on day 1 with bortezomib 1 mg/m^2 on day 1, 4, 8, and 11 every 21 days (155). In 114 evaluable patients, the response rate was 21% complete response (CR 2%), with encouraging median PFS of five months [confidence interval (CI) 3.5–5.4 months] and median overall survival of 11 months (CI 8.2–13 months). The one- and two-year survival rates were 47% and 14%, respectively. Anticipated grades 3 to 4 toxicities included neutropenia (52%), thrombocytopenia (63%), anemia (13%), and fatigue (13%). Further study of this regimen in a phase-III study is planned.

Clinical studies with bortezomib have been conducted in SCLC. In a phase-II Southwest Oncology Group study (S0327) of bortezomib as second-line therapy, patients were stratified into platinum-sensitive and refractory groups (156). Treatment consisted of bortezomib at 1.3 mg/m^2 on day 1, 4, 8, and 11 every 21 days. Of 57 evaluable patients, only one patient, in the refractory arm, had a PR. These disappointing results suggest that single-agent bortezomib is insufficiently active in SCLC, despite the promising preclinical data. Combination therapy with topotecan as salvage therapy in patients failing a first-line cisplatin regimen is being evaluated.

Critical questions of sequence, schedule, dose, and cumulative neurotoxicity of bortezomib remain to be answered in lung cancer. Whether neurotoxicity is a class phenomenon or specific to bortezomib will become apparent with clinical testing of the next generation of proteasome inhibitors such as PR-171 and NPI-0052.

SECOND-GENERATION PROTEASOME INHIBITORS

PR-171 is an epoxomicin-derived second-generation proteasome inhibitor that selectively and irreversibly inhibits the proteasome (157). Proteasome activity appears to recover rapidly in normal tissue. Antitumor activity has been demonstrated in a number of xenograft mouse models, and a phase-I clinical trial is currently underway in hematologic malignancies.

NPI-0052 (salinosporamide A) is a second-generation nonpeptide proteasome inhibitor derived from a novel marine-obligate actinomycete (158). It is orally bioavailable and differs from current inhibitors as it has activity against the chymotryptic, tryptic, and postglutamyl peptidyl hydrolytic-like activities of the proteasome. NPI-0052 acts on the FADD-caspase-8–mediated cell death signaling pathway, and, in preclinical studies, appears to be active against bortuzimab-resistant myeloma cells from patients (159). Neuropathy was not a prominent feature in mouse xenograft models treated for extended periods. Recent preclinical in vivo data show that NPI-0052 enhances the activity of biologics such as cetuximab, and chemotherapy agents such as CPT-11 and oxaliplatin, supporting its use in solid tumors including non–small lung cell carcinomas.

CONCLUSIONS

The elucidation of the mechanism of action of tyrosine kinase inhibitors of the EGFR and the presence of receptor mutations in a subgroup of patients have served to focus our attention on the heterogeneous nature of NSCLC, emphasizing the need for closer attention to specific groups of patients with possibly unique mechanisms of cancer pathogenesis.

A number of novel agents targeting the proliferative, cell cycle and apoptosis pathway are emerging. There is abundant in vitro data supporting the combination of many of these agents to affect synergistic tumor kill. Many of these studies reiterate the potential for enhancing defective apoptosis; as for example, the enhanced sensitivity to TRAIL-induced apoptosis following proteasome inhibition. Similarly, data suggest that inhibition of the Akt kinase pathway may sensitize lung cancer cells to TRAIL-induced apoptosis, providing a rationale for this combination of drugs targeting these pathways (160).

The challenge for the future treatment of lung cancer will be to achieve the most effective combination of these agents and to identify specific patients who might best benefit from such individual or combination therapy.

REFERENCES

1. Pujol JL, Barlesi F, Daures JP. Should chemotherapy combinations for advanced non-small cell lung cancer be platinum-based? A meta-analysis of phase III randomized trials. Lung Cancer 2006; 51(3):335–345.
2. Schiller JH, Harrington D, Belani CP, et al. Comparison of four chemotherapy regimens for advanced non-small-cell lung cancer. N Engl J Med 2002; 346(2):92–98.
3. Delbaldo C, Michiels S, Syz N, et al. Benefits of adding a drug to a single-agent or a 2-agent chemotherapy regimen in advanced non-small-cell lung cancer: a meta-analysis. JAMA 2004; 292(4):470–484.
4. Paccagnella A, Oniga F, Bearz A, et al. Adding Gemcitabine to Paclitaxel/Carboplatin combination increases survival in advanced non-small-cell lung cancer: results of a phase II-III study. J Clin Oncol 2006; 24(4):681–687.
5. Gatzemeier U, Pluzanska A, Szczesna A, et al. Results of a phase III trial of erlotinib (OSI-774) combined with cisplatin and gemcitabine (GC) chemotherapy in advanced non-small cell lung cancer (NSCLC). J Clin Oncol 2004; 22(14S):619s [abstr. 7010].
6. Giaccone G, Herbst RS, Manegold C, et al. Gefitinib in combination with gemcitabine and cisplatin in advanced non-small-cell lung cancer: a phase III trial—INTACT 1. J Clin Oncol 2004; 22(5):777–784.
7. Herbst RS, Giaccone G, Schiller JH, et al. Gefitinib in combination with paclitaxel and carboplatin in advanced non-small-cell lung cancer: a phase III trial—INTACT 2. J Clin Oncol 2004; 22(5):785–794.

8. Herbst RS, Prager D, Hermann R, et al. TRIBUTE: a phase III trial of erlotinib hydro-chloride (OSI-774) combined with carboplatin and paclitaxel chemotherapy in advanced non-small-cell lung cancer. J Clin Oncol 2005; 23(25):5892–5899.
9. Sandler A, Gray R, Brahmer J, et al. Randomized phase II/III Trial of paclitaxel (P) plus carboplatin (C) with or without bevacizumab (NSC# 704865) in patients with advanced non-squamous non-small cell lung cancer (NSCLC): an Eastern Cooperative Oncology Group (ECOG) Trial—E4599 [abstr. LBA4]. J Clin Oncol 2005; 23(16S):2s.
10. Shepherd FA, Dancey J, Ramlau R, et al. Prospective randomized trial of docetaxel versus best supportive care in patients with non-small-cell lung cancer previously treated with platinum-based chemotherapy. J Clin Oncol 2000; 18(10):2095–2103.
11. Hanna N, Shepherd FA, Fossella FV, et al. Randomized phase III trial of pemetrexed versus docetaxel in patients with non-small-cell lung cancer previously treated with chemotherapy. J Clin Oncol 2004; 22(9):1589–1597.
12. Shepherd FA, Rodrigues Pereira J, et al. Erlotinib in previously treated non-small-cell lung cancer. N Engl J Med 2005; 353(2):123–132.
13. Thatcher N, Chang A, Parikh P, Pemberton K, Archer V. Results of a Phase III placebo-controlled study (ISEL) of gefitinib (IRESSA) plus best supportive care (BSC) in patients with advanced non-small-cell lung cancer (NSCLC) who had received 1 or 2 prior chemotherapy regimens [abstr. #LB-6]. Proc Am Assoc Cancer Res 2005:46.
14. Herbst RS, Johnson DH, Mininberg E, et al. Phase I/II trial evaluating the anti-vascular endothelial growth factor monoclonal antibody bevacizumab in combination with the HER-1/epidermal growth factor receptor tyrosine kinase inhibitor erlotinib for patients with recurrent non-small-cell lung cancer. J Clin Oncol 2005; 23(11):2544–2555.
15. Noda K, Nishiwaki Y, Kawahara M, et al. Irinotecan plus cisplatin compared with etoposide plus cisplatin for extensive small-cell lung cancer. N Engl J Med 2002; 346(2):85–91.
16. Hanna N, Einhorn L, Sandler A, Langer C, et al. Randomized, phase III trial comparing irinotecan/cisplatin (IP) with etoposide/cisplatin (EP) in patients (pts) with previously untreated, extensive-stage (ES) small cell lung cancer (SCLC) [abstr. LBA 7004]. J Clin Oncol 2005; 23(16S):622s.
17. Danial NN, Korsmeyer SJ. Cell death: critical control points. Cell 2004; 116(2): 205–219.
18. Letai A, Bassik MC, Walensky LD, et al. Distinct BH3 domains either sensitize or activate mitochondrial apoptosis, serving as prototype cancer therapeutics. Cancer Cell 2002; 2(3):183–192.
19. Kuwana T, Bouchier-Hayes L, et al. BH3 domains of BH3-only proteins differentially regulate Bax-mediated mitochondrial membrane permeabilization both directly and indirectly. Mol Cell 2005; 17(4):525–535.
20. Wei MC, Zong WX, Cheng EH, et al. Proapoptotic BAX and BAK: a requisite gateway to mitochondrial dysfunction and death. Science 2001; 292(5517):727–730.
21. Letai A. Pharmacological manipulation of Bcl-2 family members to control cell death. J Clin Invest 2005; 115(10):2648–2455.
22. Puthalakath H, Strasser A. Keeping killers on a tight leash: transcriptional and post-translational control of the pro-apoptotic activity of BH3-only proteins. Cell Death Differ 2002; 9(5):505–512.
23. Yu J, Zhang L, Hwang PM, Kinzler KW, Vogelstein B. PUMA induces the rapid apoptosis of colorectal cancer cells. Mol Cell 2001; 7(3):673–682.

24. Oda E, Ohki R, Murasawa H, et al. Noxa, a BH3-only member of the Bcl-2 family and candidate mediator of p53-induced apoptosis. Science 2000; 288(5468): 1053–1058.

25. Luciano F, Jacquel A, Colosetti P, et al. Phosphorylation of Bim-EL by Erk1/2 on serine 69 promotes its degradation via the proteasome pathway and regulates its proapoptotic function. Oncogene 2003; 22(43):6785–6793.

26. Li H, Zhu H, Xu CJ, Yuan J. Cleavage of BID by caspase 8 mediates the mitochondrial damage in the Fas pathway of apoptosis. Cell 1998; 94(4):491–501.

27. Cheng EH, Wei MC, Weiler S, et al. BCL-2, BCL-X(L) sequester BH3 domain-only molecules preventing BAX- and BAK-mediated mitochondrial apoptosis. Mol Cell 2001; 8(3):705–711.

28. Chen L, Willis SN, Wei A, et al. Differential targeting of prosurvival Bcl-2 proteins by their BH3-only ligands allows complementary apoptotic function. Mol Cell 2005; 17(3):393–403.

29. Cuddeback SM, Yamaguchi H, Komatsu K, et al. Molecular cloning and characterization of Bif-1. A novel Src homology 3 domain-containing protein that associates with Bax. J Biol Chem 2001; 276(23):20559–20565.

30. Guo B, Zhai D, Cabezas E, et al. Humanin peptide suppresses apoptosis by interfering with Bax activation. Nature 2003; 423(6938):456–461.

31. Sawada M, Sun W, Hayes P, et al. Ku70 suppresses the apoptotic translocation of Bax to mitochondria. Nat Cell Biol 2003; 5(4):320–329.

32. Au NH, Cheang M, Huntsman DG, et al. Evaluation of immunohistochemical markers in non-small cell lung cancer by unsupervised hierarchical clustering analysis: a tissue microarray study of 284 cases and 18 markers. J Pathol 2004; 204(1):101–109.

33. Paik KH, Park YH, Ryoo BY, et al. Prognostic value of immunohistochemical staining of p53, bcl-2, and Ki-67 in small cell lung cancer. J Korean Med Sci 2006; 21(1):35–39.

34. Martin B, Paesmans M, Berghmans T, et al. Role of Bcl-2 as a prognostic factor for survival in lung cancer: a systematic review of the literature with meta-analysis. Br J Cancer 2003; 89(1):55–64.

35. Fennell DA. Bcl-2 as a target for overcoming chemoresistance in small-cell lung cancer. Clin Lung Cancer 2003; 4(5):307–313.

36. Zereu M, Vinholes JJ, Zettler CG. p53 and Bcl-2 protein expression and its relationship with prognosis in small-cell lung cancer. Clin Lung Cancer 2003; 4(5): 298–302.

37. Song L, Coppola D, Livingston S, Cress D, Haura EB. Mcl-1 regulates survival and sensitivity to diverse apoptotic stimuli in human non-small cell lung cancer cells. Cancer Biol Ther 2005; 4(3):267–276.

38. Karczmarek-Borowska B, Filip A, Wojcierowski J, et al. Estimation of prognostic value of Bcl-xL gene expression in non-small cell lung cancer. Lung Cancer 2006; 51(1):61–69.

39. Crooke ST. Molecular mechanisms of antisense drugs: RNase H. Antisense Nucleic Acid Drug Dev 1998; 8(2):133–134.

40. Dias N, Stein CA. Potential roles of antisense oligonucleotides in cancer therapy. The example of Bcl-2 antisense oligonucleotides. Eur J Pharm Biopharm 2002; 54(3):263–269.

41. Reed JC, Stein C, Subasinghe C, et al. Antisense-mediated inhibition of BCL2 protooncogene expression and leukemic cell growth and survival: comparisons of phosphodiester and phosphorothioate oligodeoxynucleotides. Cancer Res 1990; 50(20):6565–6570.

42. Hu Z, Sayeed MM. Suppression of mitochondria-dependent neutrophil apoptosis with thermal injury. Am J Physiol Cell Physiol 2004; 286(1):C170–C178.
43. Marshall J, Chen H, Yang D, et al. A phase I trial of a Bcl-2 antisense (G3139) and weekly docetaxel in patients with advanced breast cancer and other solid tumors. Ann Oncol 2004; 15(8):1274–1283.
44. Tolcher AW, Kuhn J, Schwartz G, et al. A phase I pharmacokinetic and biological correlative study of oblimersen sodium (Genasense, G3139), an antisense oligonucleotide to the Bcl-2 mRNA, and of docetaxel in patients with hormone-refractory prostate cancer. Clin Cancer Res 2004; 10(15):5048–5057.
45. Rudin CM, Kozloff M, Hoffman PC, et al. Phase I study of G3139, a Bcl-2 antisense oligonucleotide, combined with carboplatin and etoposide in patients with small-cell lung cancer. J Clin Oncol 2004; 22(6):1110–1117.
46. Rudin CM, Otterson GA, Mauer AM, et al. A pilot trial of G3139, a bcl-2 antisense oligonucleotide, and paclitaxel in patients with chemorefractory small-cell lung cancer. Ann Oncol 2002; 13(4):539–545.
47. Chanan-Khan AA, Niesvizky R, Hohl RJ, et al. Randomized multicenter phase 3 trial of high-dose dexamethasone (dex) with or without oblimersen sodium (G3139; Bcl-2 antisense; Genasense) for patients with advanced multiple myeloma (MM). ASH Annu Meeting Abstr 2004; 104(11):1477.
48. Kirkwood JM, Bedikian AY, Millward MJ, et al. Long-term survival results of a randomized multinational phase 3 trial of dacarbazine (DTIC) with or without Bcl-2 antisense (oblimersen sodium) in patients (pts) with advanced malignant melanoma (MM) [abstr. 7506]. J Clin Oncol 2005; 23(16S):711s.
49. Rai KR, Moore JO, Boyd TE, et al. Phase 3 randomized trial of fludarabine/cyclophosphamide chemotherapy with or without oblimersen sodium (Bcl-2 Antisense; Genasense; G3139) for patients with relapsed or refractory chronic lymphocytic leukemia (CLL). ASH Annu Meeting Abstr 2004; 104(11):338.
50. Simoes-Wust AP, Hopkins-Donaldson S, Sigrist B, et al. A functionally improved locked nucleic acid antisense oligonucleotide inhibits Bcl-2 and Bcl-xL expression and facilitates tumor cell apoptosis. Oligonucleotides 2004; 14(3):199–209.
51. Hansen B, Westergaard M, Frieden M, et al. SPC2996-A Bcl-2 inhibitor for treatment of chronic lymphocytic leukemia [abstr. A41]. Clin Cancer Res 2005; 11(suppl 23):66S.
52. Leech SH, Olie RA, Gautschi O, et al. Induction of apoptosis in lung-cancer cells following bcl-xL anti-sense treatment. Int J Cancer 2000; 86(4):570–576.
53. Zangemeister-Wittke U, Leech SH, Olie RA, et al. A novel bispecific antisense oligonucleotide inhibiting both bcl-2 and bcl-xL expression efficiently induces apoptosis in tumor cells. Clin Cancer Res 2000; 6(6):2547–2555.
54. Johnston JB, Paul JT, Neufeld NJ, et al. Role of myeloid cell factor-1 (Mcl-1) in chronic lymphocytic leukemia. Leuk Lymphoma 2004; 45(10):2017–2027.
55. Le Gouill S, Podar K, Harousseau JL, Anderson KC. Mcl-1 regulation and its role in multiple myeloma. Cell Cycle 2004; 3(10):1259–1262.
56. Michels J, Johnson PW, Packham G. Mcl-1. Int J Biochem Cell Biol 2005; 37(2):267–271.
57. Thallinger C, Wolschek MF, Maierhofer H, et al. Mcl-1 is a novel therapeutic target for human sarcoma: synergistic inhibition of human sarcoma xenotransplants by a combination of mcl-1 antisense oligonucleotides with low-dose cyclophosphamide. Clin Cancer Res 2004; 10(12 Pt 1):4185–4191.

58. Yu C, Bruzek LM, Meng XW, et al. The role of Mcl-1 downregulation in the proapoptotic activity of the multikinase inhibitor BAY 43-9006. Oncogene 2005; 24(46) 6861–6869.

59. Chang JS, Hsu YL, Kuo PL, Chiang LC, Lin CC. Upregulation of Fas/Fas ligand-mediated apoptosis by gossypol in an immortalized human alveolar lung cancer cell line. Clin Exp Pharmacol Physiol 2004; 31(10):716–722.

60. McGreivy JS, Marshall J, Cheson BD, et al. Initial results from ongoing phase I trials of a novel pan bcl-2 family small molecule inhibitor [abstr. 3180]. J Clin Oncol 2005; 23(16S):236s.

61. Saleh M, Pitot H, Hartung J, et al. Phase I trial of AT-101, an orally bioavailable inhibitor of BCL-2, in patients with advanced malignancies [abstr. C89]. Clin Cancer Res 2005; 11(suppl 23):9121s.

62. Bauer JA, Trask DK, Kumar B, et al. Reversal of cisplatin resistance with a BH3 mimetic, (-)-gossypol, in head and neck cancer cells: role of wild-type p53 and Bcl-xL. Mol Cancer Ther 2005; 4(7):1096–1104.

63. Benz CC, Keniry MA, Ford JM, et al. Biochemical correlates of the antitumor and antimitochondrial properties of gossypol enantiomers. Mol Pharmacol 1990; 37(6): 840–847.

64. Liu S, Kulp SK, Sugimoto Y, et al. The (−)-enantiomer of gossypol possesses higher anticancer potency than racemic gossypol in human breast cancer. Anticancer Res 2002; 22(1A):33–38.

65. Oltersdorf T, Elmore SW, Shoemaker AR, et al. An inhibitor of Bcl-2 family proteins induces regression of solid tumours. Nature 2005; 435(7042):677–681.

66. Ashkenazi A. Targeting death and decoy receptors of the tumour-necrosis factor superfamily. Nat Rev Cancer 2002; 2(6):420–430.

67. Wang S, El-Deiry WS. TRAIL and apoptosis induction by TNF-family death receptors. Oncogene 2003; 22(53):8628–8633.

68. Suliman A, Lam A, Datta R, Srivastava RK. Intracellular mechanisms of TRAIL: apoptosis through mitochondrial-dependent and -independent pathways. Oncogene 2001; 20(17):2122–2133.

69. Barnhart BC, Alappat EC, Peter ME. The CD95 type I/type II model. Semin Immunol 2003; 15(3):185–193.

70. LeBlanc HN, Ashkenazi A. Apo2L/TRAIL and its death and decoy receptors. Cell Death Differ 2003; 10(1):66–75.

71. Halpern W, Lincoln C, Sharifi A, et al. Variable distribution of TRAIL receptor 1 in primary human tumor and normal tissues [abstr. 225]. Eur J Cancer 2004; 2(suppl 8):69.

72. Halpern W, Lincoln C, Roach C, et al. TRAIL-R2 expression in normal and tumor tissue [abstr. 83P]. Ann Oncol 2004; 15(suppl 3):iii, 22.

73. Ashkenazi A, Dixit VM. Apoptosis control by death and decoy receptors. Curr Opin Cell Biol 1999; 11(2):255–260.

74. Kelley SK, Harris LA, Xie D, et al. Preclinical studies to predict the disposition of Apo2L/tumor necrosis factor-related apoptosis-inducing ligand in humans: characterization of in vivo efficacy, pharmacokinetics, and safety. J Pharmacol Exp Ther 2001; 299(1):31–38.

75. Herbst R, Mendolson D, Ebbinghaus S, et al. A phase I safety and pharmacokinetic (PK) study of recombinant Apo2L/TRAIL, an apoptosis-inducing protein in patients with advanced cancer [abstr. 3013]. J Clin Oncol 2006; 24(18S):124s.

76. Fanger NA, Maliszewski CR, Schooley K, Griffith TS. Human dendritic cells mediate cellular apoptosis via tumor necrosis factor-related apoptosis-inducing ligand (TRAIL). J Exp Med 1999; 190(8):1155–1164.

77. Griffith TS, Wiley SR, Kubin MZ, et al. Monocyte-mediated tumoricidal activity via the tumor necrosis factor-related cytokine, TRAIL. J Exp Med 1999; 189(8): 1343–1354.

78. Kayagaki N, Yamaguchi N, Nakayama M, et al. Type I interferons (IFNs) regulate tumor necrosis factor-related apoptosis-inducing ligand (TRAIL) expression on human T cells: a novel mechanism for the antitumor effects of type I IFNs. J Exp Med 1999; 189(9):1451–1460.

79. Wooldridge JE, Weiner GJ. CpG DNA and cancer immunotherapy: orchestrating the antitumor immune response. Curr Opin Oncol 2003; 15(6):440–445.

80. Kemp TJ, Moore JM, Griffith TS. Human B cells express functional TRAIL/Apo-2 ligand after CpG-containing oligodeoxynucleotide stimulation. J Immunol 2004; b173(2):892–899.

81. Chaperot L, Blum A, Manches O, et al. Virus or TLR agonists induce TRAIL-mediated cytotoxic activity of plasmacytoid dendritic cells. J Immunol 2006; 176(1):248–255.

82. Vollmer J. Progress in drug development of immunostimulatory CpG oligodeoxynucleotide ligands for TLR9. Expert Opin Biol Ther 2005; 5(5):673–682.

83. Wang H, Rayburn E, Zhang R. Synthetic oligodeoxynucleotides containing deoxycytidyl-deoxyguanosine dinucleotides (CpG ODNs) and modified analogs as novel anticancer therapeutics. Curr Pharm Des 2005; 11(22):2889–2907.

84. Vollmer J, Weeratna R, Payette P, et al. Characterization of three CpG oligodeoxynucleotide classes with distinct immunostimulatory activities. Eur J Immunol 2004; 34(1):251–262.

85. Kawarada Y, Ganss R, Garbi N, et al. NK– and CD8+ T-cell-mediated eradication of established tumors by peritumoral injection of CpG-containing oligodeoxynucleotides. J Immunol 2001; 167(9):5247–5253.

86. Droemann D, Albrecht D, Gerdes J, et al. Human lung cancer cells express functionally active Toll-like receptor 9. Respir Res 2005; 6(1):1.

87. Nokihara H, Yanagawa H, Nishioka Y, et al. Natural killer cell-dependent suppression of systemic spread of human lung adenocarcinoma cells by monocyte chemoattractant protein-1 gene transfection in severe combined immunodeficient mice. Cancer Res 2000; 60(24):7002–7007.

88. Manegold C, Leichman G, Gravenor D. Phase II randomized trial adding a toll-like receptor 9 agonist (Promune™) to first line chemotherapy shows improved response in advanced non-small cell lung cancer [abstr. PD-046]. Lung Cancer 2005; 49(suppl 2):S80.

89. Wang D, Li Y, Yu D, et al. Immunopharmacological and antitumor effects of second-generation immunomodulatory oligonucleotides containing synthetic CpR motifs. Int J Oncol 2004; 24(4):901–908.

90. Moore D, Hwang J, McGreivy J, et al. Phase I trial of escalating doses of the TLR9 agonist HYB2055 in patients with advanced solid tumors [abstr. 2503]. J Clin Oncol 2005; 23(16S):166s.

91. Humphrey R, Shepard L, Zhang Y, et al. Novel, agonistic, human anti-TRAIL receptor monoclonal antibodies, HGS-ETR1 and HGS-ETR2, are capable of potently inducing tumor regression and growth inhibition as single agents and in combination

with chemotherapeutic agents in models of human NSCLC [abstr. B72]. Clin Cancer Res 2003:9(suppl 16).

92. Pukac L, Kanakaraj P, Humphreys R, et al. HGS-ETR1, a fully human TRAIL-receptor 1 monoclonal antibody, induces cell death in multiple tumour types in vitro and in vivo. Br J Cancer 2005; 92(8):1430–1441.

93. Pacey RE, Plummer GA, Bale C, et al. Phase I and pharmacokinetic study of HGS-ETR2, a human monoclonal antibody to TRAIL R2, in patients with advanced solid malignancies [abstr. 3055]. J Clin Oncol 2005; 23(16S);205s.

94. Tolcher A, Mita M, Patnaik A, et al. A phase I and pharmacokinetic study of HGS-ETR1(TRM-1), a human monoclonal agonist-antibody to TRAIL R1, in patients with advanced solid tumors [abstr. 3060]. J Clin Oncol 2004; 22(14S):210s.

95. Bonomi P, Greco F, Crawford J, et al. Results of a phase 2 trial of HGS-ETR1 (agonistic human monoclonal antibody to TRAIL receptor 1) in subjects with relapsed/recurrent non-small cell lung cancer (NSCLC) [abstr. P-460]. Lung Cancer 2005; 49(suppl 2):S237.

96. Chow L, Eckhardt GS, Gustafson D, et al. HGS-ETR1, an antibody targeting TRAIL-R1, in combination with paclitaxel and carboplatin in patients with advanced solid malignancies: results of a phase 1 and PK study [abstr. 2515]. J Clin Oncol 2006; 24(18S):103s.

97. Salvesen GS, Duckett CS. IAP proteins: blocking the road to death's door. Nat Rev Mol Cell Biol 2002; 3(6):401–410.

98. Miller LK. An exegesis of IAPs: salvation and surprises from BIR motifs. Trends Cell Biol 1999; 9(8):323–328.

99. Joazeiro CA, Weissman AM. RING finger proteins: mediators of ubiquitin ligase activity. Cell 2000; 102(5):549–552.

100. Holcik M, Gibson H, Korneluk RG. XIAP: apoptotic brake and promising therapeutic target. Apoptosis 2001; 6(4):253–261.

101. Deveraux QL, Takahashi R, Salvesen GS, Reed JC. X-linked IAP is a direct inhibitor of cell-death proteases. Nature 1997; 388(6639):300–304.

102. Ferreira CG, van der Valk P, Span SW, et al. Expression of X-linked inhibitor of apoptosis as a novel prognostic marker in radically resected non-small cell lung cancer patients. Clin Cancer Res 2001; 7(8):2468–2474.

103. Ferreira CG, van der Valk P, Span SW, et al. Assessment of IAP (inhibitor of apoptosis) proteins as predictors of response to chemotherapy in advanced non-small-cell lung cancer patients. Ann Oncol 2001; 12(6):799–805.

104. Deveraux QL, Leo E, Stennicke HR, et al. Cleavage of human inhibitor of apoptosis protein XIAP results in fragments with distinct specificities for caspases. Embo J 1999; 18(19):5242–5251.

105. Wu TY, Wagner KW, Bursulaya B, Schultz PG, Deveraux QL. Development and characterization of nonpeptidic small molecule inhibitors of the XIAP/caspase-3 interaction. Chem Biol 2003; 10(8):759–767.

106. Li L, Thomas RM, Suzuki H, et al. A small molecule Smac mimic potentiates TRAIL- and TNF-alpha-mediated cell death. Science 2004; 305(5689):1471–1474.

107. Schimmer AD, Welsh K, Pinilla C, et al. Small-molecule antagonists of apoptosis suppressor XIAP exhibit broad antitumor activity. Cancer Cell 2004; 5(1):25–35.

108. Hu Y, Cherton-Horvat G, Dragowska V, et al. Antisense oligonucleotides targeting XIAP induce apoptosis and enhance chemotherapeutic activity against human lung cancer cells in vitro and in vivo. Clin Cancer Res 2003; 9(7):2826–2836.

109. LaCasse E, Cherton-Horvat G, Lefebvre C, et al. Anti-tumor activity of XIAP antisense compound, AEG35156, correlates with suppression of XIAP mRNA and protein levels in human cancer models [abstr. A40]. Clin Cancer Res 2005; 11(suppl 23):8975s.

110. Ranson M, Dive C, Ward T, et al. A phase I trial of AEG35156 (XIAP antisense) administered as a 7-day continuous intravenous infusion in patients with advanced tumors [abstr. C72]. Clin Cancer Res 2005; 11(suppl 23):9116s.

111. Sun C, Nettesheim D, Liu Z, Olejniczak ET. Solution structure of human survivin and its binding interface with Smac/Diablo. Biochemistry 2005; 44(1):11–17.

112. Song Z, Yao X, Wu M. Direct interaction between survivin and Smac/DIABLO is essential for the anti-apoptotic activity of survivin during taxol-induced apoptosis. J Biol Chem 2003; 278(25):23130–23140.

113. Altieri DC. Survivin, versatile modulation of cell division and apoptosis in cancer. Oncogene 2003; 22(53):8581–8589.

114. Chen J, Jin S, Tahir SK, et al. Survivin enhances Aurora-B kinase activity and localizes Aurora-B in human cells. J Biol Chem 2003; 278(1):486–490.

115. Mahotka C, Wenzel M, Springer E, Gabbert HE, Gerharz CD. Survivin-deltaEx3 and survivin-2B: two novel splice variants of the apoptosis inhibitor survivin with different antiapoptotic properties. Cancer Res 1999; 59(24):6097–6102.

116. Badran A, Yoshida A, Ishikawa K, et al. Identification of a novel splice variant of the human anti-apoptopsis gene survivin. Biochem Biophys Res Commun 2004; 314(3):902–907.

117. Caldas H, Honsey LE, Altura RA. Survivin 2alpha: a novel Survivin splice variant expressed in human malignancies. Mol Cancer 2005; 4(1):11.

118. Caldas H, Jiang Y, Holloway MP, et al. Survivin splice variants regulate the balance between proliferation and cell death. Oncogene 2005; 24(12):1994–2007.

119. Noton EA, Colnaghi R, Tate S, et al. Molecular analysis of survivin isoforms: evidence that alternatively spliced variants do not play a role in mitosis. J Biol Chem 2006; 281(2):1286–1295.

120. Altieri DC. Validating survivin as a cancer therapeutic target. Nat Rev Cancer 2003; 3(1):46–54.

121. Falleni M, Pellegrini C, Marchetti A, et al. Survivin gene expression in early-stage non-small cell lung cancer. J Pathol 2003; 200(5):620–626.

122. Monzo M, Rosell R, Felip E, et al. A novel anti-apoptosis gene: re-expression of survivin messenger RNA as a prognosis marker in non-small-cell lung cancers. J Clin Oncol 1999; 17(7):2100–2104.

123. Kren L, Brazdil J, Hermanova M, et al. Prognostic significance of anti-apoptosis proteins survivin and bcl-2 in non-small cell lung carcinomas: a clinicopathologic study of 102 cases. Appl Immunohistochem Mol Morphol 2004; 12(1):44–49.

124. Choi KS, Lee TH, Jung MH. Ribozyme-mediated cleavage of the human survivin mRNA and inhibition of antiapoptotic function of survivin in MCF-7 cells. Cancer Gene Ther 2003; 10(2):87–95.

125. Olie RA, Simoes-Wust AP, Baumann B, et al. A novel antisense oligonucleotide targeting survivin expression induces apoptosis and sensitizes lung cancer cells to chemotherapy. Cancer Res 2000; 60(11):2805–2809.

126. Ling X, Li F. Silencing of antiapoptotic survivin gene by multiple approaches of RNA interference technology. Biotechniques 2004; 36(3):450–454, 456–460.

127. Nakahara T, Takeuchi M, Isao K, et al. YM155, a novel survivin suppressant, induced downregulation of survivin and potent antitumor activities in experimental human

prostate tumor xenograft models [abstr. B203]. Clin Cancer Res 2005; 11(suppl 24):9082s.

128. Tolcher A, Antonia S, Lewis L, et al. A phase I study of YM155, a novel survivin suppressant, administered by 168 hour continuous infusion to patients with advanced solid tumors [abstr. 3014]. J Clin Oncol 2006; 24(18S):124s.

129. Heller JD, Kuo J, Wu TC, Kast WM, Huang RC. Tetra-O-methyl nordihydroguaiaretic acid induces G2 arrest in mammalian cells and exhibits tumoricidal activity in vivo. Cancer Res 2001; 61(14):5499–5504.

130. Chang CC, Heller JD, Kuo J, Huang RC. Tetra-O-methyl nordihydroguaiaretic acid induces growth arrest and cellular apoptosis by inhibiting Cdc2 and survivin expression. Proc Natl Acad Sci USA 2004; 101(36):13239–13244.

131. O'Connor DS, Grossman D, Plescia J, et al. Regulation of apoptosis at cell division by p34cdc2 phosphorylation of survivin. Proc Natl Acad Sci USA 2000; 97(24):13103–13107.

132. Park R, Chang CC, Liang YC, et al. Systemic treatment with tetra-O-methyl nordihydroguaiaretic acid suppresses the growth of human xenograft tumors. Clin Cancer Res 2005; 11(12):4601–4609.

133. Rohayem J, Diestelkoetter P, Weigle B, et al. Antibody response to the tumor-associated inhibitor of apoptosis protein survivin in cancer patients. Cancer Res 2000; 60(7):1815–1817.

134. Andersen MH, Pedersen LO, Capeller B, et al. Spontaneous cytotoxic T-cell responses against survivin-derived MHC class I-restricted T-cell epitopes in situ as well as ex vivo in cancer patients. Cancer Res 2001; 61(16):5964–5968.

135. Ichiki Y, Hanagiri T, Takenoyama M, et al. Tumor specific expression of survivin-2B in lung cancer as a novel target of immunotherapy. Lung Cancer 2005; 48(2): 281–289.

136. Bachinsky MM, Guillen DE, Patel SR, et al. Mapping and binding analysis of peptides derived from the tumor-associated antigen survivin for eight HLA alleles. Cancer Immun 2005; 5:6.

137. Fuessel S, Meye A, Schmitz M, et al. Vaccination of hormone-refractory prostate cancer patients with peptide cocktail-loaded dendritic cells: results of a phase I clinical trial. Prostate 2006; 66(8)811–821.

138. Hirschowitz EA, Foody T, Kryscio R, et al. Autologous dendritic cell vaccines for non-small-cell lung cancer. J Clin Oncol 2004; 22(14):2808–2815.

139. Tsuruma T, Hata F, Torigoe T, et al. Phase I clinical study of anti-apoptosis protein, survivin-derived peptide vaccine therapy for patients with advanced or recurrent colorectal cancer. J Transl Med 2004; 2(1):19.

140. Wobser M, Keikavoussi P, Kunzmann V, et al. Complete remission of liver metastasis of pancreatic cancer under vaccination with a HLA-A2 restricted peptide derived from the universal tumor antigen survivin. Cancer Immunol Immunother 2006; 55(10)1294–1298.

141. Schwartz AL, Ciechanover A. The ubiquitin-proteasome pathway and pathogenesis of human diseases. Annu Rev Med 1999; 50:57–74.

142. Hershko A, Ciechanover A. The ubiquitin system. Annu Rev Biochem 1998; 67:425–479.

143. Adams J. The proteasome: a suitable antineoplastic target. Nat Rev Cancer 2004; 4(5):349–360.

144. Maffei A, Papadopoulos K, Harris PE. MHC class I antigen processing pathways. Hum Immunol 1997; 54(2):91–103.

145. Tsuruta F, Sunayama J, Mori Y, et al. JNK promotes Bax translocation to mitochondria through phosphorylation of 14-3-3 proteins. Embo J 2004; 23(8):1889–1899.
146. Adams J, Behnke M, Chen S, et al. Potent and selective inhibitors of the proteasome: dipeptidyl boronic acids. Bioorg Med Chem Lett 1998; 8(4):333–338.
147. Ling YH, Liebes L, Ng B, et al. PS-341, a novel proteasome inhibitor, induces Bcl-2 phosphorylation and cleavage in association with G2-M phase arrest and apoptosis. Mol Cancer Ther 2002; 1(10):841–849.
148. Mortenson MM, Schlieman MG, Virudachalam S, Bold RJ. Effects of the proteasome inhibitor bortezomib alone and in combination with chemotherapy in the A549 non-small-cell lung cancer cell line. Cancer Chemother Pharmacol 2004; 54(4):343–353.
149. Gumerlock P, Kimura T, Holland W, et al. Differential in vivo activity of docetaxel plus PS-341 combination therapy in non-small cell lung carcinoma (NSCLC) xenografts [abstr. 7144]. J Clin Oncol 2004; 22(14S):652s.
150. Aghajanian C, Soignet S, Dizon DS, et al. A phase I trial of the novel proteasome inhibitor PS341 in advanced solid tumor malignancies. Clin Cancer Res 2002; 8(8):2505–2511.
151. Stevenson J, Nho C, Johnson S, et al. Effects of bortezomib (PS-341) on NF-kB activation in peripheral blood mononuclear cells (PBMCs) of advanced non-small lung cancer (NSCLC) patients: a phase II/pharmacodynamic trial [abstr. 7145]. J Clin Oncol 2004; 22(14S):652s.
152. Fanucchi M, Fossella F, Fidias P, et al. Bortezomib ± docetaxel in previously treated patients with advanced non-small cell lung cancer (NSCLC): a phase 2 study [abstr. 7034]. J Clin Oncol 2005;23(16S):629s.
153. Appleman L, Ryan D, Clark J, et al. Phase I dose escalation study of bortezomib and gemcitabine safety and tolerability in patients with advanced solid tumors [abstr. 839]. Proc Am Soc Clin Oncol 2003; 22:209.
154. Ma C, Alberts S, Croghan G. A phase I trial of the proteasome inhibitor, PS-341 in combination with paclitaxel and carboplatin in patients with advanced cancer [abstr. 4009]. Proc Am Assoc Cancer Res 2004:45.
155. Davies A, McCoy J, Lara P, et al. Bortezomib + gemcitabine (Gem)/carboplatin (Carbo) results in encouraging survival in advanced non-small cell lung cancer (NSCLC): results of a phase II Southwest Oncology Group (SWOG) trial (S0339) [abstr. 7017]. J Clin Oncol 2006; 24(18S):368s.
156. Johl J, Chansky K, Lara P, et al. The proteasome inhibitor PS-341 (Bortezomib) in platinum (plat)-treated extensive-stage small cell lung cancer (E-SCLC): a SWOG (0327) phase II trial. J Clin Oncol 2005; 23(16S):632s.
157. Kirk C, Bennett M, Buchholz T, et al. Pharmacokinetics, pharmacodynamics and anti-tumor efficacy of PR-171, a novel inhibitor of the 20S proteasome [abstr. 609]. Blood 2005; 106(11).
158. Williams PG, Buchanan GO, Feling RH, et al. New cytotoxic salinosporamides from the marine actinomycete salinispora tropica. J Org Chem 2005; 70(16):6196–6203.
159. Chauhan D, Catley L, Li G, et al. A novel orally active proteasome inhibitor induces apoptosis in multiple myeloma cells with mechanisms distinct from Bortezomib. Cancer Cell 2005; 8(5):407–419.
160. Kandasamy K, Srivastava RK. Role of the phosphatidylinositol 3'-kinase/PTEN/ Akt kinase pathway in tumor necrosis factor-related apoptosis-inducing ligand-induced apoptosis in non-small cell lung cancer cells. Cancer Res 2002; 62(17): 4929–4937.

8

Lung Cancer Vaccines

Cheryl Ho

*Division of Medical Oncology, British Columbia Cancer Agency,
Vancouver, British Columbia, Canada*

Oliver Gautschi, Primo N. Lara, David R. Gandara, and Angela M. Davies

*University of California Davis Cancer Center, Sacramento,
California, U.S.A.*

INTRODUCTION

Lung cancer is the leading cause of cancer-related death, accounting for over 150,000 deaths per year in the United States alone (1). More than 70% of all lung-cancer patients present with advanced disease at the time of diagnosis, and although palliative treatment with conventional cytotoxic drugs and targeted therapies can prolong the survival, the overall median survival of 10 to 12 months remains poor. Many therapeutic strategies are being explored to improve this situation.

Cancer immunotherapy is a rapidly expanding experimental field that has made great progress in the last two decades based on the advances in immunology and molecular biology (2). Two retrospective clinical studies in the early 1970s suggested a link between lung cancer and the immune system, when the presence of a postoperative empyema was found to be associated with improved survival in patients with resected disease (3,4). Later studies failed to confirm these results. Nonspecific intrapleural immune stimulation trials were also negative, leading to a decline in interest in immunotherapy for lung cancer (5–7). In the 1990s, antibodies against autologous tumor proteins were found in sera of 50% to 75% of patients with lung cancer and were associated with improved survival (8). This

Table 1 Selected Antigen Targets for Lung Cancer Immunotherapy

Class	Name	Cancer expression	Function
Over-expressed antigens	EGFR (HER1) (9)	NSCLC (up to 60%), breast, colon, head, and neck	Regulator of proliferation, survival, and apoptosis
	HER2 (9)	NSCLC (up to 40%) and breast	Proto-oncogene with function similar to EGFR
	CEA (10)	NSCLC (60%), colon, and pancreas	Adhesion
	MUC1 (11) (episialin)	NSCLC (60%), breast, colon and ovary	Blocks adhesion
	Ep-CAM (12)	Lung (60%), gastric, colon, and prostate	Adhesion
	Gangliosides: fuc-GM1, GD3, polysialic acid, and others (13)	SCLC (60–100%)	Metastasis and angiogenesis
Mutant antigens	Mutp53 (14)	SCLC (90%), NSCLC (50%), and most other cancers	Tumor-suppressor gene, regulates cell-cycle, DNA-repair, and apoptosis
	MutK-RAS (15)	NSCLC (15–30%) and pancreas	Proto-oncogene, regulates MAP kinase pathway
Cancer testis antigens	MAGE-3 (16)	NSCLC (40%) and melanoma	Cell cycle control and apoptosis
	XAGE-1 (17)	NSCLC, prostate, melanoma, and Ewing's sarcoma	Similar to MAGE
	NY-ESO-1 (18)	Lung (10–30%), breast, esophagus, bladder, and melanoma	Unknown
	SSX-4 (19)	Lung (20%) and synovial sarcoma	Transcriptional repressors

Note: A definition for cancer testis antigens is provided in the paragraph on MAGE-3.
Abbreviations: CEA, carcinoembryonic antigen; EGFR, epidermal growth factor receptor; NSCLC, non–small cell lung cancer; SCLC, small cell lung cancer.

led to the exploration of multiple antigens for lung-cancer vaccination, including p53, K-Ras, epidermal growth factor (EGF) receptor (EGFR), HER2, MUC1, carcinoembryonic antigen (CEA), MAGE, XAGE-1, and others (Table 1). At the same time, T-cell lymphocytes were detected in tumor tissue [tumor-infiltrating lymphocytes, (TIL)], lymph nodes, and peripheral blood from lung cancer patients (20). It was shown that these lymphocytes are directed against lung cancer cells, but their activity is blocked by cancer-derived factors (21,22). Unlike melanoma and renal cell cancer, lung cancer harbors relatively few TIL. Nevertheless, these findings were consistent with the presence of spontaneous, but insufficient cancer-specific immune response in lung cancer patients, providing the rationale for thera-peutic strategies aimed at triggering or boosting this process. This review provides basic knowledge in cancer immunology and immunotherapy, summarizes recent clinical results with vaccines in lung cancer, and discusses the clinical implica-tions and perspectives.

CANCER IMMUNOLOGY

The human immune system is composed of innate (constitutive) and adaptive (acquired) immunity. Innate immunity is non–antigen-specific and consists of ana-tomical and physical barriers (skin, membranes, elevation of temperature, acid), phagocytic cells [natural killer (NK) cells and macrophages], and complement (23). Adaptive immunity is antigen-specific and consists of cellular (T-cells and B-cells) and humoral immunity (antibodies) (24). Both innate and adaptive immunity are dependent on cytokines secreted by cells of the immune system or by tumor cells and include interleukins (IL), interferons (IFNs), tumor-necrosis factors (TNFs), transforming growth factors, and colony-stimulating factors (CSFs) (25).

The adaptive immune system plays an important role in tumor recognition and control. T-cells are considered the most important effectors of tumor immu-nity, particularly the cytotoxic T-lymphocytes (CTL) and the NK T-cells (26). CTL can be activated by antigen-presenting tumor cells (direct priming) or by professional antigen-presenting cells (pAPC) such as dendritic cells (DCs) (cross-priming). DCs migrate to secondary lymphatic organs, including lymph nodes and spleen, where they present tumor antigen with major histocompatibility complex (MHC) class I molecules (Fig. 1). Thereby, DC can prime naive CD8+ CTL and induce antitumor immune response. Solid tumors express relatively low amounts of MHC class II and therefore tumor-antigen–specific CD4+ T-cells are exclusively induced by pAPC. CTL priming is improved by costimulatory mole-cules that are often provided by antigen-presenting cells (APCs), including B7, CD40, and chemokine receptors (CXCR and CCR) (27).

Burnet and Thomas formulated the hypothesis of immune-surveillance in malignancy whereby constantly arising malignant cells are eliminated by a highly effective immune system, and that clinically detectable tumors will only result if the malignant cells can escape immune surveillance (28,29). This hypothesis has been disputed in the last decade because patients under immunosuppression are not at an increased risk for most types of nonhematologic solid tumors (30). According to a modern hypothesis, malignancy develops only sporadically, and epithelial tumors develop because of immunological ignorance and evasion (26). Immunological ignorance of most solid tumors is a result of insufficient antigen-presentation in secondary lymphatic organs, and it has been demonstrated that antigen dose, localization, and persistence over time are important determinants of this process (Fig. 2) (31). Most solid tumors develop in peripheral epithelial tissue and deliver insufficient doses of tumor antigen to lymphatic organs in early

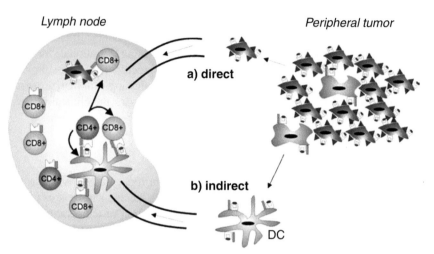

Figure 1 Induction of an antitumor CTL response. Naïve CD8+ T-cells are induced in secondary lymphoid organs either direct by tumor cells or indirect via by antigen cross-presenting professional antigen-presenting cells. Naïve CD4+ T-cells are also induced in secondary lymphoid organs; however, because most peripheral carcinomas and sarcomas are major-histocompatibility complex class II negative, only pAPCs are able to activate CD4+ T-cells. CD4+ T-cell activation provides direct help to CD8+ T-cells and, in most tumor models, CTL responses are dependent on the activation of helper T-cells. In addition, CD4+ T-cells provide signals to pAPC to induce their maturation. *Abbreviations*: CTL, cytotoxic T-lymphocytes; DC, dendritic cell; pAPCs, professional antigen-presenting cells. *Source*: From Ref. 26.

stages; only lymph-node metastasis in late stages may be sufficient to activate naïve T-cells in local lymph nodes. In addition, tumor cells can actively escape immune control by reduced expression of antigens, MHC molecules, and costimulatory factors, and by inhibition of both T-cell function (secretion of aspar-aginase and alterations in the Fas-signaling pathway) and DC function (produc-tion of nitric oxide, expression of Toll-like receptors, and upregulation of

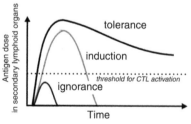

Figure 2 Antigen dose over time in secondary lymphoid organs determines the resulting CTL response (26). The *horizontal dotted line* determines the minimal amount of antigen necessary for the induction of a CTL response, threshold for CTL activation. *Abbreviation*: CTL, cytotoxic T-lymphocyte.

cyclooxygenase-2, leading to decrease of IL-10 and IFN-γ) (32). These mechanisms truly challenge the development of any effective immunotherapy in solid tumors including lung cancer.

CANCER IMMUNOTHERAPY

The term vaccination (Latin *vacca* = cow) originated from the injection of smallpox vaccine by Jenner in 1796, and it described a preparation that contains antigen in the form of killed, attenuated, or fragmented disease-causing organisms (33). Today, the terms "immunotherapy" and "vaccination" are used for almost any therapeutic intervention that activates the innate or adaptive immune system. One of the earliest documented cancer vaccines dates back to 1891, when William Coley, a young surgeon at the New York Memorial Hospital, discovered a patient with recurrent soft-tissue sarcoma, whose tumor had shrunk after erysipelas and who was healthy and tumor-free seven years after the infection (34). Coley suspected that the febrile infection was responsible for the cure of this patient, and he developed a vaccine from killed *Streptococcus pyogenes* and *Serratia marcensces*, which was used in hundreds of patients with sarcoma or carcinoma thereafter, with some reported success. Later studies identified that Coley's vaccine stimulated the immune response through the innate pathway (35).

In the 1980s, the tuberculosis vaccine Bacille Calmette-Guerin (BCG), containing live attenuated *Mycobacterium bovis,* activating the immune system in a similar way as Coley's vaccine, showed activity against superficial bladder cancer (36). At the same time, IL-2 was tested in patients with metastatic melanoma and renal-cell cancer, and tumor regressions were reported in 15% to 20% (37). These encouraging results prompted a plethora of new studies for cancer immunotherapy.

Most of today's cancer vaccine strategies are considered therapeutic. Preventive vaccines, classically directed against microorganisms causing cancer, such as *Human papilloma virus* and *Helicobacter pylori*, are important exceptions (38,39). Therapeutic vaccinations are currently being developed in lung cancer with different strategies (Table 2) (40). General immune stimulation is obtained by adjuvants such as BCG, keyhole limpet hemocyanin (KLH), and bacterial lipopolysaccharides. Specific immune stimulation includes vaccines directed against tumor antigens, idiotypes, and tumor cells and DC vaccines and DNA vaccines. Antigen vaccines make use of tumor-specific antigens such as proteins or synthetic peptides, which are processed and presented by DC. Anti-idiotype vaccines use tumor cell-binding antibodies that act as antigens themselves. DC vaccines use DC that are loaded with antigen ex vivo and then reinjected to induce immune response. DNA vaccines can encode for antigens or for cytokines that stimulate antigen production and immune response. Tumor-cell vaccines use irradiated cancer cells that are injected into the patient. Although these tumor cells are unable to proliferate, the antigens are still recognized by the immune system. Individual cytokines, including IL-2, IFN-α, and granulocyte-macrophage CSF (GM-CSF), are often used to boost the active immune reaction.

Table 2   Approaches to Lung Cancer Immunotherapy

Categories of vaccine design[a]	Characteristics	Examples	Determinants
Intent	Prophylactic	Antinicotine vaccine (41)	Knowledge of causative agent, precancerous antigen, or cancer antigen
	Therapeutic	Antigen vaccine (42)	
Immune response	Nonspecific	Bacille Calmette-Guerin (43)	Knowledge of tumor antigen, efficient antigen presentation, and T-cell activation
	Specific	Dendritic cell (44)	
Immunity	Passive (antibody)	Cetuximab (45)	Availability of effective anti-tumor antibody or antigen-based vaccination protocol
	Active (antigen)	Antigen vaccine (42)	
Active component	Noncellular	Tumor antigen (46)	Ability to induce immune response by antigen injection or generation of anticancer T-cells
	Cellular	Cytotoxic T-lymphocytes or dendritic cells injection	
Material	Tumor antigen	MUC1 (47–49)	Availability of autologous tumor cells, tumor-specific peptides, efficient gene transfer methods, and carriers
	Allogenic tumor cells	Adenocarcinoma cell lines (50)	
	Autologous tumor cells	Irradiated cryopreserved cells (51)	
	DNA	Adenoviral IL-2 (49)	

[a]Categories are not exclusive and can overlap.

NON–SMALL CELL LUNG CANCER

Multiple vaccines have been created for the treatment of non–small cell lung cancer (NSCLC) (Table 3). In the sections below, vaccines have been categorized according to their immunologic target: non–antigen-specific, tumor antigen–specific, cell-based, allogenic tumor cell- and autologous tumor cell-based vaccines.

Non–Antigen Specific Vaccines

SRL 172 (*Mycobacterium vaccae*) Vaccine

M. vaccae is an environmental saprophyte that is nonpathogenic in humans. It has been evaluated for use in the treatment of tuberculosis, asthma, and cancer because of its immune modulating properties. Vaccination with SRL 172, a suspension of heat-killed *M. vaccae*, results in activation of APC, NK cells and increased helper T-cell 1 (Th1) activity. Th1 cytokines, including TNF-α, IFN-γ,

Table 3 Non–Small Cell Lung Cancer Vaccine Trials

Vaccine type	Vaccine trial	Patient population	Number of patients	Clinical outcome
Non–antigen specific	SRL 172 with mitomycin, vinblastin, cisplatin (MVP) (52); phase III	Stage IIIB–IV; untreated	419	Response: MVP 33%: MVP + vaccine 37% NS Median survival: MVP 225 days; MVP + vaccine 223 days NS
Tumor antigen–based	MAGE 3 (42); phase II	Stage I and II; surgical resection	17	—
	MAGE 3 dexosome (53); phase I	Stage IIIA–IV; previously treated	13	Response: SD 30.1%
	Epidermal growth factor (54); pilot study	Stage IIIB–IV; previously treated	40	Response: SD 30%; median survival: 8.17 mo
	MUC1 (47); phase II	Stage IIIB–IV; one prior line of therapy	171	Median survival: best supportive care 13 mo; vaccine 17.4 mo NS
	Multi-epitope (55); phase I	Stage IIB–IIIA resected NSCLC; stage III resected colon cancer	Ongoing	—
Cell based	Dendritic cell (DC) with CEA652 (44); pilot study	Stage IV GI or NSCLC (13 GI, 5 NSCLC); previously treated	18	Response: SD 22%
	DC with irradiated 1650 cells (56); pilot study	Stage IA–IIIB; treated with curative intent	16	—

(Continued)

Table 3 Non–Small Cell Lung Cancer Vaccine Trials (*Continued*)

Vaccine type	Vaccine trial	Patient population	Number of patients	Clinical outcome
Cell based (*cont.*)	B7.1 HLA-A gene modified allogenic adenocarcinoma cell line (50); phase I	Stage IIIB–IV, recurrent; previously treated	19	Response: PR 5%; SD 26%
	A 1,3 galactosyltransferase expressing allogenic tumor cell line (57); phase I	Stage IIIB–IV; previously treated	Ongoing	—
	Autologous tumor cell with Bacille Calmette-Guerin (58); pilot study	Resected NSCLC	18	—
	Autologous tumor cell transfected with granulocyte-macrophage colony-stimulating factors containing adenovirus (59); phase I	Stage IV; previously treated	38 Enrolled; 34 received treatment	Response: mixed response 3%; SD 15%
	Autologous tumor cell with bystander GVAX (51); phase I/II	Stage IV; previously treated	86 Enrolled; 49 received treatment	Response: SD 14%

Abbreviations: GI, gastrointestinal; GVAX, GM-CSF vaccine; NS, nonsignificant; NSCLC, non–small cell lung cancer; SD, stable disease.

IL-1, and IL-2, activate cell-mediated immunity, stimulate macrophages, recruit leukocytes, and generate inflammation. Th1 and Th2 are feedback regulators of each other; consequently, SRL 172 vaccination also causes downregulation of Th2 antibody—mediated immunity. In malignancies, a predominance of the Th2 cytokine profile has been observed; SRL 172 may help restore the normal Th1 and Th2 balance. SRL 172 vaccination has been evaluated in prostate cancer and melanoma with evidence of an immunologic response. The combination of SRL 172 with chemotherapy has been hypothesized to improve delivery of the drug to the tumor because of architectural disruption generated by the immunological response.

A randomized phase II trial of SRL 172 in combination with chemotherapy was conducted in previously untreated patients with stage III to IV NSCLC or mesothelioma (60). Patients were randomized to chemotherapy (mitomycin, vinblastine, cisplatin every three weeks, maximum six cycles), with or without SRL 172 vaccine. SRL 172 was administered intradermally monthly × 3 then every three to six months thereafter. Twenty-nine patients were enrolled: 20 with NSCLC and, 9 with mesothelioma. The response rate to chemotherapy alone was 33% and with vaccine, 53% ($P=0.3$). The median survival demonstrated a trend toward improvement with SRL 172: 7.5 months versus 9.4 months ($P=0.3$). The vaccine was well tolerated.

A subsequent open-label, randomized phase III trial was conducted in patients with stage III to IV NSCLC (52). Using the same treatment randomization as the phase II, over 400 patients were enrolled with the primary endpoint of overall survival. There was no improvement in survival: chemotherapy alone 225 days versus chemotherapy with vaccine 223 days ($P=0.65$) nor progression-free survival. The response rates were also similar: 33% versus 37%, respectively ($P=0.413$). Mild injection-site reactions occurred in 17% of the SRL 172– vaccinated patients. The quality-of-life (QOL) questionnaire (QLQ), European Organisation for Research and Treatment of Cancer (EORTC) QLQ-C30, indicated an improvement with vaccine after the 15-week treatment phase with improvement in the performance status, treatment-related adverse events and cancer-related symptoms.

Tumor Antigen–Based Vaccines

MAGE-3 Vaccine

MAGE-3 belongs to the class of cancer testis (CT) antigens. CT antigens are defined by the following characteristics: predominant expression in gametogenic tissues and cancer, coding genes frequently mapping to chromosome X and existing as multigene families, immunogenic in cancer patients, heterogeneous protein expression in cancer, and in vitro activation by hypomethylation and/or histone deacetylase inhibition (61). The function of CT antigens is not fully understood, but their overexpression in lung cancer correlates with poor prognosis (62). MAGE-3 was originally described in melanoma; however, the antigen has also been identified in 40% of NSCLC. MAGE-3 has multiple epitopes recognized by cytotoxic T-cells, ideal for inducing an immune response.

In a small pilot study, 17 patients with MAGE-3-expressing resected stage I or II NSCLC were enrolled (42). The first nine patients were vaccinated with 300 µg of MAGE-3 protein intradermally, every three weeks for four injections. The remaining eight patients received four injections intramuscularly every three weeks with MAGE-3 and AS02B adjuvant, containing monophosphoryl lipid A and QS21, a saponin extracted from the *Quillaja saponaria* Molina tree, to stimulate immune response. The investigators evaluated immune response to vaccination by antibody titres, CD4+ and CD8+ T-cell response. Modest MAGE-3 antibody titres were seen in three of nine patients treated with MAGE-3 alone compared to marked increases in seven of eight patients who were vaccinated with MAGE-3 plus the AS02B adjuvant. One patient in the MAGE-3 alone vaccinated group and four of the MAGE-3 with AS02B treated patients demonstrated a strong CD4+ T-cell response to the MAGE-3 DP4 peptide (amino acid 243–258). Measurement of associated cytokines indicated an increase in TNF-α, IFN-γ, and IL-2 following exposure to activated T-cell APCs, consistent with a Th1 predominant response. MAGE-3 alone was able to elicit an immune response in vaccinated NSCLC patients however; the addition of the AS02B adjuvant clearly enhanced the immunogenicity of the tumor antigen.

Further studies have evaluated other mechanisms to augment the immune reaction to MAGE-3, including the use of dexosomes loaded with MAGE tumor antigens. Dexosomes represent lipid vesicles released by DC and have the ability to act as antigen-presenting bodies to CD4+ and CD8+ T-cells. DC process antigens and form MHC-Ag complexes that are released in the circulation with immunostimulatory factors via dexosomes. The circulating dexosomes transfer the MHC-peptide complex to naïve DC, thereby amplifying the immune response.

A phase I trial in chemotherapy-treated, unresectable stage III to IV NSCLC patients was conducted with MAGE-Ag loaded dexosomes (53). Autologous dexosomes were harvested; patients underwent leukopheresis, DC were cultured, the supernatant was harvested, and dexosomes were extracted. Dexosomes were loaded with MAGE-Ag directly, by addition of MAGE-Ag on the extracted dexosomes or indirectly, and the MAGE-Ag were placed on the cultured DCs prior to harvest. Patients received both a subcutaneous and an intradermal injection weekly for four treatments. Thirteen patients were enrolled, nine completed therapy of which six achieved stable disease. Delayed type hypersensitivity (DTH) to MAGE tumor–associated peptides was noted in three of nine patients. Two of these patients had stable disease as their best response. All formulations of the vaccine were well tolerated with the most common toxicity being injection-site reaction. Phase II studies are planned for this vaccine in advanced NSCLC.

Epidermal Growth–Factor Vaccine

EGFR (EGFR, HER1) is a member of the HER/erbB family of transmembrane receptors that also includes HER2/neu, HER3, and HER4. Ligand binding prompts homo- and heterodimerization, leading to autophosphorylation and the production of second messengers. Downstream effects of EGFR activation include cell proliferation, differentiation, and angiogenesis (63). EGFR is expressed in a number of solid tumors including NSCLC, breast, colon, prostate, head and neck (64) and is associated with a poor prognosis (65). Vaccines have been developed targeting one of the key EGFR ligands, EGF, preventing ligand receptor binding and the associated downstream signaling cascade.

Data from two pilot EGF vaccines were pooled for evaluation of safety and immunogenicity (54). Both trials were open-label, randomized studies in patients with previously treated advanced stage NSCLC. In the first study, patients were vaccinated with EGF-P64K adsorbed to alum ($n=10$) or emulsified in montanide ISA 51 ($n=10$). P64K is a *Neisseria meningitides* recombinant protein that acts as an immunologic carrier protein for weak immunogens. In the second trial, the same vaccines were used however; patients were treated with a single dose of cyclophosphamide 200 mg/m^2 three days prior to each vaccination ($n=20$) to stimulate immune response. Higher anti-EGF antibodies were noted with the montanide ISA 51 and pretreatment with cyclophosphamide. Twelve of 40 patients had radiographic stable disease after six months. The median survival was eight months. Good EGF antibody responders (titre >1:4000, or eightfold increase over baseline) had a better median survival, 9.1 months, compared to poor antibody responders, 4.5 months. Reactions to the vaccine were mild with no evidence of severe clinical toxicity. A phase II trial is underway comparing this vaccine with best supportive care (BSC) in advanced disease.

MUC1 Vaccine

MUC1 is an epithelial-associated mucin glycoprotein that is involved in cell adhesion. This cell-surface protein is overexpressed and aberrantly glycosylated in multiple malignancies including breast, lung, stomach, pancreas, ovary, and prostate cancers, making it an excellent target for vaccine immunotherapy. Approximately 60% of NSCLC are positive for MUC1.

Butts et al. conducted a randomized phase II trial of BLP25 liposome vaccine in stage IIIB and IV NSCLC patients treated with one prior line of systemic therapy (47). The L-BLP25 vaccine consisted of BLP25 lipopeptide, immunoadjuvant monophosphoryl lipid A and three lipids, forming a liposome. The vaccine was administered weekly for eight weeks, followed by maintenance vaccination every six weeks at the investigators discretion. The vaccination was preceded by three days with cyclophosphamide 300 mg/m^2 to augment the effects of immunotherapy. Patients ($n=171$) were randomized to BSC versus BSC plus vaccine. There was trend toward improved median survival in the vaccine arm, 17.4 months versus 13 months ($P=0.066$). In a subgroup analysis, the stage IIIB locoregional disease patients appeared to achieve the greatest survival benefit, adjusted hazard ratio 0.5237, although the results were not statistically significant ($P=0.0692$). The QOL analysis using the Functional Assessment of Cancer—Lung indicated an advantage for the L-BLP25 arm. The most common adverse events associated with vaccination were flu-like symptoms, injection-site reactions, and nausea related to the cyclophosphamide treatment. Future trials are being planned to evaluate the role of maintenance L-BLP25 vaccine in stage III disease.

A second vaccine designed to target MUC1 involves the use of a highly attenuated recombinant Vaccinia virus expressing MUC1 and IL-2 (TG4010) (55). Phase I studies of this vaccine in MUC1-expressing solid tumors demonstrated good tolerability with some evidence of efficacy. Squiban et al. are currently conducting a randomized phase II trial comparing cisplatin/vinorelbine with TG4010 versus upfront TG4010 alone followed by the addition of cisplatin/vinorelbine at disease progression in advanced NSCLC (IIIB and IV).

Multi-Epitope Vaccine

Malignant cells aberrantly express cell-surface markers that can be used to design tumor-associated antigen vaccines. Two epitopes from CEA, p53, HER2/neu, and MAGE-2/3 were selected to develop the EP 2101 vaccine (66). Eight epitopes were combined with CAP1-6D, the pan DR epitope (PADRE) helper T-epitope and emulsified in montanide ISA 51. CAP1-6D is a CEA epitope that stimulates cytotoxic T-cells and PADRE is a synthetic, non-natural pan HLA-DR-binding epitope that binds with high or intermediate affinity to the most common human leukocyte antigen-DR (HLA-DR) types. Patients with resected stage IIB/IIIA NSCLC and stage III colon cancer following standard treatment were eligible to receive six vaccines of EP 2101 at three weekly intervals. Preliminary data indicate that the vaccine is safe and well tolerated. Cytotoxic T-cell response, as measured by the IFN-γ Elispot assay, was observed in the majority of patients. Data on the efficacy of this vaccine are not available, but vaccination against multiple epitopes and antigens may have a promising therapeutic potential.

Cell-Based Vaccines

DC Vaccines

DCs are pAPCs that can prime and activate CTLs. Lung cancers are commonly characterized by a lack of tumor antigen presentation that DC vaccines attempt to overcome.

Ueda et al. evaluated a cancer vaccine composed of autologous DC and HLA-A24-restricted CEA-derived peptide (44). CEA is a 180 kDa glycoprotein adhesion molecule that is involved in metastasis and is expressed in over 60% of NSCLC. The vaccine was developed with CEA652, a 9 amino acid peptide that is a potent HLA-A24-restricted CTL epitope. Patients with HLA-A24-positive, stage IV, CEA-positive, gastrointestinal (GI) or lung adenocarcinoma were enrolled. Patients underwent cell mobilization by recombinant human granulocyte-CSF (G-CSF) and leukopheresis. Peripheral blood mononuclear cells were cultured with G-CSF and IL-4, growth factors for nonproliferating CD14+ progenitor cells for DC, then exposed to CEA652 for four hours. The cells were then washed and prepared as a cell suspension for the vaccine. The vaccine was administered subcutaneously every two weeks for a minimum of five vaccinations. Five patients with NSCLC and 13 with GI malignancies were enrolled in the trial. No responses were seen. Three patients with NSCLC had decreases in serum CEA levels and four patients had stable disease. Patients were evaluated for DTH to CEA652-pulsed DC prior to the first injection and after the fifth treatment. Three of 11 patients demonstrated DTH (two with NSCLC) indicating an immune response. The vaccine was well tolerated.

A second autologous DC vaccine was evaluated in stage IA to IIIB NSCLC patients treated surgically with curative intent (56). Patients underwent leukopheresis and DC was isolated using a CD14+ magnetic bead protocol. G-CSF and IL-4–stimulated DC were exposed to an apoptosed, lethally irradiated adenocarcinoma cell line (1650) that overexpressed several tumor antigens including HER-2/neu, CEA, MAGE-2, WT-1, and survivin. Sixteen patients received a vaccine prime followed by a boost one month later. Six patients demonstrated a minor Ag-specific reaction to 1650 Ag however; the immune response did not correlated with the clinical outcome, five patients had recurrent or progressive disease. The toxicities were minimal, with self-limited wheal and flare skin reaction after immunization being most common.

Allogenic Tumor Cells

B7.1 HLA-A Gene Modified Allogenic Adenocarcinoma Cell Line

B7.1 (CD80) is a transmembrane protein that provides regulatory signals to T-lymphocytes. It is expressed on APCs and interacts with costimulatory receptors CD28 and CTL-associated antigen 4 (CTLA-4) expressed on T-cells. Binding of CD28 results in upregulation of T-cell activity, associated with increased proliferation, cytokine production, and lack of tolerance induction. In contrast, CTLA-4 binding promotes T-cell suppression and induction of anergy. Tumor cells demonstrate downregulation of B7.1; it has been hypothesized that expression of B7.1 may facilitate generation of an immune response to tumor cells. Immune stimulation by B7.1 may be augmented by the coexpression of HLA-A class I antigens that activate CD8+ cytotoxic T-cells.

A phase I trial was conducted in selected stage IIIB, IV, and recurrent NSCLC patients using a B7.1 HLA-A vaccine with allogenic lung-tumor cells (50). A human lung adenocarcinoma cell line, AD100, was transfected with plasmid cDNA containing B7.1 and HLA-A1 or HLA-A2. Transfected AD100 cells were irradiated and administered intradermally every two weeks for three vaccinations. Patients who were HLA-A1 or HLA-A2 positive received the appropriately matched vaccine and if HLA-A1 and HLA-A2 negative, received HLA-A1 transfected vaccine. Of the 19 patients enrolled, 1 had a partial response, 5 had stable disease, and 13 had progression. The median survival was 18 months; longer than anticipated considering that all had prior treatment; 89% had prior chemotherapy and 50% had two or greater prior regimens. The vaccine was well tolerated with the most common toxicity being discomfort or erythema at the injection site. Immune response to vaccination was evaluated using an immunospot assay for IFN-γ, a marker of cytotoxic T-cell response. Seventeen patients were evaluated and 16 had a measurable increase in CD8 response after three vaccinations. A phase I/II study is currently being conducted to evaluate the role of allogenic vaccination with a B7.1 HLA-A gene-modified adenocarcinoma cell line in early stage NSCLC.

α1,3 Galactosyltransferase-Expressing Allogenic Tumor Cell Vaccine

Transplantation of mammalian tissues to humans results in rejection due to the presence of foreign cell-surface markers. In mammals, α1,3 galactosyltransferase adds sugar moieties to cell-membrane proteins and lipids. Humans have pre-existing anti-α gal antibodies that represent up to 1% of serum IgG. Recognizing that glycosylation by this enzyme mediates hyperacute rejection in xenografts, researchers have modified tumor cell lines to express immunogenic α1,3 galactosyltransferase.

A phase I study was conducted in NSCLC patients with a vaccine preparation containing three irradiated, genetically altered human lung cancer cell lines (HAL 1, 2, 3) containing murine α1,3 galactosyltransferase. This modification resulted in the expression of xenotransplantation antigens (HyperAcute Lung Cancer Vaccine™) (57). According to a preliminary report, of the first seven patients enrolled, four patients showed evidence of stable disease above 16 weeks. There were no severe toxicities associated with administration of the vaccine; grade 2 or lesser discomfort of injection site discomfort, local skin reaction, fatigue, and hypertension were reported. This study is ongoing through the National Cancer Institute (NCI) with a planned phase II component.

Autologous Tumor Cells

Autologous Tumor BCG Vaccine

BCG is a vaccine derived from attenuated live bovine tuberculosis bacillus, *M. bovis*. As a recognized immunomodulator, it causes increased expression of cytokines and mediators of inflammation. BCG has a long history in the treatment of lung cancer. It has been evaluated as adjuvant, intrapleural therapy for resected NSCLC with and without chemotherapy (6,67–70). No survival advantage was seen with intrapleural therapy. Intratumoral injection prior to resection has also been assessed. However, again there were no survival benefits observed although these studies were not powered to determine survival differences (71).

BCG has been evaluated in vaccine format, 18 patients with resected NSCLC received three weekly intradermal injections of 10^7 irradiated, cryopreserved, autologous NSCLC tumor cells and 10^7 BCG, one to three months after surgical resection or completion of radiotherapy (58). Thirteen evaluable patients developed delayed cutaneous reaction (DCR) to autologous tumor cells. Over half of the patients (*10*) had relapsed after a median follow follow-up of 17 months, including 7 patients who had a positive DCR. This vaccine is not being developed further although it has been suggested that the lack of benefit may have been related to the vaccine preparation.

GM-CSF Vaccine

The immune system fails to mount a response to tumor cells for multiple reasons: tolerance, suboptimal antigen presentation, imbalance of Th1 and Th2, and lack of cytokine stimulation. GM-CSF, a human cytokine, stimulates the growth and production of neutrophils, macrophages, and DCs and enhances the functional activity of mature cells, encouraging effective immune responses.

Salgia et al. conducted a phase I trial of an autologous tumor GM-CSF vaccine (GVAX) in patients with metastatic NSCLC (59). Accessible metastases were resected and processed to a single-cell suspension. Cells were cultured, infected with a replication-defective adenovirus encoding human GM-CSF, and irradiated in preparation for vaccine administration. Patients received an intradermal vaccination weekly for three weeks followed by every two weeks until the vaccine was depleted. Thirty-eight patients were enrolled; tumor tissue was obtained for 35 patients and a successful vaccine was created for 34 patients. Five patients had stable disease and one patient had a mixed response with regression of the primary tumor and lymph-node metastasis but development of a metastatic bone lesion. One patient with bronchioloalveolar carcinoma (BAC), who underwent three resections and had no evidence of disease at enrollment, remained disease-free 42 months later.

A second trial with the same autologous GVAX platform was performed by Nemunaitis et al. (48). Two cohorts of patients were enrolled: an early stage cohort (cohort A) with stage IB/II NSCLC and an advanced stage cohort (cohort B) with previously treated stage III and IV disease. Intradermal injections of vaccine were administered every two weeks for three to six vaccinations. Eighty-three patients had tumor harvested and 43 initiated vaccine therapy (cohort A, 10 and cohort B, 33). With a median follow-up of 20 months, 6 patients in cohort A have had recurrence. Among the patients who received vaccination in cohort B, the median progression-free survival was four months and the median overall survival, 12 months. Of interest, two patients with BAC in the advanced-stage cohort achieved a complete response. It has been hypothesized that this unique histological subtype of NSCLC may be more amenable to immunologic therapy than other variants of NSCLC because of a possible retroviral etiology with parallels being drawn between BAC and a retroviral-associated pulmonary disease in sheep—Jaagsietke (72,73). Based on the promise of this approach, the Southwest Oncology Group (S0310) has conducted a phase II trial of GVAX (CG8123) in patients with advanced BAC. This trial has just completed accrual and the results are anticipated in 2007.

In an effort to potentiate the effect of the vaccine, low-dose immunomodulatory cyclophosphamide has been added to GVAX therapy. A randomized phase II trial was conducted using GVAX, (CG8123) with or without cyclophosphamide (74). Although there was a trend to of improved outcomes with the addition of cyclophosphamide, it was not statistically significant and there was no improvement in progression-free survival (3.8 months without vs. 5 months with cyclophosphamide), or overall survival (5.4 months vs. 9.6 months).

Because of the challenges of an autologous vaccine platform, a "bystander GVAX" was also developed. Bystander GVAX consists of K562, a human erythroleukemia cell line, transfected with a GM-CSF containing bacterial plasmid (CG9962). In a phase I/II trial, metastatic NSCLC tumor cells were harvested and processed to a single-cell suspension (51). Autologous irradiated tumor cells were combined with CG9962 in a 2:1 ratio to generate the final vaccine; five dose levels were evaluated. Patients received an intradermal vaccination every two weeks for a total of 3 to 12 injections. Eight-six patients were enrolled and 49 proceeded to vaccine treatment. There were no responders. Seven patients had stable disease for a minimum of 12 weeks. Antibodies to autologous tumor were noted in 31% of the patients. DTH evaluated at zero weeks and four weeks were positive in 13% and 34% of patients, respectively. The immune endpoints did not correlate with the clinical endpoints of progression-free and overall survival. The vaccine was well tolerated with the most common side effects being injection-site reaction, fatigue, dyspnea, nausea, and fever. Although a bystander vaccine platform is more appealing from a practical standpoint, it was not developed further because of lack of efficacy. Although the autologous GVAX platform demonstrated preliminary efficacy, the challenges of this platform necessitated abandoning further development in lung cancer.

SMALL-CELL LUNG CANCER

Small-cell lung cancer (SCLC) is a distinct immunologic entity from NSCLC, with the expression of different cell-surface markers and proteins. The following section divides vaccines developed against SCLC based on their target: non–antigen-specific, tumor antigen–specific, and cell-based therapies (Table 4).

Non–Antigen Specific Vaccines
SRL 172 (*M. vaccae*) Vaccine

SRL 172, as a nonspecific immunologic adjuvant, was evaluated in SCLC in combination with chemotherapy. Previously untreated limited and extensive stage patients were randomized to chemotherapy alone or with SRL 172 vaccine (75). Chemotherapy was delivered at three weekly intervals for a maximum of six cycles and was either platinum based; (mitomycin, vinblastine, and cisplatin) or anthracycline based (doxorubicin, cyclophosphamide, and etoposide). The vaccination was delivered prior to the first chemotherapy followed by three monthly injections and then every three to six months thereafter. Twenty-eight patients were enrolled in the trial. The response rate with chemotherapy alone and with vaccine was identical, 57%. Although not powered for survival, the median survival showed a trend toward improvement with SRL 172, 12.9 months versus

Table 4 Small-Cell Lung Cancer Vaccine Trials

Vaccine type	Vaccine trial	Patient population	Number of patients	Clinical outcome
Non–antigen specific	SRL 172 with mitomycin, vinblastin, cisplatin (MVP) (75); phase II	Limited or extensive; untreated	28	RR MVP 57%: MVP + vaccine 57% Median survival: MVP 8.6 mo; MVP + vaccine 12.9 mo NS
Tumor antigen–based	Polysialic acid with keyhole limpet hemocyanin (76); pilot study	Limited or extensive; completed first-line therapy	13	—
	GM1 with keyhole limpet hemocyanin (77); pilot study	Limited or extensive; completed first-line therapy	16	—
	BEC2 (78); phase III	Limited; completed first-line therapy	515	Median survival: best supportive care 16.4 mo; vaccine 14.3 mo NS
Cell based	DC transduced with p53 (79); phase II	Extensive; completed first-line therapy	Ongoing	—

Abbreviations: NS, non significant; RR, response rate.

8.6 months ($P = 0.10$). The vaccine did not result in additive toxicity. A phase III trial is currently ongoing, evaluating the role of SRL 172 in limited and extensive SCLC in combination with chemotherapy.

Tumor Antigen–Based Vaccines

Polysialic Acid

The combination of polysialic acid (polySA) and KLH has been explored in SCLC. Polysialic acid contains more than 20 sialic acid residues. It modulates neural cell adhesion and exists as a polymer in embryonal tissues but is found in oligo form in adults. This large, negatively charged molecule interferes with neural cell adhesion and promotes cell motility. PolySA is also found on the surface of gram-negative bacteria including group B meningococcus. *N*-propionylation of polySA (NP polySA) boosts IgG response. There are limited amounts of polySA expressed in normal tissues (primarily the brain) however; it is overexpressed in

SCLC, rendering it a good target for immunotherapy. KLH is found in the hemo-lymph of *Megathura crenulata*, a sea mollusk. It is a copper-containing glyco-protein that is immunostimulatory and has been used to promote immune response in multiple vaccines.

A pilot study of polySA conjugated with KLH was conducted in SCLC. Patients with limited or advanced SCLC received either polySA-KLH or NP polySA-KLH vaccine 4 to 12 weeks after completing their initial therapy (76). The vaccination schedule was weekly for four treatments followed by an injection at 8 and 16 weeks. Thirteen patients were enrolled in the study; eight progressed within one to five months; two with limited-stage disease, and six with extensive-stage disease. Immunoglobulin (Ig)M and IgG titers for antibodies against polySA or NP polySA were notably higher in the latter group. The vaccine was associated with injection-site pain, swelling, erythema, fatigue, and flu-like symptoms. The immune response mounted against NP polySA suggests that it may be an appropriate addition to a polyvalent vaccine against SCLC.

GM1

KLH has also been conjugated to fucosylated monosialoganglioside GM1 (fuc-GM1) in the development of a SCLC vaccine (77). Fuc-GM1 is a carbohy-drate antigen present on SCLC cells but absent on most normal tissues. Low levels have been detected in small round cells of the thymus, spleen, small intestine, and pancreatic islet cells. Similar to the previous trial with KLH, patients with limited or advanced SCLC were vaccinated with fuc-GM1 conjugated with KLH, 4 to 12 weeks after initial treatment. Intradermal immunizations occurred on week 1, 2, 3, 4, 8, and 16. Interpatient dose escalation of 3, 10, and 30 µg was planned to determine the lowest effective dose needed to generate an antibody response. Sixteen patients were enrolled and no responses were observed; nine patients had a recurrence and four patients were free of disease after 18 months of follow-up, three were lost to follow-up. Antibody titers were measured using enzyme-linked immunosorbent assay (ELISA) and fluorescence-activated cell sorting. Patient sera was added to human SCLC cell line DMS 79 and incubated with a fluores-cent labeled antihuman IgM or IgG and evaluated using flow cytometry. Eight of 11 patients at the 10 and 30 µg dose had IgM titer 1:80 or above and 10 of 11 had an increase in the percentage of DMS 79 cells positive. The IgG responses were less robust. Not all of the patients at the 3 µg vaccine level had a significant increase in IgM or IgG, suggesting that the higher doses are better at eliciting an immune response. The fuc-GM1-KLH antigen is also planned to be a component of a polyvalent vaccine designed for treatment of SCLC.

BEC2

BEC2 is a mouse IgG2b anti-idiotypic antibody that is similar in structure to GD3. GD3 is a glycosphingolipid expressed on the cell surface of SCLC in addition to cells of neuroectodermal origin and a subset of T-lymphocytes. BCG was included in the vaccine as a nonspecific immune stimulant. Two trials were conducted using the xenogenic BEC2-BCG vaccine in limited SCLC. The vaccination schedule involved an intradermal injection at week 0, 2, 4, 6, and 10. The first trial enrolled 15 patients who had a partial or complete response after first line therapy for SCLC (78). The median time to relapse was 10.6 months with a median overall survival of 20.5 months. The longest relapse-free intervals were seen in the patients who developed detectable anti-GD3 IgG antibodies ($n=3$). All patients evaluated ($n=13$) developed IgM anti-GD3 antibodies. The associated adverse events included grade 1 fevers and local skin reaction. Of note, 14 patients had grade 3 local skin toxicity including pain, induration, and ulceration. This was attributed to the BCG administration and was less severe with lower doses of BCG.

This pilot study led to a randomized phase III trial of BEC2-BCG in limited stage SCLC (80). Patients who had a complete or partial response after concurrent chemoradiotherapy were randomized to five vaccinations with BEC2-BCG vaccine or follow-up. Prophylactic cranial irradiation (PCI) was recommended but optional. Patients were stratified by performance status, response, and institution. The primary endpoint was to detect an increase in median survival of 40%. Over 500 patients were enrolled in the study over a 4.5-year period. The results were disappointing; the median progression-free survival was not statistically significantly different nor was the overall survival; 16.4 months in the observation arm and 14.3 months in the vaccination arm, hazard ratio 1.12 ($P=0.2834$). Humoral response was measured by GD3 ELISA in 213 patients; 142 did not mount a response and 72 had a positive response. In subgroup analysis, humoral responders showed a trend toward improved survival: 19.2 months versus 13.9 months ($P=0.0851$). However, this result must be interpreted with caution because more patients in the responder group received PCI. Skin reaction was the most commonly reported toxicity and 36% of patients had toxicity of grade 3 or above. Fever, arthralgias, and lethargy were also observed. QOL, as determined using the EORTC-QOL-C30 version 3 and lung module QLC-LC13 questionnaires, was not different between the two groups. The authors have suggested several reasons for the failure of this trial, including poor choice of vaccine adjuvant and expression of GD3 in only 60% of SCLC tissues. Similar to previous trials in SCLC, the investigators advocate a multivalent vaccine for treatment of SCLC.

Cell-Based Vaccines

DC Vaccine

Autologous DC vaccines for immunostimulation have been evaluated in SCLC. In a phase II trial, patients with extensive SCLC were treated with first-line chemotherapy and then underwent leukopheresis (79). DCs were harvested and infected with an adenovirus containing wild type p53 (ADVEXIN) because mutant p53 is frequently overexpressed in SCLC. Patients received three intradermal vaccinations and if they demonstrated a response or stable disease, they went on to receive three further doses. This study is ongoing and to date 22 patients have been enrolled. Five patients had stable disease after three treatments. Of 20 patients tested, 11 demonstrated significant immunological response to vaccination as determined by p53 Elispot and staining with tetramers. There were no significant toxicities. Of the 17 patients who went on to have second-line therapy, 13 were evaluable for response. Seven patients responded to second-line chemotherapy (53.8%). The investigators have hypothesized that the DC-p53 vaccine may sensitize SCLC tumors to subsequent chemotherapy, which has yet to be demonstrated by further studies.

CONCLUSION

Cancer immunotherapy is an expanding experimental field that has made great progress in the last two decades due to advances in immunology and molecular biology (2). An increased understanding of mechanisms by which lung cancer cells can escape the immune system and recognition of key tumor antigens and components of the immune system involved in tumor ignorance have led to the development of a variety of lung cancer vaccines. Many trials have explored the potential of immunotherapy in lung cancer and although improvements in the understanding of cellular and molecular tumor immunology have been achieved, clinical success has been limited. The best response achieved is typically stable disease, and a significant improvement in overall survival has not been seen.

Evaluating immunologic correlatives of lung cancer vaccines has also proven to be a challenge. Although measurements of antibody levels, DTH, cutaneous reactions, and CD4/CD8 responses have been assessed in a number of studies, these markers do not consistently correspond to tumor response or patient survival and thus are ineffective as surrogate markers of patient outcomes.

Vaccines have been successful tools for disease prevention by augmenting the immune system to prevent the development of illness upon exposure. In the setting of malignancy, however, vaccines are expected to be therapeutic, producing a tumor response. There are significant obstacles to achieving this goal, including generating an immune response to an entity that the immune system has already developed tolerance for and addressing a significant burden of the disease. The setting in which vaccines may be best employed in lung cancer needs to be reevaluated, because most of the studies described have been in advanced stage disease. Observations from these trials suggest that vaccines may be best employed when the bulk of the disease is limited. Thus, further development of vaccines should focus on the adjuvant setting where perhaps, it is more realistic to anticipate immune control of microscopic disease. In addition, future efforts should concentrate on establishing a relationship between markers of immune stimulation and clinically relevant outcomes. Although our understanding of immune processes and malignancy has grown, it remains to be seen whether vaccine therapies will ever play a prominent role in the treatment of lung cancer.

ACKNOWLEDGMENTS

We thank Professor A.F. Ochsenbein (Clinic of Medical Oncology, Bern, Switzerland) for critical discussion and valuable comments. Cheryl Ho is supported by a Canadian Association of Medical Oncologists/Canadian Institute of Health Research grant. Oliver Gautschi is supported by the Swiss National Science Foundation and the Swiss Cancer League.

REFERENCES

1. Alberg AJ, Brock MV, Samet JM. Epidemiology of lung cancer: looking to the future. J Clin Oncol 2005; 23:3175–3185.
2. Laheru DA, Pardoll DM, Jaffee EM. Genes to vaccines for immunotherapy: how the molecular biology revolution has influenced cancer immunology. Mol Cancer Ther 2005; 4:1645–1652.
3. Ruckdeschel JC, Codish SD, Stranahan A, et al. Postoperative empyema improves survival in lung cancer. Documentation and analysis of a natural experiment. N Engl J Med 1972; 287:1013–1017.
4. Takita H. Effect of postoperative empyema on survival of patients with bronchogenic carcinoma. J Thorac Cardiovasc Surg 1970; 59:642–644.
5. Witz JP, Roeslin N. Postpneumonectomy empyema does not improve survival in bronchogenic carcinoma. Ann Thorac Surg 1983; 36:529–531.
6. The Ludwig Lung Cancer Study Group (LLCSG). Immunostimulation with intrapleural BCG as adjuvant therapy in resected non-small cell lung cancer. Cancer 1986; 58:2411–2416.
7. Di Giorgio A, Sammartino P, Arnone P, et al. Prognostic significance of postoperative empyema in lung cancer. Int Surg 1996; 81:407–411.
8. Winter SF, Sekido Y, Minna JD, et al. Antibodies against autologous tumor cell proteins in patients with small-cell lung cancer: association with improved survival. J Natl Cancer Inst 1993; 85:2012–2018.
9. Suzuki M, Shigematsu H, Hiroshima K, et al. Epidermal growth factor receptor expression status in lung cancer correlates with its mutation. Hum Pathol 2005; 36:1127–1134.
10. Veronesi G, Pelosi G, Sonzogni A, et al. Tumour CEA as predictor of better outcome in squamous cell carcinoma of the lung. Lung Cancer 2005; 48:233–240.
11. Guddo F, Giatromanolaki A, Koukourakis MI, et al. MUC1 (episialin) expression in non-small cell lung cancer is independent of EGFR and c-erbB-2 expression and correlates with poor survival in node positive patients. J Clin Pathol 1998; 51:667–671.
12. Went P, Vasei M, Bubendorf L, et al. Frequent high-level expression of the immunotherapeutic target Ep-CAM in colon, stomach, prostate and lung cancers. Br J Cancer 2006; 94:128–135.
13. Zhang S, Cordon-Cardo C, Zhang HS, et al. Selection of tumor antigens as targets for immune attack using immunohistochemistry: I. Focus on gangliosides. Int J Cancer 1997; 73:42–49.
14. Takahashi T, Nau MM, Chiba I, et al. p53: a frequent target for genetic abnormalities in lung cancer. Science 1989; 246:491–494.
15. Keohavong P, DeMichele MA, Melacrinos AC, et al. Detection of K-ras mutations in lung carcinomas: relationship to prognosis. Clin Cancer Res 1996; 2:411–418.

16. Tajima K, Obata Y, Tamaki H, et al. Expression of cancer/testis (CT) antigens in lung cancer. Lung Cancer 2003; 42:23–33.

17. Liu XF, Helman LJ, Yeung C, et al. XAGE-1, a new gene that is frequently expressed in Ewing's sarcoma. Cancer Res 2000; 60:4752–4755.

18. Jungbluth AA, Chen YT, Stockert E, et al. Immunohistochemical analysis of NY-ESO-1 antigen expression in normal and malignant human tissues. Int J Cancer 92:856–860.

19. Scanlan MJ, Altorki NK, Gure AO, et al. Expression of cancer-testis antigens in lung cancer: definition of bromodomain testis-specific gene (BRDT) as a new CT gene, CT9. Cancer Lett 150:155–164.

20. Meta M, Ponte M, Guastella M, et al. Detection of oligoclonal T-lymphocytes in lymph nodes draining from advanced non-small-cell lung cancer. Cancer Immunol Immunother 1995; 40:235–240.

21. Yoshino I, Yano T, Murata M, et al. Tumor-reactive T-cells accumulate in lung cancer tissues but fail to respond due to tumor cell-derived factor. Cancer Res 1992; 52:775–781.

22. Melioli G, Ratto G, Guastella M, et al. Isolation and in vitro expansion of lymphocytes infiltrating non-small cell lung carcinoma: functional and molecular characterisation for their use in adoptive immunotherapy. Eur J Cancer 1994; 30A:97–102.

23. Ulevitch RJ, Mathison JC, da Silva Correia J. Innate immune responses during infection. Vaccine 2004; 22(suppl 1):S25–S30.

24. Pancer Z, Cooper MD. The evolution of adaptive immunity. Annu Rev Immunol 2006; 24:497–518.

25. Dezfouli S, Hatzinisiriou I, Ralph SJ. Use of cytokines in cancer vaccines/immunotherapy: recent developments improve survival rates for patients with metastatic malignancy. Curr Pharm Des 2005; 11:3511–3530.

26. Ochsenbein AF. Immunological ignorance of solid tumors. Springer Semin Immunopathol 2005; 27:19–35.

27. Subudhi SK, Alegre ML, Fu YX. The balance of immune responses: costimulation verse coinhibition. J Mol Med 2005; 83:193–202.

28. Burnet F. Cancer: a biological approach. BMJ 1957; 1:841–847.

29. Thomas L. Discussion to PB Medawar's paper. In: Lawrence H, ed. Cellular and Humoral Aspects of the Hypersensitivity States. New York: Harper, 1959:529–534.

30. Kelly DM, Emre S, Guy SR, et al. Liver transplant recipients are not at increased risk for nonlymphoid solid organ tumors. Cancer 1998; 83:1237–1243.

31. Ochsenbein AF, Sierro S, Odermatt B, et al. Roles of tumour localization, second signals and cross priming in cytotoxic T-cell induction. Nature 2001; 411:1058–1064.

32. Mapara MY, Sykes M. Tolerance and cancer: mechanisms of tumor evasion and strategies for breaking tolerance. J Clin Oncol 2004; 22:1136–1151.

33. Gross CP, Sepkowitz KA. The myth of the medical breakthrough: smallpox, vaccination, and Jenner reconsidered. Int J Infect Dis 1998; 3:54–60.

34. Hoption Cann SA, van Netten JP, van Netten C. Dr William Coley and tumour regression: a place in history or in the future. Postgrad Med J 2003; 79:672–680.

35. Shear MJ, Turner FC. Chemical treatment of tumors; isolation of hemorrhagic-producing fraction from *Serratia marcescens* (*Bacillus prodigiosus*) culture filtrate. J Natl Cancer Inst 1943; 4:81–87.

36. Lamm DL, Thor DE, Harris SC, et al. Bacillus Calmette-Guerin immunotherapy of superficial bladder cancer. J Urol 1980; 124:38–40.

37. Rosenberg SA, Lotze MT, Muul LM, et al. Observations on the systemic administration of autologous lymphokine-activated killer cells and recombinant interleukin-2 to patients with metastatic cancer. N Engl J Med 1985; 313:1485–1492.

38. Harper DM, Franco EL, Wheeler C, et al. Efficacy of a bivalent L1 virus-like particle vaccine in prevention of infection with human papillomavirus types 16 and 18 in young women: a randomised controlled trial. Lancet 2004; 364:1757–1765.

39. Aebischer T, Schmitt A, Walduck AK, et al. Helicobacter pylori vaccine development: facing the challenge. Int J Med Microbiol 2005; 295:343–353.

40. Stevenson FK. Update on cancer vaccines. Curr Opin Oncol 2005; 17:573–577.

41. Cerny T. Anti-nicotine vaccination: where are we? Recent Results Cancer Res 2005; 166:167–175.

42. Atanackovic D, Altorki NK, Stockert E, et al. Vaccine-induced CD4+ T-cell responses to MAGE-3 protein in lung cancer patients. J Immunol 2004; 172:3289–3296.

43. Engleman EG. Dendritic cell-based cancer immunotherapy. Semin Oncol 2003; 30:23–29.

44. Ueda Y, Itoh T, Nukaya I, et al. Dendritic cell-based immunotherapy of cancer with carcinoembryonic antigen-derived, HLA-A24-restricted CTL epitope: clinical outcomes of 18 patients with metastatic gastrointestinal or lung adenocarcinomas. Int J Oncol 2004; 24:909–917.

45. Robert F, Blumenschein G, Herbst RS, et al. Phase I/IIa study of cetuximab with gemcitabine plus carboplatin in patients with chemotherapy-naive advanced non-small-cell lung cancer. J Clin Oncol 2005; 23:9089–9096.

46. Raez LE, Santos ES, Mudad R, et al. Clinical trials targeting lung cancer with active immunotherapy: the scope of vaccines. Expert Rev Anticancer Ther 2005; 5:635–644.

47. Butts C, Murray N, Maksymiuk A, et al. Randomized phase IIB trial of BLP25 liposome vaccine in stage IIIB and IV non-small-cell lung cancer. J Clin Oncol 2005; 23:6674–6681.

48. Nemunaitis J, Sterman D, Jablons D, et al. Granulocyte-macrophage colony-stimulating factor gene-modified autologous tumor vaccines in non-small-cell lung cancer. J Natl Cancer Inst 2004; 96:326–331.

49. Liu M, Acres B, Balloul JM, et al. Gene-based vaccines and immunotherapeutics. Proc Natl Acad Sci USA 2004; 101(suppl 2):14567–14571.

50. Raez LE, Cassileth PA, Schlesselman JJ, et al. Allogeneic vaccination with a B7.1 HLA-A gene-modified adenocarcinoma cell line in patients with advanced non-small-cell lung cancer. J Clin Oncol 2004; 22:2800–2807.

51. Nemunaitis J, Jahan T, Ross H, et al. Phase 1/2 trial of autologous tumor mixed with an allogeneic GVAX(R) vaccine in advanced-stage non-small-cell lung cancer. Cancer Gene Ther 2006; 13(6):555–562.

52. O'Brien ME, Anderson H, Kaukel E, et al. SRL172 (killed *Mycobacterium vaccae*) in addition to standard chemotherapy improves quality of life without affecting survival, in patients with advanced non-small-cell lung cancer: phase III results. Ann Oncol 2004; 15:906–914.

53. Morse MA, Garst J, Osada T, et al. A phase I study of dexosome immunotherapy in patients with advanced non-small cell lung cancer. J Transl Med 2005; 3:9.

54. Gonzalez G, Crombet T, Torres F, et al. Epidermal growth factor-based cancer vaccine for non-small-cell lung cancer therapy. Ann Oncol 2003; 14:461–466.

55. Squiban P, Velu T, Mennecier B, et al. MVA-MUC1-IL2 vaccine immunotherapy for advanced non small cell lung cancer (NSCLC): interim phase II data (meeting abstr). J Clin Oncol 2004; 22:2544.

56. Hirschowitz EA, Foody T, Kryscio R, et al. Autologous dendritic cell vaccines for non-small-cell lung cancer. J Clin Oncol 2004; 22:2808–2815.

57. Morris JC, Vahanian N, Janik JE, et al. Phase I study of an antitumor vaccination using {alpha}(1,3) galactosyltransferase expressing allogeneic tumor cells in patients (Pts) with refractory or recurrent non-small cell lung cancer (NSCLC) (meeting abstr). J Clin Oncol 2005; 23:2586.

58. Schulof RS, Mai D, Nelson MA, et al. Active specific immunotherapy with an autologous tumor cell vaccine in patients with resected non-small cell lung cancer. Mol Biother 1988; 1:30–36.

59. Salgia R, Lynch T, Skarin A, et al. Vaccination with irradiated autologous tumor cells engineered to secrete granulocyte-macrophage colony-stimulating factor augments antitumor immunity in some patients with metastatic non-small-cell lung carcinoma. J Clin Oncol 2003; 21:624–630.

60. O'Brien ME, Saini A, Smith IE, et al. A randomized phase II study of SRL172 (*Mycobacterium vaccae*) combined with chemotherapy in patients with advanced inoperable non-small-cell lung cancer and mesothelioma. Br J Cancer 2000; 83:853–857.

61. Scanlan MJ, Gure AO, Jungbluth AA, et al. Cancer/testis antigens: an expanding family of targets for cancer immunotherapy. Immunol Rev 2002; 188:22–32.

62. Gure AO, Chua R, Williamson B, et al. Cancer-testis genes are coordinately expressed and are markers of poor outcome in non-small cell lung cancer. Clin Cancer Res 2005; 11:8055–8062.

63. Mendelsohn J, Baselga J. The EGF receptor family as targets for cancer therapy. Oncogene 2000; 19:6550–6565.

64. Dy GK, Adjei AA. Novel targets for lung cancer therapy: part I. J Clin Oncol 2002; 20:2881–2894.

65. Hirsch FR, Varella-Garcia M, Bunn PA Jr, et al. Epidermal growth factor receptor in non-small-cell lung carcinomas: correlation between gene copy number and protein expression and impact on prognosis. J Clin Oncol 2003; 21:3798–3807.

66. Ishioka GY, Disis ML, Morse MA, et al. A phase I trial of a multi-epitope cancer vaccine (EP-2101) in non-small cell lung (NSCLC) and colon cancer patients (meeting abstr). J Clin Oncol 2004; 22:2525.

67. Macchiarini P, Hardin M, Angeletti CA. Long-term evaluation of intrapleural Bacillus Calmette-Guerin with or without adjuvant chemotherapy in completely resected stages II and III non-small-cell lung cancer. Am J Clin Oncol 1991; 14:291–297.

68. National Cancer Institute Lung Cancer Study Group. Surgical adjuvant intrapleural BCG treatment for stage I non-small cell lung cancer. Preliminary report of the National Cancer Institute Lung Cancer Study Group. J Thorac Cardiovasc Surg 1981; 82:649–657.

69. Yamamura Y, Sakatani M, Ogura T, et al. Adjuvant immunotherapy of lung cancer with BCG cell wall skeleton (BCG-CWS). Cancer 1979; 43:1314–1319.

70. Yasumoto K, Manabe H, Yanagawa E, et al. Nonspecific adjuvant immunotherapy of lung cancer with cell wall skeleton of *Mycobacterium bovis* Bacillus Calmette-Guerin. Cancer Res 1979; 39:3262–3267.

71. Matthay RA, Mahler DA, Beck GJ, et al. Intratumoral Bacillus Calmette-Guerin immunotherapy prior to surgery for carcinoma of the lung: results of a prospective randomized trial. Cancer Res 1986; 46:5963–5968.

72. Nobel TA, Perk K. Bronchiolo-alveolar cell carcinoma. Animal model: pulmonary adenomatosis of sheep, pulmonary carcinoma of sheep, pulmonary carcinoma of sheep (Jaagsiekte). Am J Pathol 1978; 90:783–786.

73. Stinson JC, Leibovitz A, Brindley GV Jr, et al. Filamentous particles in human alveolar cell carcinomas: electron microscopy studies of six cases (preliminary report). J Natl Cancer Inst 1972; 49:1483–1493.

74. Schiller J, Nemunaitis, J, Ross H, et al. GM-CSF gene-modified autologous tumor vaccine with and without low dose cyclophosphamide in advanced stage non-small cell lung cancer (NSCLC), IASLC. Barcelona, Spain, 2005.

75. Assersohn L, Souberbielle BE, O'Brien ME, et al. A randomized pilot study of SRL172 (*Mycobacterium vaccae*) in patients with small cell lung cancer (SCLC) treated with chemotherapy. Clin Oncol (R Coll Radiol) 2002; 14:23–27.

76. Krug LM, Ragupathi G, Ng KK, et al. Vaccination of small cell lung cancer patients with polysialic acid or *N*-propionylated polysialic acid conjugated to keyhole limpet hemocyanin. Clin Cancer Res 2004; 10:916–923.

77. Krug LM, Ragupathi G, Hood C, et al. Vaccination of patients with small-cell lung cancer with synthetic fucosyl GM-1 conjugated to keyhole limpet hemocyanin. Clin Cancer Res 2004; 10:6094–6100.

78. Grant SC, Kris MG, Houghton AN, et al. Long survival of patients with small cell lung cancer after adjuvant treatment with the anti-idiotypic antibody BEC2 plus Bacillus Calmette-Guerin. Clin Cancer Res 1999; 5:1319–1323.

79. Gabrilovich DI, Mirza N, Chiappori A, et al. Initial results of a phase II trial of patients with extensive stage small cell lung cancer (SCLC) immunized with dendritic cells (DC) transduced with wild-type p53 (meeting abstr.). J Clin Oncol 2005; 23:2543.

80. Giaccone G, Debruyne C, Felip E, et al. Phase III study of adjuvant vaccination with Bec2/bacille Calmette-Guerin in responding patients with limited-disease small-cell lung cancer (European Organisation for Research and Treatment of Cancer 08971-08971B; Silva Study). J Clin Oncol 2005; 23:6854–6864.

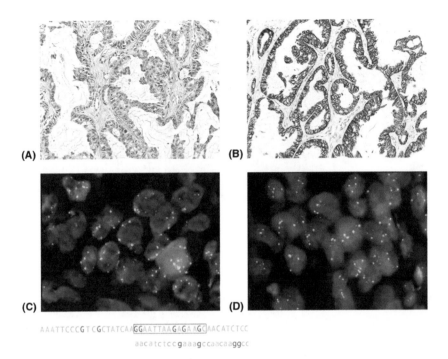

AAATTCCCGTCGCTATCAA GGAATTAAGAGAAGC AACATCTCC
aacatctccgaaagccaacaaggcc

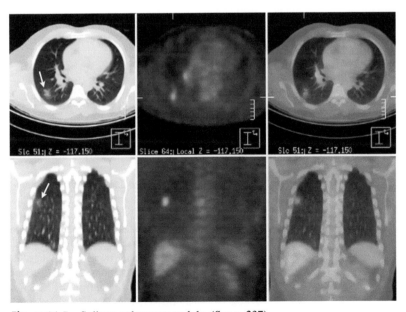

(E)

Figure 6.1 Example biomaker analysis of a lung tumor with bronchioloalveolar histology. (*See p. 101*)

Figure 11.5 Solitary pulmonary nodule. (See p. 237)

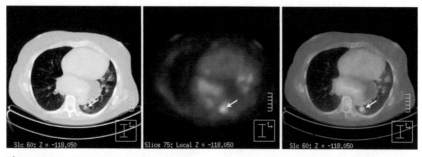

Figure 11.9 False-positive positron emission tomography (PET). (See p. 241).

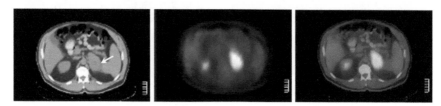

Figure 11.13 Adrenal metastasis from lung cancer. (See p. 245).

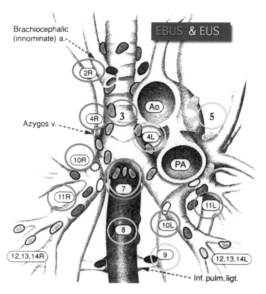

Figure 11.21 Schematic representation of the hilar and mediastinal lymph-node stations (after Mountain et al.) showing nodal stations accessible for fine needle aspiration by endobronchial ultrasound (stations: 2, 3, 4, 7, 10 and 11—*red circles*) and by EUS (L4, 5, 7, 8 and 9—*yellow circles*).

9

Advances in Chemoradiation Treatment of Locoregionally Advanced Non–Small Cell Lung Cancer

Michael T. Milano and Yuhchyau Chen

Department of Radiation Oncology, University of Rochester School of Medicine and Dentistry, Rochester, New York, U.S.A.

INTRODUCTION

Locoregionally advanced non–small-cell lung cancer (NSCLC) refers to stage IIIA and IIIB disease without clinical evidence of distant metastasis. The management of this tumor stage with aggressive therapy remains an active area of investigation due to the potential for cure by controlling the disease in the chest as well as eradicating possible subclinical distant micrometastasis. Although a combined modality approach has generally been considered the standard of care, with accepted treatment modalities including surgery, radiotherapy, chemotherapy, and nonchemotherapeutic systemic therapy (i.e., radiation sensitizers, biologic agents, molecular targeting agents, and others), radiotherapy remains the primary local treatment modality for the locoregioanlly advanced NSCLC. Although the search for the optimal combination, sequence, and chemotherapeutic agents used in the combined modality treatment for stage III NSCLC has progressed in recent years, many aspects of combining these treatment modalities remain to be defined (Fig. 1).

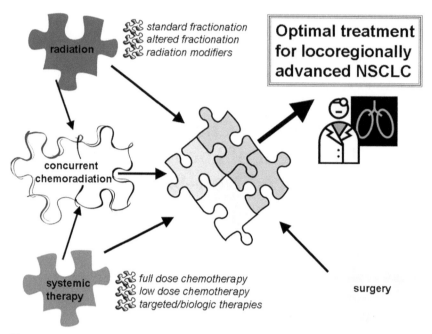

Figure 1 The modalities used to treat non–small cell lung cancer (*puzzle pieces*). The optimal treatment in a given subset of patients will achieve long-term cancer control with acceptable long-term morbidity. Which pieces of the puzzle and what sequence these pieces should be put together in (i.e., timing or treatment modality) to achieve optimal outcome is under continued investigation.

There are many clinical variables with radiation treatment as well as with chemotherapy in the management of stage III NSCLC. Chest radiotherapy can be delivered via standard fractionation or altered fractionation approaches (described in section "Advances of Radiation Fractionation"). Other radiation-related variables include the prescribed total radiation dose, treatment volume in terms of the decision of which elective nodal groups to include, and radiation technique such as conformal treatment, intensity modulated radiotherapy (IMRT), image guided radiation therapy (IGRT), and respiratory gating. Chemotherapy can be delivered prior to surgery or radiation (induction chemotherapy), concurrently during radiation therapy, and/or after radiation or surgery (adjuvant chemotherapy). The choice of systemic agents, the administered doses, and the dosing schedules are important variables. Cisplatin-based chemotherapy has traditionally been considered the most effective systemic therapy for NSCLC (1). In the past two decades, many newer agents have shown efficacy for NSCLC as well (2). Systemic agents used for definitive treatment of nonmetastatic NSCLC are generally derived from trials showing efficacy in stage IV NSCLC patients. Indeed, many recent clinical studies have enthusiastically applied third-generation chemotherapeutic agents in conjunction with radiotherapy in the treatment of stage III NSCLC (3). Within the scope of the discussion of this chapter, we will focus primarily on phase III studies and major phase II cooperative group studies in the management of locoregionally advanced NSCLC with combined modality chemotherapy and radiation. In addition, surgical resection for stage III NSCLC will be discussed in the context of its combination with chemotherapy and radiation.

ADVANCES IN RADIATION THERAPY FOR CHEST RADIATION

Technological Advances of Radiotherapy

This section will focus on the recent advances in radiotherapy technology that have impacted current radiation treatment of NSCLC. Probably the greatest radiotherapy advance in the past decade is the routine use of 3-dimensional computed tomography (CT)-based planning. In addition to providing the radiation oncologist with more accurate imaging data with which to plan the radiotherapy, CT-based planning allows for accurate quantification of volumes of tumor and volumes of normal tissue receiving a given dose of radiation. This enables optimization of the orientation and shape of the radiation beam, resulting in better sparing of normal tissues such as lung, heart, esophagus, and spinal cord, while maintaining adequate target coverage. The lungs have a relatively low threshold for radiation, with late toxicity being predicted by mean lung doses and volume of lung receiving above 20 Gy (4). Thus, a major goal of 3-dimensional planning is to accurately quantify and minimize these parameters, while maintaining adequate coverage of the target. Since the spinal-cord tolerance is in the 45 to 50 Gy range, radiation treatments for doses of above 60 Gy require multiple-beam orientations.

Recent technical radiotherapy advances include the use of positron emission tomography scans for planning purposes (5), IGRT (6), 4-dimensional radiation therapy (4DRT) (7,8), and IMRT (9). With 4DRT, chest-wall motion is monitored in real time in conjunction with patient-controlled breathing and/or respiratory gating (i.e., radiotherapy delivery synchronized with target motion). 4DRT allows for reduction of the radiation margins that are required to account for tumor motion. IGRT uses daily imaging on the treatment machine to verify patient positioning and determine any necessary adjustments to reproduce the patient setup. IGRT can also allow for modification of the radiation field to account for any tumor shrinkage that occurs, thereby potentially resulting in less normal tissue exposure. IMRT is a means of modulating the radiation beam spatially and/or temporally in an effort to better conform the full-dose isodose curves around the target volume. Its use in NSCLC is emerging. One major drawback of IMRT is the increased monitor units, which leads to a greater volume of low-dose exposure. This is a particular concern with lung radiotherapy, since the lung has a relatively low threshold (with respect to late effects) of large volume radiation dose exposure in the 10 to 20 Gy range. The addition of radioprotectors such as amifostine to IMRT may lower the risk of toxicity associated with increased low-dose exposure (9). Techniques such as 4DRT, IGRT, and IMRT will enable radiation dose escalation to desired targets.

Amifostine is a thiol-based radiation protector that chemically repairs radiation-induced DNA damage. Amifostine more readily incorporates into normal tissues than cancerous tumors and thus may protect normal tissues without sparing the cancer. Certainly amifostine use is controversial, particularly in light of the negative Radiation Therapy Oncology Group (RTOG) 9801 phase III trial, which did not demonstrate a discernable difference in acute esophagitis, the primary endpoint of that study (10). However, amifostine was given for only one of the two twice-daily fractions in this trial, which might not have been sufficient. There are some other concerns with amifostine, which include possible tumor protection (which has not been clinically demonstrated) and drug toxicity. Subcutaneous administration of amifostine (as opposed to intravenous administration as used in RTOG 9801) is better tolerated with respect to nausea and hypotension.

The optimal radiation variables such as dose, fractionation, and treatment volume are unknown. The primary concern with dose escalation is early and late toxicity (4). Early RTOG data suggests that with definitive radiation alone, dose escalation from 40 to 60 Gy results in improved local control; furthermore, survival is compromised with locoregional failure (11,12). No other cooperative group studies have explored dose escalation. In a single institution series from the University of North Carolina, induction carboplatin, irinotecan, and paclitaxel followed by weekly low-dose carboplatin and paclitaxel with concurrent 3-dimensionally planned radiation, dose escalated up to 90 Gy to gross tumor (and 40–50 Gy to the elective mediastinal nodes) was tolerable (13). The recently closed The Cancer and Leukemia Group B (CALGB) 30105 study used 3-dimensional radiation to deliver 74 Gy with concurrent low-dose chemotherapy (with the induction and concurrent chemotherapy regimen being randomized to two arms, discussed in more detail below).

An emerging trend in the radiation treatment of NSCLC is to treat gross tumor alone and forego treatment of elective nodal regions. Large field sizes increase the risk of early and perhaps late toxicity due to the increased volume of normal tissues exposed to doses above threshold. Studies using this approach without concurrent chemotherapy have shown dose escalation to be tolerable, with most series showing a risk of nodal failure below 7% outside of the treatment field (14–20).

With smaller treatment volumes, radiation dose escalation becomes more feasible, particularly when used with novel radiation technologies such as 4DRT, IGRT, and IMRT. Since chemotherapy is expected to treat regions of microscopic disease, the use of limited radiation treatment volumes with concurrent chemotherapy is certainly reasonable and can prove to be more desirable by virtue of reducing acute and late toxicity.

Advances of Radiation Fractionation

Before discussing the treatment of locoregionally advanced NSCLC, it is important to discuss the fundamentals of radiation fractionation, which is reviewed in this section. Radiation fractionation describes how the total prescribed radiation dose is divided into individual treatment doses. Daily radiation of 1.8 to 2.0 Gy has been accepted as standard fractionation for most disease sites, while there are several altered fractional schedules applied in the clinical setting. Radiobiologically, fraction sizes larger than 1.8 to 2.0 Gy are expected to result in an increased risk of "late" normal tissue toxicity. In contrast, the total cumulative dose delivered to a volume of a given organ can impact both "acute" and "late" reactions. By definition, "accelerated" fractionation regimens deliver a radiobiologically effective dose in a shorter cumulative time span. "Hypofractionated" radiation employs treatment fractions that are larger than 2.0 Gy. Larger fraction size is expected to cause worse normal tissue injury; therefore, in the treatment of NSCLC, hypofractionation has been applied in stereotactic body radiotherapy setting with limited treatment volume only. "Hyperfractionated" radiation employs the use of fraction sizes that are smaller than 1.8 to 2.0 Gy, with more than one fraction delivered per day (generally with ≥6 hours between fractions to allow for the repair of normal tissue sublethal damage). "Accelerated hyperfractionated" radiation delivers radiation over a shorter time span, with each fraction smaller than 1.8 to 2.0 Gy, delivered with more than one fraction per day. Hyperfractionated regimens with planned treatment breaks that result in no shortening of treatment duration are not considered accelerated. Generally, accelerated hyperfractionated radiation allows for more aggressive radiation delivery, with lower fraction sizes reducing the risk of late toxicity. However, with escalated daily radiation dose, severe acute reactions can lead to consequential late effects resulting from host response to acute reactions.

For example, a three-arm study by the North Central Cancer Treatment Group (NCCTG) randomized 99 patients with stage IIIA to IIIB NSCLC, comparing standard (2 Gy per day) against hyperfractionated radiation (1.5 Gy twice-daily with a planned two-week break) either with or without concurrent chemotherapy to a total of 60 Gy for all arms (21). The hyperfractionated arms fared similarly, both being better in terms of survival and disease control than the standard radiation arm, but this improvement did not reach statistical significance. The Continuous Hyperfractionated Accelerated Radiotherapy trial (CHART) randomized 563 patients with locally advanced NSCLC and demonstrated that 54 Gy in 1.5 Gy thrice-daily fractions resulted in significantly improved survival and local control rates as compared with standard radiation, with the drawback of more severe acute dysphagia and late pulmonary fibrosis (22). The improved survival with CHART suggests that radiation mediated local control can impact survival in patients not receiving chemotherapy.

No randomized data have shown altered fractionated regimens to be significantly more beneficial than standard radiation when given in conjunction with chemotherapy. The Eastern Cooperative Oncology Group (ECOG) conducted a randomized study (discussed below) suggesting that with sequential chemoradiation, hyperfractionated radiation may improve survival over standard radiation. Despite the impressive absolute benefit in survival reported in this study, the difference in survival was not significant (23). In the RTOG 9410 study (with three arms), concurrent chemoradiation with hyperfractionated radiation did not fare better than chemoradiation employing standard radiation (24,25).

COMBINATION CHEMOTHERAPY AND RADIATION FOR STAGE III NSCLC

Stage IIIA NSCLC has generally been considered marginally resectable, while stage IIIB NSCLC is generally considered surgically unresectable. Definitive radiation therapy is the standard local therapy for inoperable stages IIIA and IIIB NSCLC (11,12,26,27), particularly in stage III with bulky lymph nodes. Indeed, surgical series have shown that clinical stage IIIA fares considerably worse than pathologic stage III upgraded from clinical stage I to II disease (28,29). A multitude of trials have explored the role of combined modality chemotherapy and/or radiation with surgery (discussed in section Neoadjuvant Chemoradiation followed by Surgery), but even after resection, the prognosis of stage IIIA remains poor. The NSCLC Collaborative Group meta-analysis examined 22 randomized trials investigating definitive radiation versus definitive chemoradiation for locally advanced NSCLC (including trials with induction and/or concurrent chemotherapy); this analysis including a total of 3033 enrolled patients (1). The addition of chemotherapy resulted in a hazard ratio (HR) for death of 0.90, equating to a 10% reduction in the risk of death and 3% absolute risk reduction ($P = 0.006$). In 11 of the 22 trials that used cisplatin-based regimens, the HR was 0.87 ($P = 0.005$), with a 4% absolute benefit in survival. The HRs in the subsets of alkylating agents (five trials), vinca alkaloids or etoposide (three trials), or other agents (three trials, mainly anthracyclines) were not significant. An Italian meta-analysis of 14 randomized trials including 1887 patients treated for stage III disease also showed a significant survival benefit with the addition of chemotherapy, particularly with cisplatin-based regimens, though this benefit was not appreciated beyond three years (30).

Although meta-analyses support the benefit of adding chemotherapy to radiation for locally advanced NSCLC, uncertainties remain as to how to integrate the two modalities to maximize the therapeutic ratio. Overall, when chemotherapy and radiation are delivered concurrently, the acute toxicities of radiotherapy are exacerbated. When chemotherapy and radiation are delivered in a sequential manner, toxicities are more tolerable, but treatments lose the benefit of radiosensitization by concurrent chemotherapy, and there is a concern of delaying local therapy in the setting of induction chemotherapy followed by chest radiation. Thus the discussion of this topic will be divided into three categorical clinical settings: (*i*) studies involving induction chemotherapy followed by radiation therapy, (*ii*) studies involving concurrent chemoradiation with low-dose chemotherapy, and (*iii*) studies involving concurrent chemoradiation with full-dose chemotherapy.

STUDIES INVOLVING INDUCTION CHEMOTHERAPY FOLLOWED BY RADIATION THERAPY

The use of systemic doses of chemotherapy followed by radiation allows for systemic treatment of occult micrometastatic disease upfront as well as the potential of tumor shrinkage prior to radiation. This is termed induction or sequential chemotherapy since it precedes radiation. Table 1 summarizes the key trials discussed below.

Table 1 Summary of Actuarial Survival in Selected Trials of Sequential Induction Chemotherapy Followed by Chest Radiation: Studies that Address the Addition of Induction Chemotherapy

Trial (Refs.)	Patients	#	Treatment	MS (mo)	OS	*P* value
CALGB 8433 phase III (31,32)	Selected stage IIIA	165	RT C→RT	9.6 13.7	5 yr: 6% 5 yr: 17%	0.012
NCCTG phase III (33)	Unselected stage III	114	RT C→RT→ C	10.3 10.4	5 yr: 7% 5 yr: 5%	NS
French phase III (34,35)	Unresectable	353	RT C→RT	10 12	3 yr: 5% 3 yr: 11%	0.08
Intergroup phase III (36,37)	Selected stage II–III	452	RT C→RT HFRT	11.4 13.2 12.0	5 yr: 5% 5 yr: 8% 5 yr: 6%	0.04

Abbreviations: C, chemotherapy; HFRT, hyperfractionated radiation therapy; MS, median survival; OS, overall survival; RT, standard radiation;

Several trials have compared sequential chemotherapy and radiation versus radiation alone. CALGB conducted a landmark randomized controlled trial in 165 patients with T3 and/or N2 stage IIIA disease, with a favorable performance status and pretreatment weight loss of below 5% (31,32). Patients were randomized to receive standard radiation alone (60 Gy in daily 2 Gy fractions) versus sequential cisplatin (100 mg/m^2, days 1 and 29) and vinblastine (5 mg/m^2, days 1, 8, 15, 22, and 29) followed by standard radiation. The sequential chemotherapy arm resulted in significantly improved progression-free survival (18% vs. 8% at three years, $P = 0.012$) and overall survival (17% vs. 6% at five years).

An NCCTG trial randomized 114 patients to radiation (60 Gy in 2 Gy daily fractions) with or without sequential methotrexate (40 mg/m^2), doxorubicin (40 mg/m^2), cyclophosphamide (400 mg/m^2), and lomusitne (30 mg/m^2), with chemotherapy delivered for two cycles every 28 days before radiation and an additional two cycles after completion of the chest radiotherapy. These patients were not selected on the basis of performance status or weight. In this trial, there were no significant differences between the two arms with respect to overall survival, progression-free survival, or patterns of failure (33).

A French multicenter trial randomized 353 patients with Karnofsky Performance Score (KPS) of above 50% to radiation alone (65 Gy in daily 2.5 Gy fractions) versus the same radiation treatment with three cycles of induction chemotherapy in a sandwich schedule using vendesine (1 mg/m^2, day 1–2), lomustine (50 and 25 mg/m^2 on day 2 and 3), cisplatin (100 mg/m^2 on day 2), and cyclophosphamide (200 mg/m^2, days 2–4). Sequential chemotherapy significantly reduced the rate of distant failure (60% vs. 47% at three years, $P < 0.001$) and resulted in a trend toward improved survival (34,35).

An Intergroup trial sponsored by the RTOG (RTOG 8808 and ECOG 4588), randomized 452 favorable (KPS >70%, weight loss <5%) patients with inoperable stage II to III NSCLC to three arms: (*i*) standard radiation alone (60 Gy in 2 Gy daily fractions); (*ii*) sequential cisplatin and vinblastine followed by standard chest radiation as utilized in the CALGB trial, (*iii*) hyperfractionated radiation (69.6 Gy in 1.2 Gy twice-daily fractions) (36,37), with the hyperfractionated regimen derived from the earlier RTOG 8311 phase I/II study (a dose escalation trial from 60 to 79.2 Gy in which the 69.6 Gy dose level demonstrated the best survival) (27,38). The study results showed that the arm with sequential chemotherapy and radiation fared the best in terms of survival, further supporting the notion of improved outcome with the addition of chemotherapy to radiation.

The following discussion addresses randomized phase III studies applying induction chemotherapy as the standard for both arms and offers comparisons of the efficacy of local therapies after induction chemotherapy (Table 2). ECOG conducted a randomized trial (ECOG 2597) of 112 patients with stage III NSCLC with a KPS status of 70% and above and a weight loss of 10% and below. Both study arms of ECOG 2597 received two cycles of induction paclitaxel (200 mg/m^2) and carboplatin [area under the curve (AUC) = 6], followed by chest radiotherapy; patients were randomized to either standard radiation (64 Gy in daily 2 Gy fractions) or hyperfractionated radiation (57.6 Gy in thrice-daily—TID fractions of 1.5, 1.5, and 1.8 Gy) (23). A trend toward improved survival was seen favoring hyperfractionated radiotherapy. Statistical significance was not achieved, possibly due to early closure. Patients in the hyperfractionated arm experienced more acute grade 3 to 4 esophagitis (25.0% vs. 15.9%) and no acute grade 3 to 4 pulmonary complications (as opposed to 10.5% in the standard arm).

Retrospective data (29) as well as some randomized trials support neoadjuvant chemotherapy prior to resection in stage IIIA NSCLC (41–45). Since either surgery or radiation alone is effective locoregional treatment for stage IIIA NSCLC and neoadjuvant chemotherapy improves outcome with either approach, the question arises whether either modality (surgery vs. radiation) proves superior to the other after neoadjuvant chemotherapy. An Intergroup (ECOG and RTOG 8901) trial randomized 73 stage IIIA patients to two arms, with all patients receiving four cycles of cisplatin (120 mg/m^2, day 1) and vinblastine (4.5 mg/m^2, days 1 and 15)

Table 2 Summary of Actuarial Survival in Selected Trials of Sequential Induction Chemotherapy Followed by Chest Radiation: Studies in Which Induction Chemotherapy is Used in All Arms

Trial (Refs.)	Patients	#	Treatment	MS (mo)	OS	*P* value
ECOG 2597 phase III (23)	Selected stage III	112	C→RT C→HFRT	14.9 20.3	3 yr: 14% 3 yr: 34%	NS
Intergroup phase III (39)	Operable stage IIIA	73	C→S C→RT	19.4 17.4	1 yr: 70% 1 yr: 60%	NS
EORTC phase III (40)	Operable stage IIIA	333	C→S C→RT	16.4 17.5	5 yr: 16% 5 yr: 13%	NS

Abbreviations: C, chemotherapy; HFRT, hyperfractionated radiation therapy; MS, median survival; OS, overall survival; RT, standard radiation.

followed by the randomized local disease treatment of either surgery or radiation (64 Gy in 2 Gy daily fractions) after two cycles (39). There were no differences in outcomes between these two arms.

A European Organization for Research and Treatment of Cancer (EORTC) trial randomized 333 patients with N2 disease to platinum-based chemotherapy followed by either radiation (60 Gy) or surgery (of which 39% were offered postoperative radiation) (40). No survival differences were noted in this trial either.

In summary, large phase III clinical studies have investigated the benefit of induction chemotherapy followed by radiation and found a significant survival benefit in two studies (31,32,36,37), a trend toward a survival benefit in the French study (34,35), and no benefit in the NCCTG study (33). Other phase III studies adopted induction chemotherapy as the standard for both treatment arms while comparing the efficacy of local therapy by standard radiation, hyperfractionated radiation, or surgery. In these three studies comparing the role of local therapy after induction chemotherapy, none of the studies showed a survival difference in the study arms (Table 2). Thus systemic doses of chemotherapy upfront appear to improve survival followed by definitive radiation. For marginally respectable stage IIIA disease after induction chemotherapy, radiation therapy seems to fare as well as surgery in the bimodality approach.

CONCURRENT CHEMORADIATION WITH LOW-DOSE CHEMOTHERAPY

Select chemotherapeutic agents have known radiosensitization properties, discovered in preclinical studies and/or in other disease sites. It should be recognized that concurrent chemoradiation for stage III NSCLC invariably increases the treatment-related toxicity, particularly in the rates and severity of pneumonitis and esophagitis. Chemotherapy regimens at reduced doses delivered weekly, twice weekly, three times weekly, daily, or as continuous infusions have all been conducted with concurrent chest radiation. In this type of approach, the systemic activity of chemotherapy may not be well characterized, since the activity of these chemotherapy schedules have not been well investigated in stage IV patients (46), except for weekly low-dose chemotherapy for the elderly population (47). Thus, the primary goal of low-dose chemotherapy with concurrent radiation has been aimed at improving locoregional control via radiosensitization. Table 3 summarizes the studies discussed in this section.

Several trials have randomized radiation alone versus concurrent radiation and low-dose chemotherapy. The EORTC conducted a three-arm randomized phase II trial, which was then followed by a phase III trial, accruing a total of 331 patients with inoperable stage I to III (mostly stage III) NSCLC (with the patients being pooled for the final analysis). This study compared radiation alone (55 Gy split-course radiation) against concurrent radiation (same dose as control arm) and cisplatin at two different dose schedules (30 mg/m^2 weekly vs. 6 mg/m^2 daily) (48). The survival in the concurrent chemoradiation arms was significantly

Table 3 Summary of Actuarial Survival in Selected Trials of Concurrent Low-Dose
Chemotherapy and Radiation

Trial (Refs.)	Patients	#	Treatment	MS (mo)	OS	P value
EORTC phase II–III (48)	Inoperable	331	RT	~12	3 yr: 2%	0.009
			cRT	~12–13	3 yr: 13–16%	
Yugoslavian phase III (49)	Stage III	169	HFRT	8	3 yr: 7%	0.027 HFRT vs. best HFCRT arm
			HFCRT	13–18	3 yr: 16–23%	
Italian phase III (50)	Stage III	173	RT	10.3	3 yr: 9%	NS
			cRT	10.0	3 yr: 9%	
CALGB 39801 phase III (51)	Unresectable stage III	366	cRT	11.4	1 yr: 48%	NS
			C→cRT	14.0	1 yr: 54%	
CALGB 9130 phase III (52)	Inoperable stage III	283	C→RT	13.4	3 yr: 10%	NS
			C→cRT	13.5	3 yr: 13%	
German phase III (53)	Inoperable stage III	303	C→RT	14.6	—	NS
			C→cRT	19.2	—	
French phase III (54)	Inoperable stage III	584	C→RT	11	—	NS
			C→cRT	14	—	
French phase III (55)	Inoperable stage III	205	C→RT→C	14.5	4 yr: 14%	NS
			cRT→C	16.3	4 yr: 21%	
LAMP ran. phase II (56)	Unresectable stage III	257	C→RT	13.0	3 yr: 17%	NS
			C→cRT	12.7	3 yr: 15%	
			cRT→C	16.3	3 yr: 17%	

Abbreviations: C, chemotherapy; cRT, concurrent full-dose chemotherapy and radiation; HFRT, hyperfractionated radiation therapy; HFCRT, concurrent chemotherapy and hyperfractionated radiation therapy; MS, median survival; OS, overall survival; RT, standard radiation.

better than the radiation-alone arm, with no difference seen between the two chemoradiotherapy arms. The two-year survival rate without local failure was 30% versus 19%. Interestingly, distant failure was not significantly impacted, supporting the notion that improved local control can impact survival. A criticism of this trial is that the split-course radiation with a planned treatment break has not been considered standard radiation treatment with curative intent in the United States.

A series of phase II to III studies from Yugoslavia have examined hyperfractionated (64.8 Gy in 1.2 Gy fractions) radiation with concurrent low-dose platinum-based regimens. These studies found a significant survival benefit with the addition of concurrent low-dose chemotherapy for hyperfractionated chest radiotherapy (57–63). In a phase III randomized trial, the addition of concurrent carboplatin (100 or 200 mg, days 1–2) and etoposide (100 mg, days 1–3 or days 1–5) significantly improved median and overall survival (49).

An Italian randomized study in 173 patients with inoperable stage III NSCLC compared radiation (45 Gy in 1.8 Gy fractions) with or without concurrent low-dose cisplatin (6 mg/m^2 daily). The study resulted in similar median survival in both arms (50). The radiation dose in this study is substantially lower than the commonly accepted doses 60 Gy or above for definitive radiation.

Some studies have examined sequential chemotherapy (induction and/or consolidation) and radiation with concurrent low-dose chemotherapy versus sequential chemotherapy and radiation alone. These are discussed in the remainder of this section.

The CALGB 9130 (in collaboration with the ECOG) study randomized 283 patients with inoperable stage III NSCLC to radiation alone (60 Gy in 2 Gy fractions) or carboplatin (100 mg/m^2 weekly) concurrently with radiation, with both arms receiving induction vinblastine (5 mg/m^2 weekly for five weeks) and cisplatin (100 mg/m^2 on day 1 and 29). No significant benefit was seen with the addition of concurrent carboplatin, with both arms suffering frequent in-field (i.e., within the radiation volume) failures (69% vs. 59% favoring the chemoradiation arm, but not statistically significant) (52).

A German study randomized 303 patients with inoperable stage III NSCLC to radiation alone (60 Gy in 2 Gy fractions) or paclitaxel (60 mg/m^2 weekly) concurrently with radiation. Both arms received two cycles of induction paclitaxel (200 mg/m^2) and carboplatin (AUC = 6) every three weeks (53). The preliminary analysis suggests a nonsignificant trend toward a median survival benefit favoring the concurrent chemoradiation arm.

A French study randomized 584 patients with inoperable stage III NSCLC to radiation alone (66 Gy in 2 Gy fractions) or carboplatin (15 mg/m^2 daily) with concurrent radiation, with both arms receiving two cycles of induction vinorelbine (30 mg/m^2 weekly for nine weeks) and cisplatin (100 mg/m^2, weeks 1, 5, and 9) (54). In patients who have responded to chemotherapy, the one-year local control rate was similar in both arms, with no significant benefit seen in median survival.

Another French study randomized 205 patients with good performance status and inoperable stage III NSCLC to sequential cisplatin (120 mg/m^2 on days 1, 29, and 57) and vinorelbine (30 mg/m^2 weekly) followed by 66 Gy in 2 Gy fractions versus concurrent radiation, daily cisplatin (20 mg/m^2/day) and daily etoposide (50 mg/m^2/day) on days 1 to 5 and days 29 to 33 (55). Both arms received two cycles of consolidative cisplatin (80 mg/m^2) and vinorelbine (30 mg/m^2 weekly) after chemoradiation (as opposed to sequential induction chemotherapy as used in the trials discussed thus far). Although esophageal toxicity was worse (32% vs. 3%) in the concurrent arm, the survival favored the concurrent arm but did not reach statistical significance.

The recently published Locally Advanced Multimodality Protocol (LAMP) addressed the benefit of induction versus consolidation chemotherapy (with two of the three arms receiving low-dose chemotherapy concurrently with radiation) and also included a sequential chemotherapy and radiation arm "without" concurrent low-dose chemotherapy (56). The LAMP is a three-arm randomized phase II study (designed to compare each arm against historical controls) in which all patients received standard radiation (63 Gy in 1.8 Gy daily fractions) as well as two cycles of systemic PC: [PC is paclitaxel (200 mg/m²) and carboplatin (AUC = 6)]. In arm 1 (sequential), PC was followed by radiation; in arm 2 (induction + concurrent), PC was followed by radiation concurrently with weekly paclitaxel (45 mg/m²) and carboplatin (AUC = 2); and in arm 3 (concurrent + consolidation), PC was preceded by radiation and concurrent weekly paclitaxel (45 mg/m²) plus carboplatin (AUC = 2). There were no significant differences in survival among these three arms (three-year overall survival 17% vs. 15% vs. 17%, respectively), with the median survival favoring (not reaching statistical significance) the third arm (13.0 months vs. 12.7 months vs. 16.3 months, respectively). Arms 2 and 3, with concurrent radiation and chemotherapy, experienced significantly more grade 3 esophagitis as compared with arm 1 (4% vs. 20% vs. 28%, respectively).

In the CALGB 39801 randomized trial for unresectable stage III NSCLC, all patients received low-dose chemoradiation, treated with concurrent radiation (66 Gy in 2 Gy fractions) and weekly paclitaxel (50 mg/m²) plus carboplatin (AUC = 2). Patients were randomized to receive or not receive two cycles of induction paclitaxel (200 mg/m²) and carboplatin (AUC = 6) (51). The trial enrolled 366 patients with stage III NSCLC. A trend toward improved median survival was seen in the arm with induction chemotherapy.

The recently completed CALGB 30105 treated all patients with two cycles of induction chemotherapy followed by thoracic radiation (74 Gy in 2 Gy fractions) with concurrent low-dose chemotherapy. Arm 1 received induction carboplatin (AUC = 6) and paclitaxel (225 mg/m²) and then carboplatin (AUC = 2 per week) and paclitaxel (45 mg/m² per week) concurrent with radiation. Arm 2 received induction carboplatin (AUC = 5) and gemcitabine (1000 mg/m²) and then gemcitabine (35 mg/m² twice per week) concurrent with radiation.

Thus, trials from the EORTC and Yugoslavia demonstrated that concurrent low-dose chemotherapy with concurrent radiation is significantly superior to radiation alone, while an Italian study did not demonstrate such a difference. When systemic doses of chemotherapy are also given sequentially, the benefit of concurrent low-dose chemotherapy is not readily apparent, with some studies revealing a trend in improved survival with concurrent low-dose chemotherapy (53–55). The LAMP study suggests a trend toward a median survival benefit with consolidation versus induction chemotherapy. The question of when full-dose chemotherapy should be given then arises: prior to radiation (induction), concurrently with radiation, and/or after radiation (consolidative). The next section discusses the concurrent delivery of full-dose chemotherapy and radiation, and whether the toxicity of such an approach is acceptable.

CONCURRENT CHEMORADIATION WITH FULL-DOSE CHEMOTHERAPY

Full-dose chemotherapy given concurrently with radiation acts both as a systemic therapy (as in sequential regimens) and as a radiation sensitizer. Several trials have compared sequential chemoradiation with concurrent chemoradiation, using full doses of chemotherapy in both arms. An obvious concern with a concurrent chemoradiation approach (particularly with full-dose chemotherapy) is the exacerbation of radiation toxicities, particularly in grade 3 to 4 esophagitis. Tables 4 and 5 summarize the studies discussed in this section.

A phase III trial from the Hoosier Oncology Group, including 240 patients with unresectable and inoperable NSCLC, did not show a benefit with the addition of concurrent moderate-dose cisplatin (70 mg/m^2 every three weeks) to daily radiation (60–65 Gy in 1.8–2.0 Gy fractions) (64).

Table 4 Summary of Actuarial Survival in Selected Trials of Concurrent Full-Dose Chemotherapy and Radiation

Trial (Refs.)	Patients	#	Treatment	MS (mo)	OS	P value
HOG phase III (64)	Unresectable	240	RT	9.9	5 yr: 5%	NS
			CRT	10.6	5 yr: 2%	
Japanese phase III (65,66)	Unresectable stage III	314	C→RT→C	13.3	3 yr: 15%	0.04
			CRT→C	16.5	3 yr: 22%	
Czech phase III (67)	Unresectable stage III	102	C→RT	12.9	3 yr: 10%	0.024
			CRT	16.6	3 yr: 19%	
RTOG 9410 phase III (24,25)	Selected unresectable stage II–III	611	C→RT	14.6	4 yr: 12%	vs. arm 1
			CRT	17.0	4 yr: 21%	0.046
			HFCRT	15.2	4 yr: 17%	0.296
RTOG 9204 ran. phase II (68,69)	Inoperable stage II–III	162	HFCRT	15.5	5 yr: 13%	NS
			C→CRT	16.5	5 yr: 16%	
CALGB 9431 ran. phase II (70)	Selected stage III	175	C→CRT (PG)	18.3	3 yr: 28%	NS
			C→CRT (PT)	14.8	3 yr: 19%	
			C→CRT (PV)	17.7	3 yr: 23%	
CALGB 9534 phase II (71)	Stage III	40	C→CRT	14	3 yr: 27%	N/A
SWOG 9019 phase II (72)	Selected stage IIIB	50	CRT	15	3 yr: 15%	
SWOG 9504 phase II (73,74)	Selected stage IIIB	83	CRT→C	26	3 yr: 37% / 5 yr: 29%	
SWOG 9429 phase II (75)	Poor risk stage III	60	CRT	13	2 yr: 21%	
SWOG 9712 phase II (76)	Poor risk stage III	96	CRT→C	10.3	2 yr: 27%	

Abbreviations: C, chemotherapy; CRT, concurrent full-dose chemotherapy and radiation; C-HFCRT, concurrent chemotherapy and hyperfractionated radiation therapy; G, gemcitabine; HFRT, hyperfractionated radiation therapy; OS, overall survival; P, cisplatin; RT, standard radiation; T, paclitaxel; V, vinorelbine; MS, median survival.

Table 5 Summary of Actuarial Survival in Selected Trials of Concurrent Full-Dose Chemotherapy and Radiation Followed by Resection

Trial (Refs.)	Patients	#	Treatment	MS (mo)	OS	P value
CALGB phase II (77)	Operable stage IIIA	41	CRT→S→C	15.5	1 yr: 58%	N/A
SWOG 8805 phase II (78,79)	Select bulky stage III	126	CRT→S	13–17	6 yr: 20%	N/A
Intergroup 0139 phase III (80,81)	Select stage III	396	CRT	23.6	5 yr: 20%	NS
			CRT→S	22.2	5 yr: 27%	NS
Intergroup 0160 phase II (82,83)	T3-4N0-1 superior sulcus	111	CRT→S	33	5 yr: 41%	All patients
				71	5 yr: 53%	After complete resection
German phase III (84)	Stage III	481	C→S→RT	15	5 yr: 24%	NS
			C→HFCRT→S	17	5 yr: 23%	NS

Abbreviations: C, chemotherapy; C-HFCRT, concurrent chemotherapy and hyperfractionated radiation therapy; CRT, concurrent full-dose chemotherapy and radiation; HFRT, hyperfractionated radiation therapy; MS, median survival; OS, overall survival; RT, standard radiation.

A Japanese trial treated 314 patients with unresectable stage III disease (excluding T3N1), with ECOG (Zubrod) performance status of 0 to 2. Radiation therapy was delivered via a split course, with 56 Gy in 2 Gy fractions; chemotherapy consisted of vindesine (3 mg/m^2 on day 1 and day 8), cisplatin (80 mg/m^2 on day 1), and mitomycin C (8 mg/m^2 on day 1), with cycles repeating every 28 days (65,66). Patients were randomized to concurrent or sequential administration of chemotherapy and radiation, with both arms receiving one to two additional cycles of consolidative chemotherapy after radiotherapy. The concurrent chemoradiation arm resulted in improved survival, reduced brain metastases, and reduced supra-clavicular failure. Local failure was similar (32.7% vs. 39.3%) in the concurrent versus sequential arm, respectively. The concurrent chemoradiotherapy arm experienced significantly ($P < 0.001$) greater myelosuppression and thrombocytopenia but had similar rates of grade 3 (and no grade 4) esophageal toxicity. In fact, the rates of grade 3 esophagitis were low (<3%), which the authors attributed to the use of split course.

A Czechoslovakian phase III study also compared sequential-versus-concurrent chemoradiotherapy in 102 patients with locally advanced stage III NSCLC (67). Chemotherapy comprised up to four cycles of cisplatin (80 mg/m^2 on day 1) and vinorelbine (25 and 12.5 mg/m^2 × 3 weeks in cycles 1, 4, and 2, 3, respectively). Radiation (60 Gy in 2 Gy fractions) was randomized to start on day 4 of cycle 2 or after chemotherapy. Median survival (16.6 months vs. 12.9 months, $P = 0.023$) and median progression-free survival (11.9 months vs. 8.5 months,

$P = 0.024$) significantly favored the concurrent chemoradiotherapy arm. The three-year local control was greater in the concurrent arm as well (35% vs. 12%, $P = 0.016$), while distant control was similar.

The RTOG 9410 trial is a three-arm phase III study that enrolled 611 patients with medically inoperable stages II and IIIA or unresectable stages IIIA to IIIB NSCLC (with KPS $\geq$ 70% and weight loss $\leq$5%). The three arms were (*i*) sequential cisplatin (80 mg/m^2 on days 1 and 29) and vinblastine (5 mg/m^2 weekly $\times$ 5) followed by standard radiation (a total of 63 Gy treated with 45 Gy in 1.8 Gy fractions followed by 18 Gy in 2 Gy fractions); (*ii*) cisplatin and vinblastine concurrently with radiation (same doses as arm 1); and (*iii*) cisplatin (50 mg/m^2 on days 1, 8, 29, and 36) and oral etoposide (50 mg twice-daily for five days during weeks 1, 2, 5, and 6) concurrently with twice-daily radiation (69.6 Gy in 1.2 Gy fractions) (24,25). The first arm was similar to the CALGB trial discussed above (but with a slightly lower cisplatin dose and slightly higher radiation dose). The second arm used the same chemotherapy regimen as arm 1 but started radiotherapy and chemotherapy together on day 1. The third arm was derived from the RTOG 9106 phase II study, which was preceded by the RTOG 9015 phase II study of 69.6 Gy hyperfractionated radiation concurrently with vinblastine and cisplatin (85,86). In the RTOG 9410 three-arm study, the second arm, with concurrent chemotherapy and standard radiotherapy had the best median and overall survival, significantly better than the arm with sequential chemotherapy. Although the difference in survival was not significant between the two arms with concurrent chemoradiotherapy, the third arm using twice-daily radiation had worse acute grade 3 top 4 nonhematological toxicity (30% vs. 48% vs. 62%) with no appreciable differences in late toxicity.

The RTOG 9204 randomized phase II trial, in patients with inoperable stage II to III NSCLC, compared hyperfractionated radiation concurrently with cisplatin and etoposide (RTOG 9106 regimen: see above) against sequential cisplatin and vinblastine followed by standard radiation (63 Gy in daily 1.8 Gy fractions) concurrently with cisplatin (75 mg/m^2) (68,69). In this trial, hyperfractionated radiation with chemotherapy delayed the time to in-field failure (32% vs. 20% at 1 year, $P = 0.009$) but did not significantly impact survival. Grade 3 to 4 acute esophagitis was significantly worse in the hyperfractionated arm (37% vs. 3.3%, $P < 0.0001$).

There are innumerable phase II studies of concurrent full-dose chemotherapy and radiation for locoregionally advanced NSCLC. Selected few studies are presented here. The CALGB 9431 study was a three-arm phase II randomized study of 175 patients with stage IIIA to IIIB NSCLC with CALGB performance status of 0 to 1 and weight loss below 5% (70). All patients received four cycles (every 21 days) of induction and concurrent cisplatin (80 mg/m^2) with radiation (66 Gy in 2 Gy fractions starting with the third cycle); the three arms were randomized to one of three additional agents: arm 1-gemcitabine (2 cycles of 1250 mg/m^2 on days 1 and 8 and 2 cycles of 600 mg/m^2 on days 1 and 8); arm 2-paclitaxel (2 cycles of 225 mg/m^2 on day 1 and 2 cycles of 135 mg/m^2 on day

1); arm 3-vinorelbine (2 cycles of 25 mg/m² on days 1 and 8 and 2 cycles of 15 mg/m² on days 1 and 8). The median survival and three-year overall survival were not significantly different among the three arms. Likewise, the median failure-free survival (8.4 months vs. 9.1 months vs. 11.5 months) and patterns of first failure were similar. Grade 3 to 4 esophagitis was seen in 52%, 39% and 25% of patients in arms 1, 2, and 3, respectively.

The CALGB 9534 study enrolled 40 stage IIIA to IIIB patients (not selected for minimal weight loss) in a phase II trial of two cycles (every three weeks) of induction paclitaxel (200 mg/m²) and carboplatin (AUC = 6) followed by concurrent radiation (66 Gy in 2 Gy fractions) and weekly paclitaxel (50 mg/m²) and carboplatin (AUC = 2) (71). A three-year failure-free survival of 15% and a three-year overall survival of 27% were achieved. The ongoing ECOG 3598 protocol is randomizing carboplatin, paclitaxel, and radiation with or without thalidomide.

The Southwest Oncology Group (SWOG) has published several phase II trials utilizing etoposide and platinum-based chemotherapy with concurrent radiation. The SWOG 9019 phase II study enrolled 50 patients with a SWOG performance status of 0 to 1 and good pulmonary function [forced expiratory volume in one second (FEV_1) > 2 L or >0.8 L in contralateral lung] diagnosed with stage IIIB NSCLC, for treatment with cisplatin (2 cycles of 50 mg/m² on days 1 and 8) and etoposide (2 cycles of 50 mg/m² on days 1–5) concurrently with radiation (45 Gy in 1.8 Gy fractions), with two additional cycles of chemotherapy and additional radiation (16 Gy in 2 Gy fractions) delivered after reassessment for response to therapy (72). This study followed from the SWOG 8805 study in which patients were treated with 45 Gy with concurrent cisplatin and etoposide followed by planned resection (discussed below). Grade 3 and 4 esophagitis occurred in 12% and 8%, respectively. The median survival of 15 months and three-year overall survival rate of 15% was promising. The SWOG 9504 trial assessed the benefit of consolidative chemotherapy after radiotherapy. The study included 83 stage IIIB NSCLC patients with the same eligibility criteria as the prior SWOG 8805 and 9019 studies and the same concurrent chemoradiation as in SWOG 9019. Consolidative docetaxel (3 cycles every 3 weeks, initiated at 75 mg/m² with escalation to 100 mg/m² during cycles 2 and 3) was added in the SWOG 9504 protocol (73,74). Grade 3/4 esophagitis occurred in 12% and 5% of patients and grade 3 radiation pneumonitis occurred in 5% (with no grade 4 pneumonitis) of patients. The median survival of 26 months and five-year overall survival rate of 29% were remarkable outcomes.

The SWOG 0023 phase III trial randomized the addition of maintenance gefitinib (Iressa) to the SWOG 9504 regimen. Gefitinib is a small molecule tyrosine kinase inhibitor that targets the epidermal growth-factor receptor. More than 500 patients enrolled before closure. A preliminary toxicity analysis has demonstrated acceptable rates of radiation pneumonitis (87). The survival in SWOG 0023 has not yet been published, though an interim analysis has reportedly shown that the arm receiving Iressa did not fare better. Furthermore, survival was not as high as that reported in SWOG 9504; if this holds true in both arms, it would temper the impressive results of SWOG 9504 somewhat, since patients in the control arm of SWOG 0023 were treated the same as in SWOG 9504.

The ongoing CALGB 30106 phase II study treated patients with two cycles of induction carboplatin (AUC = 6) and paclitaxel (200 mg/m^2) followed by standard radiation (66 Gy in 2 Gy fractions) concurrent with gefitinib. Patients with a CALGB performance status of 0 to 1 and weight loss of 5% or less also received weekly carboplatin (AUC = 2) and paclitaxel (50 mg/m^2) concurrent with radiation, while poor risk patients (performance status = 2 or weight loss >5%) received only gefitinib. Preliminary analysis had demonstrated acceptable toxicity (88).

The recently completed RTOG 0324 phase II study treated stage IIIA to IIIB patients with weekly paclitaxel (50 mg/m^2), carboplatin (AUC = 2), and cetuximab (a chimeric monoclonal antibody that blocks epidermal growth-factor receptors) concurrently with radiation (63 Gy) followed by consolidation paclitaxel (200 mg/m^2), carboplatin (AUC = 6), and cetuximab. Toxicity reported in an interim analysis was acceptable (55% nonhematological grade 3 toxicity) (89).

The SWOG 9429 study enrolled 60 patients with stage III NSCLC, who were not eligible for cisplatin-based protocols because of poor risk (poor pulmonary or renal function, history of congestive heart failure, hearing loss, peripheral neuropathy, or weight loss) (75). Patients received daily radiation (61 Gy) concurrently with two cycles (every 28 days) of carboplatin (200 mg/m^2 on days 1 and 3) and etoposide (50 mg/m^2 on days 1–4). Grade 3 to 4 toxicities were as follows: esophagitis in 15%, leukopenia in 50%, and thrombocytopenia in 23%. The median survival was 13 months and two-year overall survival, 21%. These numbers approached the survival of favorable risk patients. The subsequent SWOG 9712 phase II trial enrolled 96 poor risk stage IIIA to IIIB patients treated as in SWOG 9429, with the addition of consolidation paclitaxel (76). The addition of consolidation chemotherapy improved the response rate (58% vs. 29% in SWOG 9429) whereas the median survival of 10.3 months and two-year overall survival of 27% were slightly worse than outcomes in the prior 9429 regimen. Grade 3 to 4 toxicities during radiation were as follows: esophagitis in 5%, leukopenia in 45% and thrombocytopenia in 23%. There is an ongoing SWOG 0429 study, which is a phase I study of weekly docetaxel and cetuximab for poor risk stage III NSCLC patients.

In summary, emerging data supports the use of concurrent radiation and full-dose chemotherapy for stage III NSCLC. Several randomized studies have shown that the concurrent delivery of radiation and full-dose chemotherapy yields significantly improved survival over the sequential delivery of the same chemotherapy and radiation (24,25,55,67). Since the systemic treatment of distant micrometastases should be the same with either concurrent or sequential delivery of full-dose chemotherapy, the improved survival would suggest an effect of improved locoregional control, which was demonstrated in the Czechoslovakian trial but not the French study (and is not yet reported in RTOG 9410). There is no strong evidence to support hyperfractionated radiation (with or without concurrent chemotherapy). Induction and/or consolidation chemotherapy in the setting of full-dose chemotherapy with concurrent radiation does not appear to have a well-defined role though this has not been tested in phase III trials. Nevertheless, the impressive results of the SWOG 9504 phase II study (see above) support treatment of those who are in a favorable risk subgroup with concurrent cisplatin, etoposide, and radiation followed with consolidation docetaxel.

NEOADJUVANT CHEMORADIATION FOLLOWED BY SURGERY

Several studies have demonstrated pathologic downstaging and/or improved survival with the use of induction chemotherapy followed by resection (41–45). An emerging treatment approach in stage III NSCLC is induction chemotherapy with concurrent radiation followed by resection. Several studies, discussed below, have demonstrated that neoadjuvant chemoradiation and resection is a promising approach.

The CALGB enrolled 41 stage IIIA patients in a phase II study using two cycles of cisplatin (100 mg/m^2 on day 1), vinblastine (3 mg/m^2 on days 1–3), and 5-fluorouracil (30 mg/kg on days 1–3) concurrently with 30 Gy of radiation (2 Gy fractions) followed by resection and consolidation chemotherapy (one additional cycle) concurrent with an additional 60 Gy. Of the 41 patients who had enrolled, 31 underwent surgery and 25 had a resection. The one-year overall survival rate was 58% and median survival was 15.5 months (77).

The SWOG conducted a landmark phase II study (SWOG 8805) in 126 patients with stage IIIA to B NSCLC treated with neoadjuvant cisplatin (2 cycles of 50 mg/m^2 on days 1 and 8) and etoposide (2 cycles of 50 mg/m^2 on days 1–5) concurrently with standard radiation (45 Gy in 1.8 Gy daily fractions) (78,79). Patients were selected with a SWOG performance status of 0 to 1 and good pulmonary function (FEV$_1$ >2 L or >0.8 L in the contralateral lung). Eligible T4 disease was limited to carinal, tracheal, or mediastinal invasion; eligible N3 disease included supraclavicular and/or contralateral mediastinal lymphadenopathy. After neoadjuvant chemoradiotherapy, if sampled lymph nodes were positive at thoracotomy, or if the patient was unable to undergo a curative resection, then the patient went on to receive additional chemoradiation of 14.4 Gy. Of the 107 patients eligible for thoracotomy (85% of those enrolled), 85% of stage IIIA patients underwent resection while 9% were deemed unresectable; for stage IIIB patients, 80% underwent resection, while 15% were unresectable. The median survival was 13 months among stage IIIA patients and 17 months among stage IIIB patients (not significantly different). The corresponding two-year overall survival rate was 37% and 39%, respectively. The six-year overall survival rate of those undergoing trimodality therapy was 20% with identical survival for stages IIIA and B.

The impressive results of SWOG 8805 (neoadjuvant chemoradiotherapy) in stage IIIA to B patients and SWOG 9019 (definitive chemoradiotherapy) in stage IIIB patients led to the SWOG sponsored Intergroup 0139 trial comparing neoadjuvant chemoradiotherapy and resection versus definitive chemoradiotherapy in 396 eligible patients with stage IIIA NSCLC, who had good performance status and lung function (as in the earlier studies) and technically resectable disease at the time of registration (80,81). In this trial, patients were randomized to definitive chemoradiation as in SWOG 9019 versus neoadjuvant chemoradiation as in SWOG 8805. Grade 3 to 4 esophagitis was significantly greater in the definitive chemoradiation arm (44% vs. 20%, $P = 0.0006$), while other toxicities were similarly prevalent. The neoadjuvant chemoradiotherapy arm resulted in significantly improved local control (10% vs. 22%, $P = 0.002$) and progression-free survival (five-year progression-free survival of 22.4% vs.11.1% and median progression-free survival 12.8 vs. 10.5 months, $P = 0.017$). Survival at two years was similar in both arms, with a median survival of 23.6 versus 22.2; after 18 months the actuarial curves crossed, beyond which there was a trend ($P = 0.1$) toward improved survival beyond five years (five-year overall survival 27.2% vs. 20.3%) in patients undergoing resection. Patients in the neoadjuvant chemoradiotherapy arm, who underwent pneumonectomy, had a 26% perioperative mortality in contrast with 1% of patients undergoing lobectomy, suggesting that a trimodality approach is not recommended in patients who would require pneumonectomy. Randomized patients who underwent lobectomy, compared with a matched pair cohort of randomized patients treated with definitive chemoradiation, had a significantly improved five-year overall survival rate (36% vs. 18%, $P = 0.002$).

The Intergroup 0160 phase II trial, sponsored by the SWOG (9416), enrolled 111 patients with mediastinoscopy-negative T3-4 N0-1 superior sulcus NSCLC, treated with two cycles of cisplatin and etoposide chemotherapy concurrently with 45 Gy radiation (as in SWOG 8805), followed by resection and two additional cycles of consolidation cisplatin and etoposide chemotherapy. Of 95 patients eligible for surgery, 88 underwent thoracotomy and 83 had a complete resection. The median survival was 33 months for all patients and 71 months in those undergoing complete resection. The corresponding five-year overall survival rate was 41% and 53%, respectively (82,83).

The RTOG 0229 study is an ongoing phase II study enrolling patients with stage IIIA to B NSCLC, to be treated with induction chemotherapy with weekly carboplatin (AUC = 2) and paclitaxel (50 mg/m²) concurrently with full-dose chest radiation (50.4 Gy + 10.8 Gy boost to tumor) followed by planned resection; all patients (resectable or not) will receive consolidation carboplatin (AUC = 6) and paclitaxel (200 mg/m²) chemotherapy every three weeks. The novel aspect of this study is the relatively higher preoperative radiation dose used.

A German study randomized 481 eligible patients with stage IIIA to B NSCLC to neoadjuvant chemoradiation versus neoadjuvant chemotherapy. Patients in the chemoradiation arm were treated with three cycles cisplatin (55 mg/m² on days 1 and 4) and etoposide (100 mg/m², days 1–4), followed by hyperfractionated radiation (45 Gy in 1.5 Gy twice-daily fractions) with concurrent weekly carboplatin (100 mg/m²) and vindesin (3 mg) followed by surgery. Patients in the chemotherapy-alone arm received three cycles of cisplatin and etoposide followed by surgery, which was followed by postoperative radiation (54 Gy in 1.8 Gy fractions). Patients who did not undergo a complete resection would receive a total of 69 Gy in arm 1 and 68.4 Gy in arm 2. Patients in the chemoradiation arm experienced significantly more grade 3 to 4 esophagitis (15% vs. 4%, $P < 0.0001$), with no appreciable differences in response rate, rate of resection (45% vs. 50%), treatment-related deaths, progression-free survival, median survival (15 months vs. 17 months), and three-year overall survival (24% vs. 23%). Because of the relatively small percentage of patients undergoing resection (as compared with the SWOG studies), it is difficult to interpret these results (84).

The recently closed SWOG 0332/RTOG 0412 randomized controlled trial sought to compare induction chemotherapy with two cycles (every three weeks) of cisplatin (75 mg/m^2 on day 1) and docetaxel (75 mg/m^2 on day 1) followed by resection versus induction chemoradiotherapy with two cycles (every three weeks) of cisplatin (50 mg/m^2 on days 1 and 8) and docetaxel (20 mg/m^2 on days 1, 8, and 15) concurrently with radiation (50.4 Gy in 1.8 Gy fractions) followed by resection. Three cycles (every three weeks) of consolidation docetaxel (75 mg/m^2 on day 1) were offered after resection. Eligible patients must have had a single parenchymal lesion, stage IIIA disease with ipsilateral involved mediastinal lymph nodes measuring ≤3 cm and separate from primary tumor. The trial was closed due to poor accrual.

In summary, neoadjuvant chemoradiation followed by resection has shown promising results in stage III NSCLC patients. Preliminary data suggests that trimodality therapy with surgery and chemoradiation results in improved disease control as well as improved survival as compared with definitive chemoradiation, particularly if patients are selected with minimal gross disease (i.e., nonbulky stage IIIA) who require only a lobectomy. The ongoing SWOG/RTOG study will help determine the benefit, if any, of radiation in the neoadjuvant approach for marginally resectable stage III NSCLC.

ADJUVANT CHEMORADIATION FOLLOWING RESECTION OF NSCLC

Following resection of NSCLC lung cancer, treatment options include observation, adjuvant chemotherapy, adjuvant radiation, or adjuvant chemoradiation (delivered either concurrently or sequentially). In order to properly discuss adjuvant chemoradiation, it is necessary to first briefly discuss adjuvant chemotherapy and adjuvant radiation separately.

Postoperative Chemotherapy After Resection

For stage IB to III NSCLC, randomized data and a meta-analysis support the addition of platinum-based systemic chemotherapy as a component of therapy along with resection (1). The recent International Adjuvant Lung Cancer Trial (IALT) demonstrated a significant disease-free survival and overall survival benefit with adjuvant cisplatin-based chemotherapy (90). In the subset of stage III patients, this benefit remained significant, while in the subset of stage II patients, a trend toward an overall survival benefit was observed. In the recently published Adjuvant Navelbine International Trialist Association (ANITA) trial, similar results were observed in patients receiving adjuvant vinorelbine plus cisplatin (91). A recent Intergroup trial, sponsored by the National Cancer Institute of Canada, demonstrated a significant median survival and overall survival advantage in stage IB to II patients randomized to adjuvant cisplatin and vinorelbine chemotherapy (92). The CALGB 9633 randomized study in resected stage IB demonstrated a survival advantage with the addition of adjuvant carboplatin and paclitaxel (93).

Postoperative Radiation After Resection

Postoperative radiation in the setting of completely resected NSCLC is somewhat controversial. It is generally accepted that radiation should be offered to patients with positive surgical margins, inadequate resection of the primary lung cancer, and/or inadequate mediastinal lymph-node dissection. In addition, postoperative mediastinal radiation is often offered in patients with resected N2 lymph nodes, though the role of postoperative radiation remains controversial. There have been several retrospective analyses assessing the benefit of adjuvant radiation with conflicting results. For resected N2 disease, large retrospective studies from Massachusetts General Hospital and the Mayo Clinic have demonstrated an improvement in disease control in the chest as well as overall survival with the addition of postoperative radiation (94–96). However, the postoperative radiation therapy (PORT) meta-analysis of randomized studies of postoperative radiation in stage I to III patients has suggested that postoperative radiation is detrimental to survival, though this was not the case in the subset analysis of stage III patients or patients with N2 disease (97). Nonetheless, the trials included in this meta-analysis had many flaws, which are discussed well elsewhere (98–100). In fact, in the IALT (randomizing adjuvant chemotherapy after resection), postoperative radiation was offered to patients following chemotherapy based on individual institutional policy (90). Overall, 30.6% of all patients, 1.9% of N0, 33.7% of N1, and 64.3% of N2 received postoperative radiation following chemotherapy.

In a randomized trial from the Lung Cancer Study Group (LCSG), 210 patients with resected stage II to III squamous-cell carcinoma were randomized to receive or not receive postoperative mediastinal radiation. Postoperative radiation reduced locoregional failure from 41% without radiation to 3%, but did not impact survival (101). On subset analysis by N stage, only patients with N2 disease derived a significant benefit ($P = 0.03$) in disease control. Randomized studies from China and from the British Medical Research Council have also demonstrated a significant local control benefit with the addition of postoperative radiation (102,103). It should be recognized that these studies did not include systemic chemotherapy.

In a recent Surveillance, Epidemiology, and End Results (SEER) database retrospective study, the use of postoperative radiation in patients with N2 disease resulted in a significantly improved overall survival (hazard ratio of 0.86, $P = 0.0077$) (104). The individual patient data on the use of adjuvant chemotherapy was not available in the SEER database. The extent to which radiation improves local disease control in patients also receiving systemic chemotherapy has not been widely studied. In randomized studies comparing resection with or without induction chemotherapy, chemotherapy does reduce distant failures but does not seem to impact locoregional control. In fact, radiation may play a more important role for patients receiving postoperative systemic chemotherapy, since chemotherapy reduces rates of distant failure, and thus omitting radiotherapy may shift the patterns of failure to more locoregional failures. No modern cooperative group study has randomized postresection radiation versus no radiation in patients receiving systemic chemotherapy (pre- or postoperative). Retrospective data from M.D. Anderson Cancer Center suggests that radiation improves local control in stage IIB to IIIA patients treated with induction chemotherapy followed by resection, with five-year local control (LC) rates of 81% versus 54% ($P = 0.07$) in all patients, and 82% versus 35% ($P = 0.01$) in the subset of stage IIIA patients (105). In the recently published ANITA trial, each participating institution decided whether or not to use postoperative radiation (as was done in the IALT). The subset of N2 patients in the ANITA study who received postoperative radiation had a significant survival benefit versus those not treated with radiation, regardless of whether or not the patient was randomized to receive chemotherapy (91).

Postoperative Chemoradiation

A few studies have examined the concurrent administration of chemotherapy and radiation after surgery. An Intergroup study, sponsored by the ECOG, randomized 488 patients with stage II to IIIA NSCLC to postoperative radiation (50.4 Gy plus a boost of 10.8 Gy to sites of nodal extracapsular extension) with or without concurrent and adjuvant cisplatin (60 mg/m^2, day 1) and etoposide (120 mg/m^2, days 1–3) chemotherapy for four planned cycles every 28 days (106). All patients with lymph nodes over 1.5 cm were required to undergo mediastinoscopy, and patients with over 1 mediastinal lymph-node level were not eligible. The median survival (38–39 months), five-year overall survival (~40%), and patterns of failure were similar in both arms.

The RTOG recently published a phase II study (RTOG 9705, initiated before the Intergroup trial was published) in which 88 patients were treated with radiation (similar to Intergroup study) and four cycles (every three weeks) of concurrent and adjuvant carboplatin (AUC = 5 day 1 concurrent with radiation, AUC = 6 postradiation) and paclitaxel (135 mg/m^2 on day 1 concurrent with radiation, 225 mg/m^2 postradiation) (107). The three-year overall survival, progression-free survival, and local failure rates were 61%, 50%, and 15%, respectively.

An LCSG trial compared postoperative radiation with postoperative chemoradiation in patients with stage I to IIIA NSCLC left with positive surgical margins and/or metastasis in the highest sampled paratracheal lymph node (108,109). In this study, 164 patients were randomized to a 40-Gy split course of radiation with or without concurrent and adjuvant cytoxan (400 mg/m^2), adriamycin (40 mg/m^2), and cisplatin (40 mg/m^2) chemotherapy (six cycles every four weeks). Chemoradiation significantly improved the three-year disease-free survival (28% vs. 13%), while overall survival was not significantly affected. A local control benefit was only seen in patients with macroscopic residual.

In summary, after resection of stage II to III NSCLC, recent results from large phase III studies support that chemotherapy should be offered in the adjuvant setting. Postoperative radiation should be offered to patients with positive surgical margins, inadequate resection of the primary lung cancer, and/or inadequate mediastinal lymph-node dissection. In patients with completely resected stage III NSCLC, mediastinal radiation may be offered in order to reduce locoregional failure. Based on the recent SEER and ANITA studies, mediastinal radiation may also confer a survival benefit, though confirmation from a phase III study would be needed to solidify this recommendation.

CONCLUSIONS

Undoubtedly, progress has been made in the treatment of locally advanced NSCLC over the past decades, with disease control and survival improving as chemotherapy has been added to radiation therapy for curative treatment. How to best integrate different modalities to achieve optimal outcome is under continued investigation; at the current state, full-dose chemotherapy with concurrent radiation is proving to result in better disease control and survival as compared with sequential chemoradiotherapy.

Despite advances, the optimal treatment approach has yet to be determined. A highly effective regimen with minimal toxicity is the ideal goal. As discussed above, the radiation dose, fractionation, and treatment volume are areas of continued investigation. At this time, the optimal chemotherapy agents, doses, and dose schedules are not known. Except for two large phase III trials (48,49), most other clinical studies found that low-dose chemotherapy with concurrent radiotherapy did not seem to significantly improve efficacy above radiotherapy alone, particularly in patients who underwent induction and/or consolidative chemotherapy. However, in patients who cannot tolerate systemic doses of chemotherapy, a low-dose radiosensitizing chemoradiotherapy regimen may be warranted, particularly since most trials do show at least a trend toward survival benefit with low-dose chemotherapy with concurrent radiation. Also, most of the cooperative group studies employing systemic doses of chemotherapy did not include elderly patients and/or patients with poor performance status (with the notable exception of the SWOG 9429 and 9712 studies) and, therefore, the results from these studies do not necessarily apply to this population.

Although third-generation chemotherapeutic agents, in full dose or low-dose administration, have not been fully investigated in combination with radiation, they may have the potential of surpassing cisplatin-based chemoradiation (3). Certainly with stage IV NSCLC, there is an abundance of trials comparing chemotherapeutic regimens, which is unfortunately not the case with stage III NSCLC. Biologic agents that affect angiogenesis (110,111) inhibit growth-factor receptors or downstream effectors of growth-factor receptors (89,112,113) and/or alter the cell cycle may prove to be successful additions to standard chemotherapeutic agents and/or radiation. Radiation modifiers (i.e., radiation protectors and nonchemotherapeutic radiation sensitizers) have not shown great potential, but warrant further study. Surgery preceded by chemoradiation has shown great promise, primarily in patients with stage IIIA NSCLC with minimal disease burden but also in some patients with initially inoperable stage IIIB NSCLC. Without doubt, the continued investigation of multimodality curative treatment approaches to NSCLC will result in future improvements in disease control, patient survival, and treatment tolerability.

REFERENCES

1. Non-small Cell Lung Cancer Collaborative Group. Chemotherapy in non-small cell lung cancer: a meta-analysis using updated data on individual patients from 52 randomised clinical trials. BMJ 1995; 311:899–909.
2. Schiller JH, Harrington D, Belani CP, et al. Comparison of four chemotherapy regimens for advanced non-small-cell lung cancer. N Engl J Med 2002; 346:92–98.
3. Chen Y, Okunieff P. Radiation and third-generation chemotherapy. Hematol Oncol Clin North Am 2004; 18:55–80.
4. Mehta V. Radiation pneumonitis and pulmonary fibrosis in non-small-cell lung cancer: pulmonary function, prediction, and prevention. Int J Radiat Oncol Biol Phys 2005; 63:5–24.
5. Bradley JD, Perez CA, Dehdashti F, et al. Implementing biologic target volumes in radiation treatment planning for non-small cell lung cancer. J Nucl Med 2004; 45 (suppl)1:96S–101S.
6. Ramsey CR, Langen KM, Kupelian PA, et al. A technique for adaptive image-guided helical tomotherapy for lung cancer. Int J Radiat Oncol Biol Phys 2006.
7. Berson AM, Emery R, Rodriguez L, et al. Clinical experience using respiratory gated radiation therapy: comparison of free-breathing and breath-hold techniques. Int J Radiat Oncol Biol Phys 2004; 60:419–426.
8. Rosenzweig KE, Yorke E, Amols H, et al. Tumor motion control in the treatment of non small cell lung cancer. Cancer Invest 2005; 23:129–133.
9. Chang JY, Liu HH, Komaki R. Intensity modulated radiation therapy and proton radiotherapy for non-small cell lung cancer. Curr Oncol Rep 2005; 7:255–259.
10. Movsas B, Scott C, Langer C, et al. Randomized trial of amifostine in locally advanced non-small-cell lung cancer patients receiving chemotherapy and hyperfractionated radiation: radiation therapy oncology group trial 98-01. J Clin Oncol 2005; 23:2145–2154.
11. Perez CA, Bauer M, Edelstein S, et al. Impact of tumor control on survival in carcinoma of the lung treated with irradiation. Int J Radiat Oncol Biol Phys 1986; 12:539–547.
12. Perez CA, Pajak TF, Rubin P, et al. Long-term observations of the patterns of failure in patients with unresectable non-oat cell carcinoma of the lung treated with definitive radiotherapy. Report by the Radiation Therapy Oncology Group. Cancer 1987; 59:1874–1881.

13. Socinski MA, Morris DE, Halle JS, et al. Induction and concurrent chemotherapy with high-dose thoracic conformal radiation therapy in unresectable stage IIIA and IIIB non-small-cell lung cancer: a dose-escalation phase I trial. J Clin Oncol 2004; 22:4341–4350.
14. Hayman JA, Martel MK, Ten Haken RK, et al. Dose escalation in non-small-cell lung cancer using three-dimensional conformal radiation therapy: update of a phase I trial. J Clin Oncol 2001; 19:127–136.
15. Rosenzweig KE, Sim SE, Mychalczak B, et al. Elective nodal irradiation in the treatment of non-small-cell lung cancer with three-dimensional conformal radiation therapy. Int J Radiat Oncol Biol Phys 2001; 50:681–685.
16. Senan S, Burgers S, Samson MJ, et al. Can elective nodal irradiation be omitted in stage III non-small-cell lung cancer? Analysis of recurrences in a phase II study of induction chemotherapy and involved-field radiotherapy. Int J Radiat Oncol Biol Phys 2002; 54:999–1006.
17. Marks LB, Garst J, Socinski MA, et al. Carboplatin/paclitaxel or carboplatin/vinorelbine followed by accelerated hyperfractionated conformal radiation therapy: report of a prospective phase I dose escalation trial from the Carolina Conformal Therapy Consortium. J Clin Oncol 2004; 22:4329–4340.
18. Kong FM, Ten Haken RK, Schipper MJ, et al. High-dose radiation improved local tumor control and overall survival in patients with inoperable/unresectable non-small-cell lung cancer: long-term results of a radiation dose escalation study. Int J Radiat Oncol Biol Phys 2005; 63:324–333.
19. Bradley J, Graham MV, Winter K, et al. Toxicity and outcome results of RTOG 9311: a phase I-II dose-escalation study using three-dimensional conformal radiotherapy in patients with inoperable non-small-cell lung carcinoma. Int J Radiat Oncol Biol Phys 2005; 61:318–328.
20. Bradley J. A review of radiation dose escalation trials for non-small cell lung cancer within the Radiation Therapy Oncology Group. Semin Oncol 2005; 32: S111–S113.
21. Bonner JA, McGinnis WL, Stella PJ, et al. The possible advantage of hyperfractionated thoracic radiotherapy in the treatment of locally advanced nonsmall cell lung carcinoma: results of a North Central Cancer Treatment Group Phase III Study. Cancer 1998; 82:1037–1048.
22. Saunders M, Dische S, Barrett A, et al. Continuous hyperfractionated accelerated radiotherapy versus conventional radiotherapy in non-small-cell lung cancer: a randomised multicentre trial. CHART Steering Committee. Lancet 1997; 350: 161–165.
23. Belani CP, Wang W, Johnson DH, et al. Phase III study of the Eastern Cooperative Oncology Group (ECOG 2597): induction chemotherapy followed by either standard thoracic radiotherapy or hyperfractionated accelerated radiotherapy for patients with unresectable stage IIIA and B non-small-cell lung cancer. J Clin Oncol 2005; 23:3760–3767.
24. Curran WJ, Scott CB, Langer J, et al. Long-term benefit is observed in a phase III comparison of sequential vs concurrent chemo-radiation for patients with unresected stage III NSCLC: RTOG 9410. Proc Am Soc Clin Oncol (IL) 2003; 22:621.
25. Komaki R, Seiferheld W, Curran W, et al. Sequential vs. concurrent chemotherapy and radiation therapy for inoperable non-small cell lung cancer (NSCLC): analysis of

failures in a phase III study (RTOG 9410) Proc Am Soc Ther Radiat Oncol 2000; 48:113.

26. Curran WJ Jr, Stafford PM. Lack of apparent difference in outcome between clinically staged IIIA and IIIB non-small-cell lung cancer treated with radiation therapy. J Clin Oncol 1990; 8:409–415.

27. Cox JD, Azarnia N, Byhardt RW, et al. A randomized phase I/II trial of hyperfractionated radiation therapy with total doses of 60.0 Gy to 79.2 Gy: possible survival benefit with greater than or equal to 69.6 Gy in favorable patients with Radiation Therapy Oncology Group stage III non-small-cell lung carcinoma: report of Radiation Therapy Oncology Group 83-11. J Clin Oncol 1990; 8:1543–1555.

28. Martini N, Flehinger BJ. The role of surgery in N2 lung cancer. Surg Clin North Am 1987; 67:1037–1049.

29. Andre F, Grunenwald D, Pignon JP, et al. Survival of patients with resected N2 non-small-cell lung cancer: evidence for a subclassification and implications. J Clin Oncol 2000; 18:2981–2989.

30. Marino P, Preatoni A, Cantoni A. Randomized trials of radiotherapy alone versus combined chemotherapy and radiotherapy in stages IIIa and IIIb nonsmall cell lung cancer. A meta-analysis. Cancer 1995; 76:593–601.

31. Dillman RO, Seagren SL, Propert KJ, et al. A randomized trial of induction chemotherapy plus high-dose radiation versus radiation alone in stage III non-small-cell lung cancer. N Engl J Med 1990; 323:940–945.

32. Dillman RO, Herndon J, Seagren SL, et al. Improved survival in stage III non-small-cell lung cancer: seven-year follow-up of cancer and leukemia group B (CALGB) 8433 trial. J Natl Cancer Inst 1996; 88:1210–1215.

33. Morton RF, Jett JR, McGinnis WL, et al. Thoracic radiation therapy alone compared with combined chemoradiotherapy for locally unresectable non-small cell lung cancer. A randomized, phase III trial. Ann Intern Med 1991; 115:681–686.

34. Le Chevalier T, Arriagada R, Quoix E, et al. Radiotherapy alone versus combined chemotherapy and radiotherapy in nonresectable non-small-cell lung cancer: first analysis of a randomized trial in 353 patients. J Natl Cancer Inst 1991; 83: 417–423.

35. Le Chevalier T, Arriagada R, Quoix E, et al. Radiotherapy alone versus combined chemotherapy and radiotherapy in unresectable non-small cell lung carcinoma. Lung Cancer 1994; 10(suppl 1):S239–S244.

36. Komaki R, Scott CB, Sause WT, et al. Induction cisplatin/vinblastine and irradiation vs. irradiation in unresectable squamous cell lung cancer: failure patterns by cell type in RTOG 88-08/ECOG 4588. Radiation Therapy Oncology Group. Eastern Cooperative Oncology Group. Int J Radiat Oncol Biol Phys 1997; 39:537–544.

37. Sause W, Kolesar P, Taylor SI, et al. Final results of phase III trial in regionally advanced unresectable non-small cell lung cancer: Radiation Therapy Oncology Group, Eastern Cooperative Oncology Group, and Southwest Oncology Group. Chest 2000; 117:358–364.

38. Cox JD, Azarnia N, Byhardt RW, et al. N2 (clinical) non-small cell carcinoma of the lung: prospective trials of radiation therapy with total doses 60 Gy by the Radiation Therapy Oncology Group. Int J Radiat Oncol Biol Phys 1991; 20:7–12.

39. Johnstone DW, Byhardt RW, Ettinger D, et al. Phase III study comparing chemotherapy and radiotherapy with preoperative chemotherapy and surgical resection in patients with non-small-cell lung cancer with spread to mediastinal lymph nodes

(N2); final report of RTOG 89-01. Radiation Therapy Oncology Group. Int J Radiat Oncol Biol Phys 2002; 54:365–369.

40. van Meerbeeck JP, Kramer G, Van Schil PE, et al. A randomized trial of radical surgery (S) versus thoracic radiotherapy in patients (pts) with stage IIIA-N2 non-small cell lung cancer after response to induction chemotherapy (ICT) (EORTC 08941). Proc Am Soc Clin Oncol (FL) 2005 [abstr. 7015].

41. Rosell R, Gomez-Codina J, Camps C, et al. A randomized trial comparing preoperative chemotherapy plus surgery with surgery alone in patients with non-small-cell lung cancer. N Engl J Med 1994; 330:153–158.

42. Roth JA, Fossella F, Komaki R, et al. A randomized trial comparing perioperative chemotherapy and surgery with surgery alone in resectable stage IIIA non-small-cell lung cancer. J Natl Cancer Inst 1994; 86:673–680.

43. Rosell R, Gomez-Codina J, Camps C, et al. Preresectional chemotherapy in stage IIIA non-small-cell lung cancer: a 7-year assessment of a randomized controlled trial. Lung Cancer 1999; 26:7–14.

44. Depierre A, Milleron B, Moro-Sibilot D, et al. Preoperative chemotherapy followed by surgery compared with primary surgery in resectable stage I (except T1N0), II, and IIIa non-small-cell lung cancer. J Clin Oncol 2002; 20:247–253.

45. Pisters K, Vallieres E, Bunn P, et al. S9900: a phase III trial of surgery alone or surgery plus preoperative (preop) paclitaxel/carboplatin chemotherapy in early stage non-small cell lung cancer: preliminary results. Proc Am Soc Clin Oncol (FL) 2005 [abstr. 7012].

46. Vokes EE. Optimal therapy for unresectable stage III non-small-cell lung cancer. J Clin Oncol 2005; 23:5853–5855.

47. Effects of vinorelbine on quality of life and survival of elderly patients with advanced non-small-cell lung cancer. The Elderly Lung Cancer Vinorelbine Italian Study Group. J Natl Cancer Inst 1999; 91:66–72.

48. Schaake-Koning C, van den Bogaert W, Dalesio O, et al. Effects of concomitant cisplatin and radiotherapy on inoperable non-small-cell lung cancer. N Engl J Med 1992; 326:524–530.

49. Jeremic B, Shibamoto Y, Acimovic L, et al. Randomized trial of hyperfractionated radiation therapy with or without concurrent chemotherapy for stage III non-small-cell lung cancer. J Clin Oncol 1995; 13:452–458.

50. Trovo MG, Minatel E, Franchin G, et al. Radiotherapy versus radiotherapy enhanced by cisplatin in stage III non-small cell lung cancer. Int J Radiat Oncol Biol Phys 1992; 24:11–15.

51. Vokes EE, Herndon JE, Kelley MJ, et al. Induction chemotherapy followed by concomitant chemoradiotherapy (CT/XRT) versus CT/XRT alone for regionally advanced unresectable non-small cell lung cancer (NSCLC): initial analysis of a randomized phase III trial. Proc Am Soc Clin Oncol (LA) 2004 [abstr. 7005].

52. Clamon G, Herndon J, Cooper R, et al. Radiosensitization with carboplatin for patients with unresectable stage III non-small-cell lung cancer: a phase III trial of the Cancer and Leukemia Group B and the Eastern Cooperative Oncology Group. J Clin Oncol 1999; 17:4–11.

53. Huber RM, Schmidt M, Flentje M, et al. Induction chemotherapy and following simultaneous radio/chemotherapy versus induction chemotherapy and radiotherapy alone in inoperable NSCLC (Stage IIIA/IIIB) Proc Am Soc Clin Oncol 2003; 22:622.

54. Gervais R, Ducolone A, Lechevalier T, et al. Conventional radiation (RT) with daily carboplatin (Cb) compared to RT alone after induction chemotherapy (ICT) [vinorelbine (Vr)-cisplatin (P)]: final results of a randomized phase III trial in stage III unresectable non small cell lung (NSCLC) cancer. Study CRG/BMS/NPC/96 of the French Lung Cancer Study Group FNCLCC and IFCT. Proc Am Soc Clin Oncol 2005 [abstr. 7016].

55. Fournel P, Robinet G, Thomas P, et al. Randomized phase III trial of sequential chemoradiotherapy compared with concurrent chemoradiotherapy in locally advanced non-small-cell lung cancer: Groupe Lyon-Saint-Etienne d'Oncologie Thoracique-Groupe Francais de Pneumo-Cancerologie NPC 95-01 Study. J Clin Oncol 2005; 23:5910–5917.

56. Belani CP, Choy H, Bonomi P, et al. Combined chemoradiotherapy regimens of paclitaxel and carboplatin for locally advanced non-small-cell lung cancer: a randomized phase II locally advanced multi-modality protocol. J Clin Oncol 2005; 23:5883–5891.

57. Jeremic B, Jevremovic S, Mijatovic L, et al. Hyperfractionated radiation therapy with and without concurrent chemotherapy for advanced non-small cell lung cancer. Cancer 1993; 71:3732–3736.

58. Jeremic B, Shibamoto Y, Milicic B, et al. Concurrent radiochemotherapy for patients with stage III non-small-cell lung cancer: long-term results of a phase II study. Int J Radiat Oncol Biol Phys 1998; 42:1091–1096.

59. Jeremic B, Shibamoto Y, Acimovic L, et al. Hyperfractionated radiation therapy and concurrent low-dose, daily carboplatin/etoposide with or without weekend carboplatin/etoposide chemotherapy in stage III non-small-cell lung cancer: a randomized trial. Int J Radiat Oncol Biol Phys 2001; 50:19–25.

60. Jeremic B, Milicic B, Dagovic A, et al. Interfraction interval in patients with stage III\ non-small-cell lung cancer treated with hyperfractionated radiation therapy with or without concurrent chemotherapy: final results in 536 patients. Am J Clin Oncol 2004; 27:616–625.

61. Jeremic B, Milicic B, Dagovic A, et al. Stage III non-small-cell lung cancer treated with high-dose hyperfractionated radiation therapy and concurrent low-dose daily chemotherapy with or without weekend chemotherapy: retrospective analysis of 301 patients. Am J Clin Oncol 2004; 27:350–360.

62. Jeremic B, Milicic B, Acimovic L, et al. Concurrent hyperfractionated radiotherapy and low-dose daily carboplatin/paclitaxel in patients with early-stage (I/II) non-small-cell lung cancer: long-term results of a phase II study. J Clin Oncol 2005; 23:6873–6880.

63. Jeremic B, Milicic B, Acimovic L, et al. Concurrent hyperfractionated radiotherapy and low-dose daily carboplatin and paclitaxel in patients with stage III non-small cell lung cancer: long-term results of a phase II study. J Clin Oncol 2005; 23: 1144–1151.

64. Blanke C, Ansari R, Mantravadi R, et al. Phase III trial of thoracic irradiation with or without cisplatin for locally advanced unresectable non-small-cell lung cancer: a Hoosier Oncology Group protocol. J Clin Oncol 1995; 13:1425–1429.

65. Furuse K, Fukuoka M, Kawahara M, et al. Phase III study of concurrent versus sequential thoracic radiotherapy in combination with mitomycin, vindesine, and cisplatin in unresectable stage III non-small-cell lung cancer. J Clin Oncol 1999; 17:2692–2699.

66. Furuse K, Hosoe S, Masuda N, et al. Impact of tumor control on survival in unresectable stage III non-small cell lung cancer treated with concurrent thoracic radiotherapy (TRT) and chemotherapy (CT). Proc Am Soc Clin Oncol 2000; 19. [abstract 1893].

67. Zatloukal P, Petruzelka L, Zemanova M, et al. Concurrent versus sequential chemoradiotherapy with cisplatin and vinorelbine in locally advanced non-small cell lung cancer: a randomized study. Lung Cancer 2004; 46:87–98.

68. Komaki R, Scott C, Ettinger D, et al. Randomized study of chemotherapy/radiation therapy combinations for favorable patients with locally advanced inoperable non-small cell lung cancer: Radiation Therapy Oncology Group (RTOG) 92-04. Int J Radiat Oncol Biol Phys 1997; 38:149–155.

69. Komaki R, Seiferheld W, Ettinger D, et al. Randomized phase II chemotherapy and radiotherapy trial for patients with locally advanced inoperable non-small-cell lung cancer: long-term follow-up of RTOG 92-04. Int J Radiat Oncol Biol Phys 2002; 53:548–557.

70. Vokes EE, Herndon JE 2nd, Crawford J, et al. Randomized phase II study of cisplatin with gemcitabine or paclitaxel or vinorelbine as induction chemotherapy followed by concomitant chemoradiotherapy for stage IIIB non-small-cell lung cancer: cancer and leukemia group B study 9431. J Clin Oncol 2002; 20:4191–4198.

71. Akerley W, Herndon JE Jr, Lyss AP, et al. Induction paclitaxel/carboplatin followed by concurrent chemoradiation therapy for unresectable stage III non-small-cell lung cancer: a limited-access study—CALGB 9534. Clin Lung Cancer 2005; 7:47–53.

72. Albain KS, Crowley JJ, Turrisi AT 3rd, et al. Concurrent cisplatin, etoposide, and chest radiotherapy in pathologic stage IIIB non-small-cell lung cancer: a Southwest Oncology Group phase II study, SWOG 9019. J Clin Oncol 2002; 20:3454–3460.

73. Gandara DR, Chansky K, Albain KS, et al. Consolidation docetaxel after concurrent chemoradiotherapy in stage IIIB non-small-cell lung cancer: phase II Southwest Oncology Group Study S9504. J Clin Oncol 2003; 21:2004–2010.

74. Gandara DH, Chansky K, Gaspar LE, et al. Long term survival in stage IIIb non-small cell lung cancer (NSCLC) treated with consolidation docetaxel following concurrent chemoradiotherapy (SWOG S9504). Proc Am Soc Clin Oncol (FL) 2005 [abstr. 7059].

75. Lau DH, Crowley JJ, Gandara DR, et al. Southwest oncology group phase II trial of concurrent carboplatin, etoposide, and radiation for poor-risk stage III non-small-cell lung cancer. J Clin Oncol 1998; 16:3078–3081.

76. Davies AM, Lau DH, Crowley J, et al. Concurrent carboplatin/etoposide and radiation followed by paclitaxel consolidation for poor risk stage III non-small cell lung cancer: a Southwest Oncology Group (SWOG) phase II trial (S9712). Proc Am Soc Clin Oncol 2002 [abstr. 1191].

77. Strauss GM, Herndon JE, Sherman DD, et al. Neoadjuvant chemotherapy and radiotherapy followed by surgery in stage IIIA non-small-cell carcinoma of the lung: report of a Cancer and Leukemia Group B phase II study. J Clin Oncol 1992; 10: 1237–1244.

78. Albain KS, Rusch VW, Crowley JJ, et al. Concurrent cisplatin/etoposide plus chest radiotherapy followed by surgery for stages IIIA (N2) and IIIB non-small-cell lung cancer: mature results of Southwest Oncology Group phase II study 8805. J Clin Oncol 1995; 13:1880–1892.

79. Albain K, Rusch VW, Crowley J, et al. Long-term survival after concurrent cisplatin/ etoposide (PE) plus chest radiotherapy (RT) followed by surgery in bulky, stages

IIIA(N2) and IIIB non-small cell lung cancer: 6-year outcomes from Southwest Oncology Group Study 8805. Proc Am Soc Clin Oncol; 1999 [abstr. 1801].

80. Albain KS, Scott CB, Rusch VR, et al. Phase III comparison of concurrent chemotherapy plus radiotherapy (CT/RT) and CT/RT followed by surgical resection for stage IIIA(pN2) non-small cell lung cancer: initial results from intergroup trial 0139 (RTOG 93-09). Proc Am Soc Clin Oncol (IL) 2003; 22:621.

81. Albain KS, Swann RS, Rusch VR, et al. Phase III study of concurrent chemotherapy and radiotherapy (CT/RT) vs CT/RT followed by surgical resection for stage IIIA(pN2) non-small cell lung cancer: outcomes update of North American Intergroup 0139 (RTOG 9309). Proc Am Soc Clin Oncol (FL) 2005 [abstr. 7014].

82. Rusch VW, Giroux DJ, Kraut MJ, et al. Induction chemoradiation and surgical resection for non-small cell lung carcinomas of the superior sulcus: initial results of Southwest Oncology Group trial 9416 (Intergroup trial 0160). J Thorac Cardiovasc Surg 2001; 121:472–483.

83. Rusch VR, Giroux DJ, Kraut MJ, et al. Induction chemoradiotherapy and surgical resection for non-small cell lung carcinomas of the superior sulcus (pancoast tumors): mature results of Southwest Oncology Group trial 9416 (Intergroup trial 0160) Proc Am Soc Clin Oncol (IL) 2003; 22 [abstr. 2548].

84. Thomas M, Macha HN, Ukena D, et al. Cisplatin/etoposide (PE) followed by twice-daily chemoradiation (hfRT/CT) versus PE alone before surgery in stage III non-small cell lung cancer: a randomized phase III trial of the German Lung Cancer Cooperative Group (GLCCG). Proc Am Soc Clin Oncol (LA) 2004; 22 [abstr. 7004].

85. Byhardt RW, Scott CB, Ettinger DS, et al. Concurrent hyperfractionated irradiation and chemotherapy for unresectable nonsmall cell lung cancer. Results of Radiation Therapy Oncology Group 90-15. Cancer 1995; 75:2337–2344.

86. Lee JS, Scott C, Komaki R, et al. Concurrent chemoradiation therapy with oral etoposide and cisplatin for locally advanced inoperable non-small-cell lung cancer: radiation therapy oncology group protocol 91-06. J Clin Oncol 1996; 14: 1055–1064.

87. Kelly K, Gaspar LE, Chansky K, et al. Low incidence of pneumonitis on SWOG 0023: a preliminary analysis of an ongoing phase III trial of concurrent chemoradiotherapy followed by consolidation docetaxel and Iressa/placebo maintenance in patients with inoperable stage III non-small cell lung cancer. Proc Am Soc Clin Oncol (FL) 2005 [abstr. 7058].

88. Ready N, Herndon JE, Vokes EE, et al. Initial cohort toxicity evaluation for chemoradiotherapy (CRT) and ZD1839 in stage III non-small cell lung cancer (NSCLC): a CALGB stratified phase II trial. Proc Am Soc Clin Oncol (LA) 2004; 22 [abstr. 7078].

89. Komaki R, Swann RS, Curran W, et al. A phase II study of cetuximab (C225) in combination with chemoradiation (CRT) in patients (PTS) with stage IIIA/B non-small cell lung cancer (NSCLC): an interim overall toxicity report of the RTOG 0324 trial. Int J Radiat Oncol Biol Phys 2005; 63:S44.

90. Arriagada R, Bergman B, Dunant A, et al. Cisplatin-based adjuvant chemotherapy in patients with completely resected non-small-cell lung cancer. N Engl J Med 2004; 350:351–360.

91. Douillard J-Y, Rossell R, De Lena M, et al. Adjuvant vinorelbine plus cisplatin versus observation in patients with completely resected stage IB-IIIA non-small-cell lung

cancer (Adjuvant Navelbine International Trialist Association [ANITA]): a randomized controlled trial. Lancet Oncol 2006; 7:719–727.

92. Winton T, Livingston R, Johnson D, et al. Vinorelbine plus cisplatin vs. observation in resected non-small-cell lung cancer. N Engl J Med 2005; 352:2589–2597.

93. Strauss GM, Herndon J, Maddaus MA, et al. Randomized clinical trial of adjuvant chemotherapy with paclitaxel and carboplatin following resection in Stage IB non-small cell lung cancer: report of Cancer and Leukemia Group B (CALGB) Protocol 9633. Proc Am Soc Clin Oncol (LA) 2004; 22 [abstr. 7019].

94. Choi NC, Grillo HC, Gardiello M, et al. Basis for new strategies in postoperative radiotherapy of bronchogenic carcinoma. Int J Radiat Oncol Biol Phys 1980; 6:31–35.

95. Sawyer TE, Bonner JA, Gould PM, et al. Effectiveness of postoperative irradiation in stage IIIA non-small cell lung cancer according to regression tree analyses of recurrence risks. Ann Thorac Surg 1997; 64:1402–1407; discussion 1407–1408.

96. Sawyer TE, Bonner JA, Gould PM, et al. The impact of surgical adjuvant thoracic radiation therapy for patients with nonsmall cell lung carcinoma with ipsilateral mediastinal lymph node involvement. Cancer 1997; 80:1399–1408.

97. Postoperative radiotherapy in non-small-cell lung cancer: systematic review and meta-analysis of individual patient data from nine randomised controlled trials. PORT Meta-analysis Trialists Group. Lancet 1998; 352:257–263.

98. Kal HB, El Sharouni SY, Struikmans H. Postoperative radiotherapy in non-small-cell lung cancer. Lancet 1998; 352:1385–1386.

99. Machtay M. Postoperative radiotherapy in non-small-cell lung cancer. Lancet 1998; 352:1384–1385 (author reply 1385–1386).

100. Munro AJ. What now for postoperative radiotherapy for lung cancer? Lancet 1998; 352:250–251.

101. The Lung Cancer Study Group. Effects of postoperative mediastinal radiation on completely resected stage II and stage III epidermoid cancer of the lung. N Engl J Med 1986; 315:1377–1381.

102. Stephens RJ, Girling DJ, Bleehen NM, et al. The role of post-operative radiotherapy in non-small-cell lung cancer: a multicentre randomised trial in patients with pathologically staged T1-2, N1-2, M0 disease. Medical Research Council Lung Cancer Working Party. Br J Cancer 1996; 74:632–639.

103. Feng QF, Wang M, Wang LJ, et al. A study of postoperative radiotherapy in patients with non-small-cell lung cancer: a randomized trial. Int J Radiat Oncol Biol Phys 2000; 47:925–929.

104. Lally BE, Zelterman D, Colasanto JM. Postoperative radiotherapy for stage II or III non-small-cell lung cancer using the surveillance, epidemiology, and end results database. J Clin Oncol 2006; 24:2998–3006.

105. Taylor NA, Liao ZX, Stevens C, et al. Postoperative radiotherapy increases locoregional control of patients with stage IIIA non-small-cell lung cancer treated with induction chemotherapy followed by surgery. Int J Radiat Oncol Biol Phys 2003; 56:616–625.

106. Keller SM, Adak S, Wagner H, et al. A randomized trial of postoperative adjuvant therapy in patients with completely resected stage II or IIIA non-small-cell lung cancer. Eastern Cooperative Oncology Group. N Engl J Med 2000; 343: 1217–1222.

107. Bradley JD, Paulus R, Graham MV, et al. Phase II trial of postoperative adjuvant paclitaxel/carboplatin and thoracic radiotherapy in resected stage II and IIIA

non-small-cell lung cancer: promising long-term results of the Radiation Therapy Oncology Group—RTOG 9705. J Clin Oncol 2005; 23:3480–3487.

108. Lad T. The comparison of CAP chemotherapy and radiotherapy to radiotherapy alone for resected lung cancer with positive margin or involved highest sampled paratracheal node (stage IIIA). LCSG 791. Chest 1994; 106:302S–306S.

109. Sadeghi A, Payne D, Rubinstein L, et al. Combined modality treatment for resected advanced non-small cell lung cancer: local control and local recurrence. Int J Radiat Oncol Biol Phys 1988; 15:89–97.

110. Sandler AB. Targeting angiogenesis in lung cancer. Semin Oncol 2005; 32: S16–S22.

111. Sandler AB, Johnson DH, Herbst RS. Anti-vascular endothelial growth factor monoclonals in non-small cell lung cancer. Clin Cancer Res 2004; 10:4258s–4262s.

112. Shepherd FA, Tsao MS. Unraveling the mystery of prognostic and predictive factors in epidermal growth factor receptor therapy. J Clin Oncol 2006; 24:1219–1220 (author reply 1220–1211).

113. Sridhar SS, Seymour L, Shepherd FA. Inhibitors of epidermal-growth-factor receptors: a review of clinical research with a focus on non-small-cell lung cancer. Lancet Oncol 2003; 4:397–406.

10

Advances in the Treatment of Brain Metastases

Malika L. Siker and Minesh P. Mehta

Department of Human Oncology, University of Wisconsin School of Medicine and Public Health, Madison, Wisconsin, U.S.A.

INTRODUCTION

Brain metastases are the most common intracranial tumor in adults, developing in 10% to 30% of adult cancer patients (1). It is estimated that 100,000 to 300,000 new cases are diagnosed in the United States each year (2). The incidence is believed to be rising due to an aging population at a higher risk of breast and lung cancer; better treatment of invasive malignancies, thus extending the survival of patients that may have otherwise succumbed to extracranial disease; improved imaging modalities with better sensitivity for detecting occult disease; and earlier use of magnetic resonance imaging (MRI) in staging asymptomatic patients (3).

Although our ability to detect brain metastases has greatly improved over the past decades, survival remains poor. Median survival with symptomatic treatment and supportive care is only one to two months (4). Definitive treatment may increase survival to a median of four months (5). The Radiation Therapy Oncology Group (RTOG) has identified and validated important prognostic factors in patients with brain metastases, resulting in a three-tiered prognostic classification, using recursive partitioning analysis (RPA) (Table 1) (6,7). Favorable prognostic factors include good performance status, control of the primary tumor, age less than 65 years, and metastases located in the brain only (6). Other factors such as

Table 1 Recursive Partitioning Analysis Classes for Brain Metastases

	Characteristics	Months
Class I	KPS ≥70, primary tumor controlled, age <65 yr, metastases in brain only	7.1
Class II	KPS ≥70, primary tumor uncontrolled, age ≥65yr, metastases in brain and other sites	4.2
Class III	KPS <70	2.3

Abbreviations: KPS, Karnofsky performance status; MOS, median overall survival.

treatment modality, response to steroids, and serum lactate dehydrogenase are also considered prognostic (8).

Patients may present with significant neurologic, cognitive, and emotional difficulties; therefore, outcomes such as neurologic and neurocognitive function are also important to consider, in addition to survival (9). Presenting symptoms may include headache (24–53%), focal weakness (16–40%), altered mental status (24–31%), seizures (15%), and ataxia (9–20%) (10). The extent and severity of symptoms depend on the size, number, and location of the lesions. Metastases may be found in the cerebral hemispheres (80%), cerebellum (15%), and brain-stem (<5%). Furthermore, one-third of all patients with brain metastases may be asymptomatic at diagnosis.

Lung cancer is the source of one-half of all patients with brain metastases (11). Other important contributors are breast cancer (15%), melanoma (10%), renal-cell carcinoma, and, less frequently, gastrointestinal or genitourinary malignancies (12). Patients with melanoma, lung cancer, and breast cancer have a higher tendency toward developing multiple metastases (13). More than 25% of the patients with lung cancer develop brain metastases and it is often the first site of recurrence (14,15).

Despite the development of new treatment approaches, improvement in survival compared to standard treatment has only been found in a subset of patients (16–18). The mainstay of treatment remains whole-brain radiation therapy (WBRT) for the majority of patients, which has been shown to improve survival and local control as well as provide palliation of neurologic symptoms (6,19). Surgical resection and stereotactic radiosurgery (SRS) have emerged as treatment alternatives. Newer management strategies include the application of innovative radiosensitizing agents and chemotherapy regimens. This chapter will review the current treatment options for patients with brain metastases while focusing on recent advances.

MEDICAL MANAGEMENT

A vital task in approaching a patient with brain metastases is assessing neurologic stability. An unstable patient may present with symptoms suggesting uncontrolled intracranial pressure, epileptic status, or both. Relief of increased intracranial pressure may be achieved with intravenous mannitol and dexamethasone and ventilatory support if needed. Seizures may exacerbate intracranial hypertension; so, it is critical to begin immediate anticonvulsants in a patient with seizures.

Once a patient is stable, medical treatment with anticonvulsants, steroids, or both may be considered. The role of anticonvulsants as seizure prophylaxis in patients with brain tumors has historically been controversial. After thorough review of the medical literature, the Quality Standards Subcommittee of the American Academy of Neurology determined that anticonvulsants were ineffective in preventing the development of seizures in patients with brain tumors (20). Furthermore, they concluded that prophylactic treatment with anticonvulsants is only indicated in patients who have previously had seizures (20). Exceptions may include patients with metastases in areas of high epileptogenicity, multiple melanoma metastases, and both brain and leptomeningeal metastases. The use of anticonvulsants should be approached cautiously because they are associated with significant drug interactions and substantial toxicities (21). Despite these guidelines, a significant proportion of physicians continue to prescribe anticonvulsants for seizure prophylaxis in patients with brain metastases (22).

Steroids are given to symptomatic patients to reduce peritumoral edema by decreasing capillary permeability in patients that show neurologic impairment. Dexamethasone is the most commonly prescribed steroid because it has less of a mineralocorticoid effect and is less protein binding than prednisone. Once the patient is clinically stable, steroids should be tapered or discontinued because prolonged use is associated with a high frequency of side effects. Concomitant use of steroids and anticonvulsants such as phenytoin should be managed judiciously because they may interact to alter hepatic metabolism and bioavailability (23).

Future directions in the medical management of brain metastases include the development of new agents with less toxicity than the standard approach of anticonvulsants and steroids. Long-term use of steroids is associated with myopathies, muscle wasting, weight gain, osteoporosis, and gastrointestinal bleeding. Furthermore, preclinical studies have suggested that dexamethasone may interfere with apoptotic death of glioma cells and induce resistance to chemotherapeutic agents and radiotherapy (24–26). One agent currently being evaluated in an ongoing study is corticorelin acetate, which is human corticotropin-releasing factor (hCRF). This agent functions like the naturally occurring neuropeptide that stimulates the hypothalamic–pituitary–adrenal axis. Administration of hCRF has been shown to reduce vasogenic peritumoral brain edema in animal models, independent of adrenal function with 100-fold greater potency and reduced weight gain (27). A prospective phase III trial is currently enrolling patients who are randomized to receive hCRF or placebo after a 50% reduction in baseline dexamethasone dose. Results from this trial are awaited.

SURGERY

Due to mortality rates of greater than 38% associated with surgery in patients with brain metastases during the 1950s and 1960s, surgery was not typically recommended in the treatment of brain metastases (28,29). With the decline in mortality

Table 2 Prospective Studies of Surgery Plus WBRT vs. WBRT Alone in Patients with a Single Brain Metastasis

Study	Treatment	n	MOS	P
Patchell et al.,	Surgery + WBRT 36 Gy vs.	25	40 wk	<0.1
1990 (16)	WBRT 36 Gy	23	15 wk	
Noordjik et al.,	Surgery + WBRT 40 Gy vs.	32	10 mo	0.04
1994 (17)	WBRT 40 Gy	31	6 mo	
Mintz et al.,	Surgery + WBRT 30 Gy vs.	41	5.6 mo	0.24
1996 (30)	WBRT 30 Gy	43	6.3 mo	

Abbreviations: MOS, median overall survival; *n*, number of patients; WBRT, whole brain radiation therapy.

rates to less than 5% in the 1990s due to improved surgical technique and postoperative care, surgery has made a significant contribution in the management of brain metastases (16). Surgery is indicated when a craniotomy or stereotactic biopsy is needed to establish diagnosis and for resection in patients where tumor removal will provide immediate palliation. Additionally, surgery followed by WBRT has been shown to benefit patients with a single brain metastasis in two prospective randomized controlled studies but not in one Canadian trial (Table 2) (16,17,30).

Patchell et al. randomized 48 patients with a single brain metastasis to resection or biopsy followed by WBRT or WBRT alone ($n = 25$ and 23) (16). The WBRT dose was 36 Gy in 12 fractions. Overall survival (40 weeks vs. 15 weeks, $P < 0.01$) and freedom from local recurrence (local failure: 20% vs. 52%, $P < 0.02$) were significantly better in patients undergoing surgery plus WBRT. The duration of functional independence was also superior in resected patients (38 weeks vs. 8 weeks, $P < 0.005$). There was no increase in mortality associated with surgery. Interestingly, despite having evidence of systemic malignancy, 6 out of 54 patients (11%) were found not to have brain metastases (three astrocytomas, two abscesses, and one sterile inflammatory lesion).

The results of the above trial are further supported by a Dutch multi-institutional study in which 63 patients were randomized to resection followed by WBRT (40 Gy in 2 Gy fractions given twice daily over two weeks) or WBRT alone ($n = 32$ and 31) (17). Median survival was significantly longer in the surgery plus WBRT group compared to WBRT alone (10 months vs. 6 months, $P = 0.04$). There was a nonsignificant trend toward longer duration of functional independence in the surgically treated patients (7.5 months vs. 3 months, $P = 0.06$). No data on local recurrence were described. Stratification for progressive-versus-stable disease revealed that the largest difference in median survival favored those with stable systemic disease treated with surgery plus WBRT compared to WBRT alone (12 months vs. 7 months, $P = 0.02$). Resection did not improve median survival in patients with progressive disease. Age less than 60 was found to be a strong positive prognostic factor.

In contrast to the trials described above, Mintz et al. did not find a significant survival benefit in patients with a single brain metastasis treated with surgery plus WBRT versus WBRT alone (30). In this trial, 84 patients were randomized to resection with WBRT (30 Gy in 10 fractions) or WBRT alone ($n = 41$ and 43). Patients treated with resection and WBRT failed to demonstrate an improvement in median survival compared to WBRT alone (5.6 months vs. 6.3 months, $P = 0.24$). There was no difference in duration of functional independence (nine weeks vs. eight weeks, $P = 0.98$). The contradictory results of this trial may be explained by the high proportion of patients who had disseminated systemic disease (45%) compared to the previous two trials (38% and 32%, respectively), underscoring the importance of selecting patients who are most likely to benefit from surgery.

The value of surgery in patients with more than one metastasis has yet to be evaluated in a prospective randomized controlled study. A retrospective case-control study by Bindal et al. of M.D. Anderson compared 56 patients with multiple metastases, who underwent resection (31). Of this population, 30 and 26 patients had incomplete and complete resections, respectively. These groups were compared to 26 matched patients who had complete resection of a single brain metastasis. The median survival was 6, 14, and 14 months, respectively. This study suggests that complete resection in patients with multiple brain metastases may result in a significant improvement in survival with a prognosis similar to that of patients with a resected single metastasis. These data are obviously exploratory and not conclusive.

The use of intraoperative guidance capabilities such as ultrasound, neuronavigation systems, and MRI represent an exciting new approach to the surgical treatment of brain metastases. These imaging techniques can improve the safety and effectiveness of neurosurgical procedures by providing better localization and characterization of targeted lesions to the surgeon before, during, and after the operation. The potential benefits of these modalities and the associated cost effectiveness need to be further evaluated (32,33).

Neurosurgical procedures such as awake-state craniotomies in the outpatient setting have been performed over the past decade and a half for the treatment of intracranial malignancies. Early studies have shown it to be a safe and effective option for selected patients. Benefits include the cost effectiveness associated with a shorter hospital stay and a psychologically less traumatic experience for patients (34). Prospective trials are needed for further assessment.

In summary, surgical resection followed by WBRT is the current standard of care in patients with a single brain metastasis because it has demonstrated a significant improvement in survival compared to WBRT alone. This benefit may be greatest in patients with stable disease, minimal systemic dissemination, younger age, and good performance status. Although preliminary data suggests that surgical resection may increase survival in patients with more than one brain metastasis, there is no level-1 evidence to justify surgical resection as the standard of care. The incorporation of intraoperative imaging and the practice of outpatient neurosurgery is an area of future research.

RADIOTHERAPY

The use of radiotherapy in the treatment of brain metastases includes WBRT, either as definitive treatment or as adjuvant to surgical resection or radiosurgery, and radiosurgery. Although definitive WBRT remains the standard of care for most patients, adjuvant WBRT with radiosurgery and surgical resection has been shown to improve local control (35). The goals of treatment are to provide symptomatic relief, improve neurologic status, and prolong survival while taking into account the toxicities of radiotherapy (19,36). Neurocognitive function impairment, which may also be related to the tumor itself, surgery, and systemic agents, is one of the potential sequelae of radiotherapy. Managing and preventing neurocognitive function impairment is an area of active research.

Definitive WBRT

Definitive WBRT is indicated in patients who have multiple or diffuse metastases, lesions that impinge on eloquent areas, or medical conditions that preclude them from surgical procedures. Multiple metastases are found in approximately 80% of patients with brain metastases, making definitive WBRT the treatment of choice for the majority of patients (37). The use of WBRT in patients with brain metastases was first described in 1954 by Chao et al. who documented that 63% of patients had relief of symptoms and proposed the optimal dose at 30 Gy (19). Several different doses, timings, and fractionation schemes have been investigated since then; however, none of these trials have demonstrated superior survival compared to conventional treatment (38–45). Furthermore, accelerated hyperfractionated schedules have not shown any benefit compared to standard treatment (45,46). Although the optimal schedule is still debated, typical WBRT regimens given in the United States for the treatment of brain metastases are 10 fractions of 3 Gy (30 Gy) over three weeks or 15 fractions of 2.5 Gy (37.5 Gy) over three weeks.

According to some reports, 60% of patients achieve a complete response (CR) or partial response (PR) to WBRT, but these are pre-MRI data that have not been adequately validated. Response may depend on histology. CT-determined response rates (CR plus PR) to WBRT for small-cell lung cancer (81%) and breast cancer (65%) have been found to be superior to those for renal-cell carcinoma (46%) and melanoma (0%) based on an institutional analysis of 108 patients (47). However, actuarial local control at one year after WBRT alone has been found to be 0% to 14% in randomized trials, suggesting that long-term control of brain metastases following conventional treatment occurs in only a minority (48,49). Because of the poor outcome following WBRT alone, newer approaches involving surgery, radiation, and chemotherapy have been tried with modestly promising results. Patients with recurrent brain metastases typically succumb to central nervous system (CNS) disease, whereas the majority of patients who achieve local control die of extracranial disease (50).

Complications of WBRT may occur acutely or in the long term. Acute toxicities, occurring less than 90 days after treatment, associated with WBRT include alopecia, dermatitis, otitis externa, otitis media, nausea or vomiting, and somnolence. Late toxicities, occurring more than 90 days after treatment, may involve necrosis, personality changes, memory loss, cerebellar dysfunction, cataracts, and neurocognitive deterioration.

In addition to the toxicities of WBRT, some have suggested that the survival is too short and meaningful palliation is not achieved by enough patients to justify WBRT in all patients, although these data are relatively sparse and not reproduced by others (51). Nevertheless, when weighing the potential benefits of symptomatic relief, improvement in neurologic status and increased survival with the limited toxicities and poor outcome without definitive treatment, WBRT remains the standard of care for patients with multiple brain metastases.

Radiosurgery

SRS is a technique that delivers precise, conformal radiation to a defined target in a single large dose. It is able to deliver a high dose of radiation to the lesion while sparing the maximum amount of normal tissue. Radiosurgery may be delivered using a Gamma Knife, modified or dedicated linear accelerator, or proton beam. It has been used to treat small lesions (<4 cm) that are not accessible surgically and residual disease after surgical resection. It is minimally invasive and well tolerated by patients who are not surgical candidates. It is best suited for patients with good performance status and limited extracranial disease (52). Local control rates range from 25% to 100% with a mean of 81% and response rates vary from 30% to 100% with an average of 69% (53,54).

Maximum tolerated doses for radiosurgery in the treatment of brain metastases were established in a prospective trial from the RTOG (55). In this dose-escalation trial, 156 patients, 100 (64%) of whom had recurrent brain metastases, underwent dose escalation in 3 Gy increments until unacceptable toxicity was reached. Investigators were unwilling to continue dose escalation to 27 Gy. The maximum tolerated doses (deemed maximum, without actually reaching toxicity) were 24, 18, and 15 Gy, for tumors less than 20, 21 to 30, and 31 to 40 mm, respectively, in maximum diameter.

The first prospective randomized trial examining the use of radiosurgery with WBRT in patients with brain metastases was published by Kondziolka et al. from the University of Pittsburgh (56). In this trial, patients with two to four brain metastases were randomized to WBRT alone to 30 Gy in 12 fractions ($n = 14$) or WBRT followed by 16 Gy radiosurgery within one month ($n = 13$). The study was stopped at interim analysis (60% accrual) due to the superior local control rate in the radiosurgery arm (8% vs. 100%, $P = 0.0016$). Median time to local failure was six months in the WBRT-alone group compared to 36 months in the radiosurgery group ($P = 0.0005$). Median time to any brain failure was also improved in the radiosurgery group (34 months vs. 5 months, $P = 0.002$). There was no difference in survival between the two groups. This trial has been criticized for the small sample size and "nonstandard" endpoints, making it difficult to interpret.

A second prospective randomized trial was reported by Chougule et al. from Brown University in abstract form (57). In this three arm trial, 96 patients with 3 or fewer lesions were randomized to radiosurgery alone, radiosurgery plus WBRT, or WBRT alone. Overall median survival was seven, five, and nine months, respectively, and local control was 87%, 91%, and 62%, respectively. Although the authors of this study concluded that radiosurgery enhanced local control, the proportion of patients who underwent surgical resection prior to receiving radiation was not balanced among the three arms, thus confounding the results.

The largest and most recent trial was published by Andrews et al. (18). In this multi-institutional RTOG trial, 333 patients with one to three brain metastases were randomized to receive WBRT alone to 37.5 Gy in 15 fractions ($n = 164$) or WBRT followed by radiosurgery ($n = 167$). Although there was no significant improvement in overall survival between the two arms (6.5 months vs. 5.7 months, $P = 0.13$), patients with a single brain metastasis (a prespecified subgroup at the time of trial design for separate analysis from the two to three brain metastases cohort) demonstrated a survival advantage when treated with WBRT plus radiosurgery compared to radiosurgery (6.5 months vs. 4.9 months, $P = 0.04$). At six months followup, patients in the radiosurgery arm were more likely to have stable or improved performance status (43% vs. 37%, $P = 0.03$). Results from this trial provide level-1 evidence supporting the use of radiosurgery in patients with a single metastasis.

A multi-institutional retrospective review suggests that WBRT with radiosurgery may improve survival in patients with brain metastases in all three RPA classes (58). Five hundred and two patients were stratified by RPA class and survival was calculated using Kaplan–Meier estimates and proportional hazard regression analysis. The addition of radiosurgery to WBRT resulted in improved median survival in all three RPA classes: A higher performance status, controlled primary absence of extracranial metastases, and lower RPA predicted for improved survival.

Based on these trials, there is level-1 evidence to support the use of radiosurgery as a boost to WBRT in patients with a single brain metastasis to maximize local control and survival. Radiosurgery offers an alternative to surgical resection and may be especially useful in patients who have a single lesion that impinges on an eloquent area or those who are unable to tolerate surgery. The role of radiosurgery and WBRT in patients with more than one brain metastasis has yet to be defined because radiosurgery in these patients improves local control without a significant survival benefit.

Adjuvant WBRT

Even in the best of circumstances with focal treatments such as surgical resection and radiosurgery, microscopic disease may remain. The aim of adjuvant WBRT following these focal treatments is to eradicate any residual disease in the tumor bed or elsewhere in the brain to improve local control. The utility of adjuvant WBRT has been called into question with the increasing efficacy of focal treatments.

Only one prospective randomized controlled trial has examined adjuvant WBRT following resection. Patchell et al. randomized 95 patients with a single brain metastasis to resection with postoperative WBRT ($n = 49$) to a total dose of 50.4 Gy in 28 fractions or no postoperative WBRT ($n = 46$) (49). Overall intracranial failure was significantly lower in patients receiving WBRT (18% vs. 70%, $P < 0.001$). Postoperative WBRT also prevented recurrence at the site of the original tumor bed (10% vs. 46%, $P < 0.001$) and elsewhere in the brain (14% vs. 37%, $P < 0.01$). Patients receiving WBRT were less likely to die of a neurologic death (14% vs. 44%, $P = 3$). There was no difference between the two arms in regard to overall survival (48 weeks vs. 43 weeks, $P = 0.39$) or duration of functional independence (37 weeks vs. 35 weeks, $P = 0.61$), further emphasizing the importance of systemic control. The trial was never powered to detect a change in the survival endpoint. It is important to note that 61% of patients in the surgery-only arm received WBRT at recurrence and that patients who received both surgery and WBRT had a survival of 12 months nearly two to three times greater than historical values (35). Although half of those patients who received surgery alone and WBRT at relapse died of CNS recurrence, only 14% of patients treated with surgery followed by WBRT had CNS recurrence as a cause of death.

In a series of retrospective reviews investigating the use of adjuvant WBRT with radiosurgery, intracranial failures were reduced in patients treated with radiosurgery followed by adjuvant WBRT compared to radiosurgery alone, but median survival was not significantly increased (59–62). However, these studies were retrospective and treatment assignment was not randomized, resulting in a patient selection bias.

These results were recently corroborated by a randomized clinical trial. The Japanese Radiotherapy Oncology Group presented preliminary results from a trial comparing radiosurgery with or without adjuvant WBRT in patients with four or fewer brain metastases (63). In this report, 120 patients were randomized to receive radiosurgery alone ($n = 61$) or radiosurgery followed by WBRT to a total dose of 30 Gy in 10 fractions ($n = 59$). At median followup of six months, there was no significant survival difference between the two arms. However, 49% of patients in the arm receiving WBRT had new brain metastases at six months compared to 82% in the radiosurgery-only arm ($P = 0.003$). The actuarial one-year local tumor control rate was better in the group receiving radiosurgery plus adjuvant WBRT (88% vs. 70%, $P = 0.019$).

Although adjuvant WBRT has not been shown to prolong life, none of the trials were designed to measure this endpoint. Further, the results of these trials provide evidence favoring the use of adjuvant WBRT to improve local and intracranial control. A small phase II prospective study of the Eastern Cooperative Oncology Group investigated the use of radiosurgery alone in patients with tumors considered radioresistant, melanoma, renal-cell carcinoma, and sarcoma (64).

Median survival was found to be 8.2 months in the 31 assessable patients. More importantly, significant rates of local and intracranial relapse were identified, suggesting that withholding WBRT maybe detrimental.

Those in favor of omitting immediate adjuvant WBRT propose that patients with a limited amount of disease (3–10 lesions, depending on institution) be treated with radiosurgery alone and be subsequently followed by frequent MRI. If a new intracranial metastasis appears, it is treated with radiosurgery again. This approach dramatically increases the overall cost of managing these patients because imaging studies can cost at least $2000 per study and radiosurgical procedures cost approximately $20,000 to $40,000 (65). The intent of this strategy is to delay treatment with WBRT for as long as possible to avoid the putative significant neurotoxicity associated with WBRT.

WBRT has been associated with an 11% risk of developing dementia in long-term survivors (greater than 12 months) based on a retrospective report of 47 patients (66). However, 4 of the 11 patients who developed dementia were treated with higher daily fractions (>3 Gy) and one patient received a radiosensitizer that may have increased normal tissue damage. Fifteen patients in this report were treated with regimens similar to those used today; none of those patients developed dementia. Furthermore, recent evidence suggests that WBRT alone does not result in significant neuropsychological decline and that the majority of deficits are present before cranial irradiation (67). Additional clinical evidence is provided in a recent Japanese trial that showed that patients randomized to radiosurgery plus WBRT had no differences in performance and neurologic functional status (using RTOG criteria) compared to patients treated with radiosurgery alone (63).

The prevention of recurrent or progressive disease is important for the preservation of neurocognitive status and may outweigh the potential toxicities associated with WBRT. Recurrent brain metastases have been found to result in a substantial decrease in mental performance and increase in neurological deficits, further supporting the use of adjuvant WBRT following focal treatment (68,69). A recent trial has shown that patients with progressive disease on MRI have increased deterioration in neurocognitive function compared to responders (70).

In conclusion, although omitting adjuvant WBRT with focal treatment may not decrease survival, especially in patients at high risk of dying from systemic progression, concern remains that in patients with controlled systemic disease, intracranial progression may enhance mortality. Further, local control is superior in those who receive adjuvant WBRT. In the absence of evidence to substantiate claims that omission of WBRT results in decreased toxicity and improved quality of life, adjuvant WBRT should remain the standard of care with focal treatment. The importance of neurocognitive function and subsequent management and prevention strategies are discussed below.

NEUROCOGNITIVE FUNCTION

With the advent of newer treatments prolonging survival in subsets of patients, neurocognitive function, and quality of life have become increasingly important.

This was reflected in a recent survey where a majority (74%) of medical and radiation oncologists responded that managing neurologic and neurocognitive function was more important than prolonging survival in patients with brain metastases (9). Furthermore, only 11% of respondents indicated that extending survival was their sole reason for providing treatment.

Comprehensive data defining the incidence of neurocognitive deficits in patients with brain metastases are limited and variable due to the differences in radiation regimens, treatment, and patient characteristics. A report by DeAngelis of 47 patients showed that 11% of one-year survivors after WBRT showed dementia; however, this study has been criticized due to a large portion of patients receiving greater than standard dose per fraction (66). None of the patients who received radiation regimens similar to standard therapy showed evidence of dementia. An analysis of neurocognitive function in a large phase III trial of 401 patients showed baseline cognitive impairment in 91% of patients (70). This is consistent with previous trials reporting that cognitive dysfunction was present in a majority of patients before receiving radiotherapy (67,71,72).

Neurocognitive dysfunction may be caused by the tumor, radiotherapy, surgery, systemic treatment such as chemotherapy and endocrine therapy, and adjuvant medications. Neurocognitive defects following radiotherapy are divided into acute, subacute, and late toxicities. Acute toxicities occur within the first few weeks of treatment and are caused by cerebral edema resulting in drowsiness, headache, nausea, vomiting, and focal defects. Appearing one to six months after treatment are subacute effects, which are thought to be the result of diffuse demyelination, manifesting as headache, somnolence, and fatigability clinically. Late effects appear after six months, secondary to vascular injury, demyelination, and necrosis. Clinically, patients may show mild lassitude, memory impairment, or dementia that may be irreversible and progressive.

Neurocognitive function has been found to be linked to survival and progression of disease. Baseline neurocognitive function has been demonstrated to be predictive of survival, with memory test score being highly related by multivariate analysis (70,73). Investigators observed that cognitive deterioration occurred around six weeks prior to radiographic failure, suggesting that neurocognitive function may be predictive of failure (74).

Strategies have been developed to treat or prevent neurocognitive deficits. Methylphenidate, a dopamine agonist used to treat narcolepsy and attention deficit disorder, is a stimulant that has been investigated in primary brain tumors (75). In a small series of 30 patients, methylphenidate at 30 mg twice daily was found to improve energy, concentration, mood, and ambulation with minimal toxicity. It is hypothesized that dopaminergic innervation of the mesolimbic system from methylphenidate would result in increased motivation and drive. Further trials are necessary to assess its applicability in brain metastases.

Agents used to treat Alzheimer disease have been proposed due to the radiographic and clinical similarity between Alzheimer disease and radiation-induced injury to the cerebrum. Donepezil, a cholinesterase inhibitor, was tested in a small trial from Wake Forest where 24 patients treated with prior irradiation for brain tumors received 24 weeks of donepezil (76). Evaluation of neurocognitive function found an improvement in scores at 24 weeks compared to baseline. Improved cognitive ability, memory, and executive function at one year were demonstrated in a small trial of 29 patients who chose among vitamin E, another treatment used in Alzheimer disease, or observation (77). Larger randomized controlled studies are needed for validation of these treatments.

It has been hypothesized that radiation-induced damage has similar pathophysiology to vascular dementia. Therefore, there is interest in treating irradiated brain tumor patients with agents such as memantine, an *N*-methyl-D-aspartate receptor agonist, which are used in the treatment of vascular dementia. Preclinical data suggest that memantine may be neuroprotective and prevent neuronal injury induced by radiation (78,79). The RTOG is planning a clinical trial to further investigate the use of memantine as prophylaxis for neurocognitive dysfunction after cranial irradiation.

Another potential therapy, erythropoietin has been shown to be neuroprotective in a blinded, randomized control study in rats given 100 Gy to the right striatum (80). Less motor impairment was found in rats treated with erythropoietin compared to saline. This finding has also been observed in a similar study with mice that were given erythropoietin one hour after WBRT to 17 Gy in a single fraction (81). Its effect is thought to be mediated by preventing neurotoxicity caused by reactive oxygen and nitrogen intermediates. However, administration of erythropoietin in women with metastatic breast cancer has recently been found to decrease survival (82). Treatment with erythropoietin in this setting remains experimental and should be approached with caution.

Modifications to the delivery of WBRT have been pursued to decrease the risk of neurotoxicity. It has been shown that patients given fraction doses of greater than 3 Gy are at higher risk of developing dementia; so, hypofractionation regimens should be avoided (66). A preclinical in vivo study in rats demonstrated that doses as low as 2 Gy or less can damage the hippocampus (83). Therefore, avoidance of the hippocampus using intensity-modulated radiotherapy is currently under investigation (Fig. 1). This technology allows for full dose to the majority of the brain while limiting the dose to the hippocampus.

In conclusion, because some patients with brain metastases are surviving longer, interest in preserving neurocognitive function has grown. Treatments such as methylphenidate, those that are used to treat dementia, and variations in radiotherapy are being investigated. Further data are needed before these agents become the standard of care.

CHEMOTHERAPY

It has been traditionally believed that most chemotherapeutic agents provide little benefit in brain tumors due to their inability to cross the blood–brain barrier. However, recent evidence has shown that metastatic tumor growth causes upregulation of angiogenic factors, resulting in neovascularization disrupting the blood–brain barrier (84). This finding along with the development of new agents

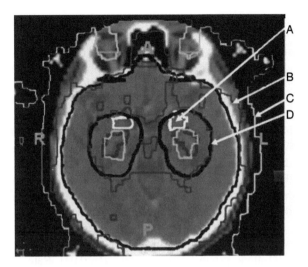

Figure 1 Hippocampus avoidance plan with intensity modulated radiotherapy via helical tomotherapy: (A) Avoidance region (*white*); (B) 30 Gy (*dark gray*); (C) 6 Gy (*light gray*); (D) 3 Gy (*black*).

with improved penetration of the blood–brain barrier has led to a renewed interest in the development of chemotherapeutic approaches.

Temozolomide is an oral alkylating agent that effectively penetrates the blood–brain barrier due to its small molecular size and lipophilic property. It has 100% bioavailability and can achieve cerebrospinal concentrations that are approximately 30% of plasma concentrations (85–87). Toxicity is mainly hematologic and low, with less than 5% incidence of myelosuppression (88). It has shown a significant survival benefit and minimal toxicities when given concomitantly and adjuvantly with radiotherapy in patients with grade IV gliomas (89). When used alone, it has shown activity in patients with both recurrent and newly diagnosed brain metastases (90–95).

Sensitivity to temozolomide may depend on the tumor histology. In a phase II study by Siena et al. released in abstract form, patients with breast cancer, non–small-cell lung cancer and melanoma were treated with a dose-intense, alternating weekly regimen of temozolomide (95). Response rates were 19%, 24%, and 40%, respectively. In a single arm trial by Dardoufas, 20 patients (55% lung cancer) with newly diagnosed brain metastases received chemoradiotherapy with temozolomide (96). Patients with lung cancer had a superior response rate (86%) compared to the group as a whole (55%). In patients with grade IV gliomas, methylation of the promoter region of the *O*6-methylguanine DNA *methyl-transferase* (MGMT) gene has been shown to increase survival (97). Patients with squamous-cell carcinoma and adenocarcinoma have been found to have a 36% and 42% incidence of MGMT promoter methylation, respectively (98). The role of the MGMT in patients with brain metastases with various histologies is unknown.

Temozolomide has been found to have synergistic effect with radiation in preclinical studies (99). Concomitant chemoradiotherapy with temozolomide has been examined in phase II and III trials (100–102). In a phase II trial by Antonadou, 52 patients with brain metastases from solid tumors were randomized to receive WBRT (40 Gy in 20 fractions) or WBRT with concomitant temozolomide (75 mg/ m^2/day) followed by six cycles of adjuvant temozolomide (200 mg/m^2/day on days one to five every 38 days) (100). Overall response rate was significantly superior in the temozolomide arm (96%, of which 38% CR, 58% PR) compared to the WBRT alone arm (66%, of which 33% CR, 33% PR) with $P = 0.017$. The treatment was well tolerated, with no grade 3 or 4 myelosuppression. Verger et al. published a phase II study that randomized 82 patients to WBRT alone (30 Gy in 10 fractions) or WBRT with concurrent temozolomide followed by two cycles of temozolomide at the doses described above (101). Temozolomide was found to be well tolerated. There was no significant difference in radiographic response. However, progression-free survival at 90 days was superior in the temozolomide group compared to the WBRT-alone group (72% vs. 54%, $P = 0.03$). Rate of neurologic death was improved in the temozolomide arm as well (41% vs. 69%, $P = 0.029$). The largest study is a phase III trial by Antonadou et al. that randomized 134 patients to WBRT alone (30 Gy in 10 fractions) or WBRT with concomitant and adjuvant temozolomide at the doses described above (102). Response rate was significantly improved in the temozolomide arm (53% vs. 33%, $P = 0.039$). The benefit was more pronounced in patients less than 60 years of age (77% vs. 32%, $P = 0.003$) and those with a Karnofsky Performance Status of 90 or greater (71% vs. 32%, $P = 0.003$). There was no significant difference in survival (8.3 months vs. 6.3 months, $P = 0.179$). These trials suggest a benefit with the addition of concomitant and adjuvant temozolomide to WBRT, but further data are needed to warrant treatment with temozolomide as standard practice.

Other chemotherapeutic agents have been explored and preliminary data are equivocal. Topotecan, a selective topoisomerase inhibitor, is an established treatment in small-cell lung cancer that has been shown to have single-agent and combined activity with WBRT (103,104). Gliadel wafer, biodegradable polymer containing 3.85% carmustine [1,3-*bis*(2-*chloroethyl*)-1-*nitrosourea*], which is a type of interstitial chemotherapy placed in the surgical bed following surgery, combined with surgery and WBRT has been evaluated in patients with brain metastases with encouraging results (105). However, in a phase II randomized study of 42 patients randomized to receive WBRT alone (20 Gy in 5 fractions) or WBRT plus concomitant carboplatin, median survival (4.4 months vs. 3.7 months, $P = 0.64$) and objective response (10% vs. 29%, $P = 0.24$) remained extremely poor and a significant improvement was not found in either arm (106).

The use of multidrug chemotherapeutic regimens in the treatment of brain metastases is another approach currently under investigation. Studies examining regimens such as paclitaxel/cisplatin/gemcitabine or vinorelbine, vinorelbine/ temcitabine, and cisplatin/etoposide as first-line treatment in brain metastases have provided promising results (107–109). The timing of combination chemotherapy with WBRT has been evaluated in a small phase III study by Robinet et al. (110). In this trial, 176 patients with brain metastases from non–small-cell lung cancer were randomized to receive chemotherapy with cisplatin and vinorelbine followed by delayed or early WBRT. Investigators found no significant difference in survival between the two arms (24 weeks vs. 21 weeks, $P = 0.83$), which is not surprising due to the high rate of death due to extracranial progression in these patients. However, response rates of brain metastases in these trials are similar to the expected response rates for the primary tumor (108–110).

Gefininib, an epidermal growthfactor receptor tyrosine kinase that has been shown to enhance the cytocidal effects of radiation, has demonstrated single-agent activity in previously treated patients with brain metastases with minimal toxicities (111). In a recent prospective trial, 76 patients with advanced non–small-cell lung cancer irrespective of performance status, number of prior treatments, and presence of brain metastases received single-agent gefitinib (112). Objective response was found to be 33.3% and median survival was 9.9 months. There was no survival difference between patients with and patients without brain lesions. Interestingly, severity of skin toxicity was associated with tumor response and patient survival ($P = 0.007$ and 0.001, respectively). Further data from large prospective randomized controlled studies are needed.

A unique new drug in development, MPC-6827, is a novel small molecular inhibitor of microtubule formation. It has shown preclinical efficacy in ovarian, breast, pancreatic and prostate cancer, and melanoma. In particular, it demonstrates activity in multiple drug-resistant cancers, and uniquely, in mice studies, it has been found to efficiently cross the blood–brain barrier, with intracranial concentrations 14-fold higher than in plasma, a level that represents an 800-fold increase in the dose necessary to activate caspase. Its brain clearance mimics blood pharmacokinetics. This drug, therefore, may be uniquely suited for testing in brain metastases patients, and early phase clinical trials are ongoing (113).

Although surgery and radiotherapy have traditionally been the modalities for local control, chemotherapeutic agents have been shown to enhance this effect. Early trials with temozolomide have generated promising results and further trials are awaited. The use of temozolomide and other chemotherapeutic agents is still investigational and more data are needed before it is considered standard practice.

Radiosensitizers

Radiosensitizers are designed to increase the efficacy of radiotherapy in tumors with no added damage to normal tissue. Historically, radiosensitizers have demonstrated little value in patients with brain metastases. Misonidazole, bromodeoxyuridine, lonidamine, nimustine, fluorouracil, and others have failed to show significant benefit in randomized trials (114,115). The development of two new compounds, motexafin gadolinium (MGd) and efaproxaril, has renewed interest in this domain.

MGd is a redox modulator that selectively concentrates in malignant tissue as shown by MRI (Fig. 2) (70,116). It works by generating reactive oxygen species, thus depleting the stores of reducing agents needed for repair of cytotoxic damage, enhancing radiotherapy-induced apoptosis (117). Early studies showed response rates of 68% to 72% in patients with brain metastases treated with MGd and WBRT (116,118). A phase III prospective randomized controlled trial compared WBRT alone (30 Gy in 10 fractions) to WBRT with MGd (5 mg/kg/day) in 401 patients (119). Patients were stratified according to tumor type, RPA class, and study center. There was no significant difference in the primary endpoints of median survival (5.2 months vs. 4.9 months, $P = 0.48$) and median time to neurologic progression (9.5 months vs. 8.3 months, $P = 0.95$). When tumor type was examined, an increased time to neurologic progression was found in the 251 patients (63%) with non–small-cell lung cancer treated with MGd compared to those who received WBRT alone (median not reached vs. 7.4 months, $P = 0.048$). A significant improvement in the secondary endpoints of death by CNS causes and memory and executive function was also demonstrated in the MGd arm for patients with non–small-cell lung cancer. Administration of MGd did not interfere with delivery of radiotherapy and adverse events were mild to moderate and easily manageable. A confirmatory phase III trial investigating the use of MGd in patients with brain metastases and NSCLC primaries has recently been completed and results are awaited.

Efaproxaril (RSR-13) is an allosteric modifier that noncovalently binds to hemoglobin and decreases its oxygen binding affinity, thereby increasing tissue pO_2. By binding directly to hemoglobin, it is able to circumvent the blood–brain barrier. Efaproxaril with WBRT was examined in 57 patients with brain metastases who received WBRT (30 Gy/fx) and efaproxaril (100 mg/kg) (120). Supplemental

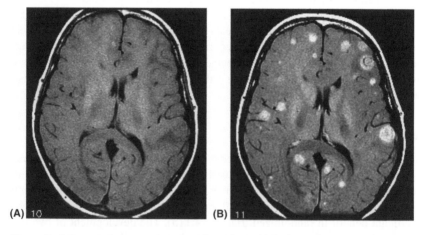

Figure 2   Magnetic resonance imaging of a patient with brain metastases. (**A**) Noncontrast scan at baseline. (**B**) Noncontrast scan after administration of motexafin gadolinium.

oxygen at 4 L was given before, during, and after delivery of fraction. These patients were compared retrospectively to a matched cohort from the RTOG RPA brain metastases database. Median survival was found to be significantly improved for the efaproxaril-treated patients (6.4 months vs. 4.1 months, $P = 0.0174$). A prospective randomized phase III study in 538 patients did not confirm this survival benefit. Patients with brain metastases in RPA class 1 or 2 were randomized to WBRT (30 Gy in 10 fractions) or WBRT with efaproxaril (121). No significant difference in the primary endpoint of survival was shown (5.3 months vs. 4.5 months, $P = 0.17$). Interestingly, on further analysis of tumor type, patients with breast cancer (21%) demonstrated improved survival when treated with efaproxaril compared to WBRT alone (8.7 months vs. 4.6 months, $P = 0.061$). Further investigation of this observation is underway with the enhancing whole brain radiation therapy in patients with breast cancer and hypoxic brain metastases (ENRICH) trial, which is currently enrolling women with breast cancer.

The development of MGd and efaproxaril has revived interest in the use of radiosensitizers. Although early clinical studies have found these agents to be putatively beneficial, there is no level-1 evidence to justify giving these agents to all patients with brain metastases. Results from future trials are awaited.

CONCLUSION

While innovative approaches and novel agents have been developed in the treatment of brain metastases, survival remains poor. WBRT continues to be the standard of care in most patients with brain metastases. Level-1 evidence supports the use of surgery followed by WBRT in the treatment of patients with a single metastasis. WBRT followed by radiosurgery as a boost is also considered standard practice for patients with a single metastasis. The omission of WBRT after local treatment such as surgery and radiosurgery has been shown to decrease local control and is not recommended. Neurocognitive function has become an increasingly important issue for patients with prolonged survival. As such, prophylaxis and treatment of neurocognitive deficits are the focus of current research. The results of preclinical and clinical trials using systemic agents such as chemotherapy and radiosensitizers are promising. Although further investigation is needed before they become the standard of care, they represent an exciting area of research.

REFERENCES

1. Larson DA, Rubenstein JL, McDermott MW. Treatment of metastatic cancer. In: DeVita VT, Hellman S, Rosenberg SA, eds. Cancer Priniples & Practice of Oncology. 7th ed. Philadelphia: Lippincott Williams & Wilkins, 2005:2323–2336.
2. Mehta MP, Tremont-Lukats I. Radiosurgery for single and multiple metastasis. In: Sawaya R, ed. Intracranial Metastases: Current Management Strategies. London: Futura Publishing, 2002.
3. Schellinger PD, Meinck HM, Thron A. Diagnostic accuracy of MRI compared to CT in patients with brain metastases. J Neurooncol 1999; 44(3):275–281.

4. Lang EF, Slater J. Metastatic brain tumors. Results of surgical and nonsurgical treatment. Surg Clin North Am 1964; 44:865–872.

5. Sundstrom JT, Minn H, Lertola KK, et al. Prognosis of patients treated for intracranial metastases with whole-brain irradiation. Ann Med 1988; 30:296–299.

6. Gaspar L, Scott C, Rotman M, et al. Recursive partitioning analysis (RPA) of prognostic factors in three Radiation Therapy Oncology Group brain metastases trials. Int J Radiat Oncol Biol Phys 1997; 37:745–751.

7. Gaspar LE, Scott C, Murray K, et al. Validation of the RTOG recursive partitioning analysis classification for brain metastases. Int J Radiat Oncol Biol Phys 2000; 47:1001–1006.

8. Lagerwaard FJ, Levendag PC, Nowak PJ, et al. Identification of prognostic factors in patients with brain metastases: a review of 1292 patients. Int J Radiat Oncol Biol Phys 1999; 43:795–803.

9. Renschler MF, Mehta MP, Donald DM, et al. Treatment intent for brain metastases: surveys of medical and radiation oncologists indicate that maintaining neurologic and neurocognitive function is more important than prolonging survival. Proc Am Soc Clin Oncol 2003; 22:552.

10. Nussbaum ES, Djalilian HR, Cho K, et al. Brain metastases, histology, multiplicity, surgery and survival. Cancer 1996; 78(8):1781–1788.

11. Yawn BP, Wollan PC, Schroeder C, et al. Temporal and gender-related trends in brain metastases from lung and breast cancer. Minn Med 2003; 86:32–37.

12. Patchell RA. The management of brain metastases. Cancer Treat Rev 2003; 29: 533–540.

13. Delattre JY, Krol G, Thaler HT, et al. Distribution of brain metastases. Arch Neurol 1988; 45:741–744.

14. Sheehan JP, Sun M-H, Kondziolka D, et al. Radiosurgery for NSCLC metastatic to the brain: long-term outcomes and prognostic factors influencing patient survival time and local tumor control. J Neurosurg 2002; 97:1276–1281.

15. Grossi F, Scolaro T, Tixi L, et al. The role of systemic chemotherapy in the treatment of brain metastases from small cell lung cancer. Crit Rev Oncol Hematol 2001; 37:61–67.

16. Patchell RA, Tibbs PA, Walsh JW, et al. A randomized trial of surgery in the treatment of single metastases to the brain. N Eng J Med 1990; 322(8):494–500.

17. Noordjik EM, Vecht CJ, Haaxma-Reiche H, et al. The choice of treatment of single brain metastases should be based on extracranial tumor activity and age. Int J Radiat Oncol Biol Phys 1994; 29:711–717.

18. Andrews DW, Scott CB, Sperduto PW, et al. Whole brain radiation therapy with or without stereotactic radiosurgery boost for patients with one to three brain metastases: phase III results of the RTOG 9508 randomised trial. Lancet 2004; 363: 1665–1672.

19. Chao JH, Phillips R, Nickson JJ. Roentgen-ray therapy of cerebral metastases. Cancer 1954; 7:682–689.

20. Glantz MF, Cole BF, Forsyth PA, et al. Practice parameter: anticonvulsant prophylaxis in patients with newly diagnosed brain tumors. Report of the Quality Standards Subcommittee of the American Academy of Neurology. Neurology 2000; 54:1886–1893.

21. Cohen N, Strauss G, Lew R, et al. Should prophylactic anticonvulsants be administered to patients with newly-diagnosed cerebral metastases? A retrospective analysis. J Clin Oncol 1988; 6:1621–1624.

22. Siomin V, Angelov L, Li L, et al. Results of a survey of neurosurgical practice patterns regarding the prophylactic use of anti-epilepsy drugs in patients with brain tumors. J Neuro Onc 2005; 74:211–215.
23. Werk EE, Choi Y, Sholiton Z, et al. Interference in the effect of dexamethasone by diphenylhydantoin. N Engl J Med 1969; 281:32.
24. Wolff JEA, Jurgens H. Dexamethasone induced partial resistance to methotrxate in C6-glioma cells. Anticancer Res 1994; 14:1585–1588.
25. Wolff JEA, Denecke J, Jurgens H. Dexamethasone induces partial resistance to cisplatinum in C6-glioma cells. Anticancer Res 1996; 16:805–810.
26. Weller M, Malipiero U, Aguzzi A, et al. Protooncogene BCL-2 gene transfer abrogates FAS/APO-1 antibody-mediated apoptosis of human malignant glioma cells and confers resistance to chemotherapeutic drugs and therapeutic irradiation. J Clin Invest 1995; 95:2633–2643.
27. Tjuvajev J, Uehara H, Desai R, et al. Corticotropin-releasing factor decreases vasogenic brain edema. Cancer Res 1996; 56:1352–1360.
28. Richards P, Mc KW. Intracranial metastases. Br Med J 1963; 5322:15–18.
29. Simionescu MD. Metastatic tumors of the brain: a follow-up study of 195 patients with neurosurgical considerations. J Neurosurg 1960; 17:361–373.
30. Mintz AH, Kestle J, Rathbone MP, et al. A randomized trial to assess the efficacy of surgery in addition to radiotherapy in patients with a single cerebral metastasis. Cancer 1996; 78:1470–1476.
31. Bindal RK, Sawaya R, Leavens ME, et al. Surgical treatment of multiple brain metastases. J Neurosurg 1993; 79:210–216.
32. Schulz T, Puccini S, Schneider JP, et al. Interventional and intraoperative MR: review and update of techniques and clinical experience. European Radiology 2004; 14:2212–2227.
33. Sosna J, Barth MM, Kruskal JB, et al. Intraoperative sonography for neurosurgery. J Ultrasound Med 2005; 24:1671–1682.
34. Bernstein M. Outpatient craniiotomy for brain tumor: a pliot feasibility study in 46 patients. Can J Neurol Sci 2001; 28:120–124.
35. Patchell RA, Regine WF. The rationale for adjuvant whole brain radiation therapy with radiosurgery in the treatment of single brain metastases. Technol Cancer Res Treat 2003; 2:111–115.
36. Order SE, Hellman S, Von Essen CF, et al. Improvement in quality of survival following whole-brain irradiation for brain metastasis. Radiology 1968; 91:149–153.
37. Sze G, Mehta M, Schultz CJ, et al. Radiologic response evaluation of brain metastases: unidimensional World Health Organization response evaluation criteria in solid tumors vs bidmensional or 3-dimensional criteria. Proc Am Soc Clin Oncol 2001; 20:59a.
38. Harwood AR, Simson WJ. Radiation therapy of cerebral metastases: a randomized prospective clinical trial. Int J Radiat Oncol Biol Phys 1977; 2:1091–1094.
39. Borgelt B, Gelber R, Kramer S, et al. The palliation of brain metastases: final results of the first two studies by the Radiation Therapy Oncology Group. Int J Radiat Oncol Biol Phys 1980; 6:1–9.
40. Borgelt B, Gelber R, Larson M, et al. Ultra-rapid high dose irradiation schedules for the palliation of brain metastases: final results of the first two studies by the Radiation Therapy Oncology Group. Int J Radiat Oncol Biol Phys 1981; 7:1633–1638.

41. Kurtz JM, Gelber R, Brady LW, et al. The palliation of brain metastases in a favorable patient population: a randomized clinical trial by the Radiation Therapy Oncology Group. Int J Radiat Oncol Biol Phys 1981; 7:891–895.

42. Chatani M, Teshima T, Hata K, et al. Prognostic factors in patients with brain metastases from lung carcinoma. Strahlenther Onkol 1986; 162:157–161.

43. Chatani M, Matayoshi Y, Masaki N, et al. Radiation therapy for brain metastases from lung carcinoma. Prospective randomized trial according to the level of lactate dehydrogenase. Strahlenther Onkol 1994; 170:155–161.

44. Haie-Meder C, Pellae-Cosset B, Laplanche A, et al. Results of a randomized clinical trial comparing two radiation schedules in the palliative treatment of brain metastases. Radiother Oncol 1993; 26:111–116.

45. Murray KJ, Scott C, Greenberg HM, et al. A randomized phase III study of accelerated hyperfractionation versus standard in patients with unresected brain metastases: a report of the Radiation Therapy Oncology Group (RTOG) 9104. Int J Radiat Oncol Biol Phys 1997; 39:571–574.

46. Sause WT, Scott C, Krisch R, et al. Phase I/II trial of accelerated fractionation in tbrain metastases RTOG 85–28. Int J Radiat Oncol Biol Phys 1993; 26:653–657.

47. Nieder C, Berberich W, Schnabel K. Tumor-related prognostic factors for remission of brain metastases after radiotherapy. Int J Radiat Oncol Biol Phys 1997; 39: 25–30.

48. Kondzoilka D, Patel A, Lunsford LD, et al. Stereotactic radiosurgery plus whole brain radiotherapy versus radiotherapy alone for patients with multiple brain metastases. Int J Radiat Oncol Biol Phys 1999; 45(2):427–434.

49. Patchell RA, Tibbs PA, Regine WF, et al. Postoperative radiotherapy in the treatment of single metastases to the brain: a randomized trial. JAMA 1998; 280: 1485–1489.

50. Arbit E, Wronski M, Burt M, et al. The treatment of patients with recurrent brain metastases. A retrospective analysis of 109 patients with nonsmall cell lung cancer. Cancer 1995; 76:765–773.

51. Bezjak A, Adam J, Barton R, et al. Symptom response after palliative radiotherapy for patients with brain metastases. Eur J Cancer 2002; 38:487–496.

52. Auchter RM, Lamond JP, Alexander E, et al. A multiinstitutional outcome and prognostic factor analysis of radiosurgery for resectable single brain metastasis. Int J Radiat Oncol Biol Phys 1996; 35:27–35.

53. Mehta MP, Patel RR. Radiotherapy and radiosurgery for brain metastases. In: Black PM, Loeffler JS, eds. Cancer of the Central Nervous System. 2nd ed. Philadelphia: Lippincott Williams & Wilkins, 2001.

54. Alexander E, Moriarty TM, Davis RB, et al. Stereotactic radiosurgery for the definitive, noninvasive treatment of brain metastases. J Natl Cancer Inst 1995; 87:34–40.

55. Shaw E, Scott C, Souhami L, et al. Single dose radiosurgical treatment of recurrent previously irradiated primary brain tumors and brain metastases: final report of RTOG protocol 90-05. Int J Radiat Oncol Biol Phys 2000; 47(2):291–298.

56. Kondziolka D, Patel A, Lunsford LD, et al. Stereotactic radiosurgery plus whole brain radiotherapy versus radiotherapy alone for patients with multiple brain metastases. Int J Radiat Oncol Biol Phys 1999; 45:427–434.

57. Chougule PB, Burton-Williams M, Saris S, et al. Randomized treatment of brain metastasis with gamma knife radiosurgery, whole brain radiotherapy or both. Int J Radiat Oncol Biol Phys 2000; 48:114.

58. Sanghavi SN, Miranpuri SS, Chappell R, et al. Radiosurgery for patients with brain metastases: a multi-institutional analysis, stratified by the RTOG recursive partitioning analysis method. Int J Radiat Oncol Biol Phys 2001; 51:426–434.

59. Sneed PK, Suh JH, Goetsch SJ, et al. A multi-institutional review of radiosurgery alone vs. radiosurgery with whole brain radiotherapy as the initial management of brain metastases. Int J Radiat Oncol Biol Phys 2002; 53:519–526.

60. Hoffman R, Sneed PK, McDermott MW, et al. Radiosurgery for brain metastases from primary lung carcinoma. Cancer J 2001; 7:121–131.

61. Pirzkall A, Debus J, Lohr F, et al. Radiosurgery alone or in combination with whole-brain radiotherapy for brain metastases. J Clin Oncol 1998; 16:3563–3569.

62. Sneed PK, Lamborn KR, Forstner JM, et al. Radiosurgery for brain metastases: is whole brain radiotherapy necessary? Int J Radiat Oncol Biol Phys 1999; 43: 549–558.

63. Aoyama H, Shirato H, Nakagawa K, et al. Interim report of the JRSOG99-1 multi-institutional randomized trial, comparing radiosurgery alone vs. radiosurgery plus whole brain irradiation for 1-4 brain metastasis. Proc Am Soc Clin Oncol 2004; 23:108.

64. Manon RR, Oneil A, Mehta M, et al. Phase II trial of radiosurgery (RS) for 1 to 3 newly diagnosed brain metastases from renal cell, melanoma, and sarcoma: an Eastern Cooperative Oncology Group Study (#6397). Proc Am Soc Clin Oncol 2004; 23:108.

65. Khuntia D, Brown P, Li J, et al. Whole brain radiation in the management of brain metastasis. J Clin Oncol 2006; 24:1295–1304.

66. DeAngelis LM, Delattre JY, Posner JB. Radiation-induced dementia in patients cured of brain metastases. Neurology 1989; 39:789–796.

67. Penitzka S, Steinvorth S, Sehlleier S, et al. Assessment of cognitive function after preventive and therapeutic whole brain irradiation using neuropsychological testing. Strahlenther Onkol 2002; 178:252–258.

68. Regine WF, Scott C, Murray K, et al. Neurocognitive outcome in brain metastases patients treated with accelerated-fraction vs. accelerated-hyperfracionated radiotherapy: an analysis from Radiation Therapy Oncology Group Study 91-04. Int J Radiat Oncol Biol Phys 2001; 51:711–717.

69. Regine WF, Huhn JL, Patchell RA, et al. Risk of symptomatic brain tumour recurrence and neurologic deficit after radiosurgery al in patients with newly diagnosed brain metastases: results and implications. Int J Radiat Oncol Biol Phys 2002; 52:333–338.

70. Meyers CA, Smith JA, Bezjak A, et al. Neurocognitive function and progression in patients with brain metastases treated with whole-brain radiation and motexafin gadolinium: results of a randomized phase III trial. J Clin Oncol 2004; 22: 157–165.

71. Gregor A, Cull A, Stephens RJ, et al. Prophylactic cranial irradiation is indicated following complete response to induction therapy in small cell lung cancer: results of a multicentre randomised trial. United Kingdom Coordinating Committee for Cancer Research (UKCCCR) and the European Organization for Research and Treatment of Cancer (EORTC). Eur J Cancer 1997; 33:1752–1758.

72. Komaki R, Meyers CA, Shin DM. et al. Evaluation of cognitive function in patients with limited small cell lung cancer prior to and shortly following prophylactic cranial irradiation. Int J Radiat Oncol Biol Phys 1995; 33(1):179–182.

73. Meyers CA, Hess KR, Yung WK, et al. Cognitive function as a predictor of survival in patients with recurrent malignant glioma. J Clin Oncol 2000; 18:646–650.

74. Meyers CA, Hess KR. Multifaceted end points in brain tumor clinical trials: cognitive deterioration precedes MRI progression. Neuro-Oncology 2003; 5:89–95.

75. Meyers CA, Weitzner MA, Valentine, et al. Methylphenidate therapy improves cognition, mood, and function of brain tumor patients. J Clin Oncol 1998; 16(7):2522–2527.

76. Rapp SR, Rosdhal R, D'Agostino RB, et al. Improving cognitive functioning in brain irradiated patients: a phase II trial of an acetylcholinesterase inhibitor (donepezil). Neuro Oncol 2004; 6:357.

77. Chan AS, Cheung MC, Law SC, et al. Phase II study of alpha-tocopherol in improving the cognitive function of patients with temporal lobe radionecrosis. Cancer 2004; 100:398–404.

78. Pellegrini JW, Lipton SA. Delayed administration of memantine prevents N-methyl-D-aspartate receptor-mediated neurotoxicity. Ann Neurol 1993; 33:403–407.

79. Chen HS, Pellegrini JW, Aggarwal SK, et al. Open-channel block of N-methyl-D-aspartate (NMDA) responses by memantine: therapeutic advantage against NMDA receptor-mediated neurotoxicity. J Neurosci 1992; 12:4427–4436.

80. Knisely JP, de Lotbiniere AC, de Lotbiniere NC, et al. Randomized trial of erythropoietin as a central nervous system radioprotectant. Int J Radiat Oncol Biol Phys 2004; 60:343–344.

81. Hossain M, Wong CS. Erythropoietin improves learning and memory impairment after whole brain irradiation, 95th American Association for Cancer Research Annual Meeting, Orlando, Florida, Mar 27–31:2001 [Abstr. No. 3125].

82. Leyland-Jones B, Semiglazov V, Pawlicki M, et al. Maintaining normal hemoglobin levels with epoetin alfa in mainly nonanemic patients With metastatic breast cancer receiving first-line chemotherapy: a survival study. J Clin Oncol 2005; 23: 5960–5972.

83. Peissner W, Kocher M, Treuer H, et al. Ionizing radiation-induced apoptosis of proliferating stem cells in the dentate Gyrus of the adult rat hippocampus. Brain Res Mol Brain Res 1999; 71:61–68.

84. van den Bent MJ. The role of chemotherapy in brain metastases. Eur J Cancer 2003; 39:2114–2120.

85. Agarwala SS, Kirkwood JM. Temozolomide, a novel alkylating agent with activity in the central nervous system, may improve the treatment of advanced metastatic melanoma. Oncologist 2000; 5:144–151.

86. Reid JM, Stevens DC, Rubin J, et al. Pharmacokinetics of 3-methyl-(triazen-1–yl) imidazole-4-carboximide following administration of temozolomide to patients with advanced cancer. Clin Cancer Res 1997; 3:2393–2398.

87. Patel M, McCully C, Godwin K, et al. Plasma and cerebrospinal fluid pharmacokinetics of intravenous temozolomide in non-human primates. J Neurooncol 2003; 61:203–207.

88. Stupp R, Gander M, Leyvraz S, et al. Current and future developments in the use of temozolomide for the treatment of brain tumours. Lancet Oncol 2001; 2:552.

89. Stupp R, Mason WP, van den Bent MJ, et al. Radiotherapy plus concomitant and adjuvant temozolomide for glioblastoma. N Engl J Med 2005; 352:987–996.

90. Abrey LE, Olson JD, Raizer JJ, et al. A phase II trial of temozolomide for patients with recurrent or progressive brain metastases. J Neurooncol 2001; 53:259–265.

91. Christodoulou C, Bafaloukos D, Kosmidis P, et al. Phase II study of temozolomide in heavily pretreated cancer patients with brain metastases. Ann Oncol 2001; 12:249–254.
92. Agarwala SS, Kirkwood JM, Gore M, et al. Temozolomide for the treatment of brain metastases associated with metastatic melanoma: a phase II study. J Clin Oncol 2004; 22:2101–2107.
93. Friedman HS, Evans B, Reardon D, et al. Phase II trial of temozolomide for patients with progressive brain metastases. Proc Am Soc Clin Oncol 2003; 22:102.
94. Dziadziusko R, Ardizzoni A, Postmus PE. et al. Temozolomide in patients with advanced non-small cell lung cancer with and without brain metastases: a phase II study of the EORTC Lung Cancer Group (08965). Eur J Cancer 2003; 39:1271–1276.
95. Siena S, Landonia G, Baietta E, et al. Multicenter phase II study of temozolomide therapy for brain metastasis in patients with malignant melanoma, breast cancer, and non-small cell lung cancer. Proc am Soc Cllin Oncol 2003; 22:102.
96. Dardoufas C, Miliadou A, Skarleas C, et al. Concomitant temozolomide (TMZ) and radiotherapy (RT) followed by adjuvant treatment with temozolomide in patients with brain metastases from solid tumours. Proc Am Soc Clin Oncol 2001; 20:75b.
97. Hegi ME, Diserens AC, Gorlia T, et al. MGMT gene silencing and benefit from temozolomide in glioblastoma. N Eng J Med 2005; 352:997–1003.
98. Furonaka O, Takeshima Y, Awaya H, et al. Aberrant methylation and loss of expression of O-methylguanine-DNA methyltransferase in pulmonary squamous cell carcinoma and adenocarcinoma. Pathol Int 2005; 55:303–309.
99. Wedge SR, Porteous JK, Glaser MG, Marcus K, Newlands ES. In vitro evaluation of temozolomide combined with X-irradiation. AntiCancer Drugs 1997; 8:92–97.
100. Antonadou D, Paraskevaidis M, Sarris G, et al. Phase II randomized trial of temozolomide and concurrent radiotherapy in patients with brain metastases. J Clin Oncol 2002; 20:3644–3650.
101. Verger E, Gil M, Yaya R, et al. Temozolomide and concomitant whole brain radiotherapy in patients with brain metastases: a phase II randomized trial. Int J Radiat Oncol Biol Phys 2005; 61:185–191.
102. Antonadou D, Coliarakis N, Paraskevaidis M, et al. Whole brain radiotherapy alone or in combination with temozolomide for brain metastases. A phase III study. Int J Radiat Oncol Biol Phys 2002; 54:93.
103. Hedde JP, Ko Y, Metzler U, et al. A phase I/II trial of topotecan and radiation therapy for CNS-metastases of patients with solid tumors. Proc Am Soc Clin Oncol 2003; 22:111.
104. Korfel A, Oehm C, von Pawel J, et al. Response to topotecan of sympomatic brain metastases of small-cell lung cancer also after whole-brain irradiation: a multicentre phase II study. Eur J Cancer 2002; 38:1724–1729.
105. Brem S, Staller A, Wotoczek-Obadia M. Interstitial chemotherapy for local control of CNS metastases. Neuro Oncol 2004; 6:370–371.
106. Guerrieri M, Wong K, Ryan G, et al. A randomised phase III study of palliative radiation with concomitant carboplatin for brain metastases from non-small cell carcinoma of the lung. Lung Cancer 2004; 46:107–111.
107. Cortes J, Rodrigues J, Aramendia JM, et al. Front-line paclitaxel/cistpatin-based chemotherapy in brain metastases from non-small-cell lung cancer. Oncology 2003; 64:28–35.

108. Bernardo G, Cuzzoni Q, Strada MR, et al. First-line chemotherapy with vinorelbine, gemcitabine, and carboplatin in the treatment of brain metastases from non-small-cell lung cancer: a phase II study. Cancer Invest 2002; 20:293–302.

109. Franciosi V, Cocconi G, Michiara M, et al. Front-line chemotherapy with cisplatin and etoposide for patients with brain metastases from breast carcinoma, nonsmall cell lung carcinoma, or malignant melanoma: a prospective study. Cancer 1999; 85:1599–1605.

110. Robinet G, Thomas P, Breton JL, et al. Results of a phase III study of early versus delayed whole brain radiotherapy with concurrent cisplatin and vinorelbine combination in inoperable brain metastasis of non-small-cell lung cancer: Groupe Francais de Pneumo-Cancerologie (GFPC) Protocol 95-1. Ann Oncol 2001; 12:59–67.

111. Ceresoli GL, Cappuzzo F, Gregorc V, et al. Gefitinib in patients with brain metastases from non-small-cell lung cancer: a prospective trial. Ann Oncol 2004; 15:1042–1047.

112. Chiu CH, Tsai CM, Chen YM, et al. Gefitinib is active in patients with brain metastases from non-small cell lung cancer and response is related to skin toxicity. Lung Cancer 2005; 47:129–138.

113. Pleiman CM, Von Hoff D, DeMie L, et al. Antitumor Activity of MPC-6827 in Human Breast, Colon, Pancreatic, Ovarian and Mouse Melanoma Tumor Xenografts in Athymic Mice. 95th American Association for Cancer Research Annual Meeting, Orlando, Florida, 2004 Mar 27–31.

114. Komarnicky LT, Phillips TL, Martz K, et al. A randomized phase III protocol for the evaluation of misonidazole combined with radiation in the treatment of patients with brain metastases (RTOG-7916). Int Radiat Oncol Biol Phys 1991; 20:53–58.

115. Phillips TL, Scott CB, Leibel SA, et al. Results of a randomized comparison of radiotherapy and bromodeoxyuridine with radiotherapy alone for brain metastases: report of RTOG trial 89-05. Int J Radiat Oncol Biol Phys 1995; 33:339–348.

116. Carde P, Timmerman R, Mehta MP, et al. Multicenter phase Ib/II trial of the radiation enhancer motexafin gadolinium in patients with brain metastases. J Clin Oncol 2001; 19:2074–2083.

117. Khuntia D, Mehta M. Motexafin gadolinium: a clinical review of a novel radio-enhancer for brain tumors. Expert Rev Anticancer Ther 2004; 4:981–989.

118. Mehta MP, Shapiro WR, Glantz MJ, et al. Lead-in phase to randomized trial of motexafin gadolinium and whole-brain radiation for patients with brain metastases: centralized assessment of magnetic resonance imaging, neurocognitive, and neurologic end points. J Clin Oncol 2002; 20:3445–3453.

119. Mehta MP, Rodrigus P, Terhaard CH, et al. Survival and neurologic outcomes in a randomized trial of motexafin gadolinium and whole-brain radiation therapy in brain metastases. J Clin Oncol 2003; 21:2529–2536.

120. Shaw E, Scott C, Suh J, et al. RSR13 plus cranial radiation therapy in patients with brain metastases: comparison with the Radiation Therapy Oncology Group Recursive Partitioning Analysis Brain Metastases Database. J Clin Oncol 2003; 21: 2364–2371.

121. Suh J, Stea B, Nabid A, et al. Standard whole brain radiation therapy (WBRT) with supplemental oxygen (O2), with or without RSR13 (efaproxiral) in patients with brain metastases: results of the randomized REACH (RT-009) study. Proc Am Soc Clin Incol 2004; 22:115S.

11

Recent Advances in Imaging for Lung Cancer

Shweta Bhatt

Department of Imaging Sciences, University of Rochester School of Medicine and Dentistry, Rochester, New York, U.S.A.

Kristopher M. Skwarski

Department of Respiratory Medicine, Royal Infirmary of Edinburgh, Edinburgh, Scotland, U.K.

Vikram S. Dogra

Department of Imaging Sciences, University of Rochester School of Medicine and Dentistry, Rochester, New York, U.S.A.

INTRODUCTION

Cross-sectional modalities of imaging such as ultrasound (US), computed tomography (CT), and magnetic resonance (MR) imaging (MRI) are an integral part of cancer care, playing an important role in every phase, from screening and diagnosis to staging and to treatment planning and follow-up. With further advances in imaging and the introduction of modalities such as positron emission tomography (PET) and endobronchial US (EBUS) imaging has made a significant impact in lung cancer care, particularly in staging lung cancer and determining the prognosis. The recent development of molecular imaging further promises to open up new horizons in earlier cancer detection and assessment of tumor characteristics by imaging.

There are five basic functions of imaging for lung cancer (or any other type of cancer)—screening, characterization, staging, assessment of therapeutic efficacy, and detection of recurrence after treatment.

This chapter presents recent advances in lung-cancer imaging, with emphasis on the latest developments in lung-cancer imaging such as PET, EBUS, and molecular imaging.

COMPUTED TOMOGRAPHY

With the advent of multidetector CT (MDCT), there has been considerable improvement in the scanning techniques that allow scanning of the whole chest within a single breath-hold using a thin-section, high-resolution technique. Problem-adapted sections in arbitrary directions have become available to the radiologist to provide an excellent spatial resolution (1). New techniques such as three-dimensional (3D) reconstruction, including volume rendering and virtual bronchoscopy, have added considerably to the CT imaging of lung cancer. These techniques can be helpful in the evaluation and demonstration of pathology within the central tracheobronchial tree and in the guidance of bronchoscopic biopsies. MDCT can now produce excellent images comparable to MRI in all desired planes and thus has become the primary modality for image interpretation.

Tumor Detection

MDCT, with its multiplanar reconstruction, has become the modality of choice for the initial detection of tumor in the lungs (Fig. 1). It has been observed that with axial and coronal maximum-intensity projection images, the ability of CT to detect nodules smaller than 5 mm is much superior to the standard axial CT images and other modalities that are able to detect nodules greater than 5 mm with ease (2,3). Further, reduced slice thickness (<1.5 mm) as compared to 5 mm thickness leads to an improvement of small nodule detection, confidence levels, and interobserver agreement, thus raising the sensitivity of MDCT in the detection of lung tumors (4). The utility of computer-aided detection (CAD) of lung nodules

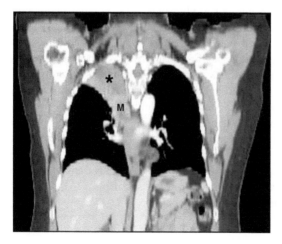

Figure 1 Coronal multiplanar reformatted image of contrast-enhanced image in a 53-year-old female demonstrates a right hilar mass (M) that obstructs the right upper lobe bronchus resulting in collapse of the right upper lobe of lung (*).

using different reconstruction slice-thickness protocols in MDCT has been found to be superior to the reading by radiologists, especially in nodules less than 10 mm, with an added advantage of a shorter evaluation time (5). Therefore, CAD can be considered a second reading for detection of lung nodules (6–8). Use of automated detection on low-dose CT scans has also been studied in the detection of lung cancers with favorable results (9,10). Chances of missing some cancers exists on such a detection system if they are very subtle and appear as small faint nodules, are overlapping normal structures, or appear in a complex background of other pulmonary disease (11).

Staging of Lung Cancer

An accurate clinical tumor, nodes, and metastasis (TNM) staging of lung cancer is essential for the determination of the extent of the disease so that an optimal therapeutic strategy can be planned. Overstaging as well as understaging can have adverse results on the patient. The current staging system for lung cancer, the American Joint Committee on Cancer TNM staging (12), relies on the pathological evaluation of the primary tumor (T), regional nodes (N), and distant metastasis (M). CT is still the cornerstone of imaging studies in the preoperative staging (Fig. 2)

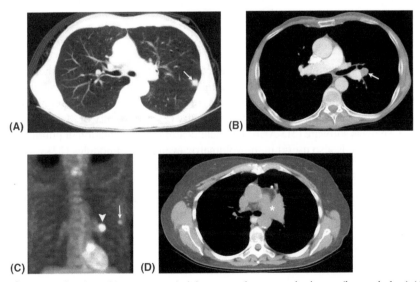

(A) (B)

(C) (D)

Figure 2 Staging of lung cancer. Axial computed tomography image (lung window) (**A**) demonstrates a 2.3 cm peripheral nodule (*arrow*) with an ipsilateral hilar lymph node (*arrow*) in the mediastinal window (**B**). Corresponding maximum intensity projection positron emission tomography image (**C**) in the coronal plane demonstrates hypermetabolic peripheral nodule (*arrow*) with metastatic hilar node (*arrowhead*) suggestive of stage IIA (T1N1M0) (surgically resectable) lung cancer. Nonenhanced CT of the lung (**D**) in another patient with a left hilar mass that encases the left pulmonary artery and shows mediastinal invasion, suggestive of stage IIIB (T4, N0M0) (surgically unresectable) lung cancer.

and posttherapeutic evaluation of lung cancer (13). It is particularly useful in the assessment of the extent of regional tumors (14) and in delineating the relation of the primary lesion to fissures and the diaphragm (15). CT-enhancement character-istics can help to predict hilar or mediastinal nodal metastasis in patients with stage T1 lung cancer. In a study by Shim et al. (16), stage T1 lung cancers showing peak enhancement of 110 Hounsfield units (HU) or greater or net enhancement of 60 HU or greater on dynamic CT indicated a high likelihood of hilar or mediasti-nal nodal metastasis.

PET/CT Imaging

Integrated PET and CT is a new imaging modality offering both anatomic local-ization and metabolic information of lesions. Combined PET/CT is a more accurate test than either of its individual components and is better than simultaneous viewing of images from both modalities (Figs. 3 and 4) (17). It is found to be useful for staging of lung cancer, therapy planning and evaluation, response evaluation during and after chemotherapy, restaging after neoadjuvant therapy, planning of radiotherapy, and detection of recurrent disease staging wherever available (18,19). Quantitative assessment using fused single-photon emission CT (SPECT)-CT images is also useful for the diagnosis of lymph-node metastasis in patients with non-small cell lung carcinoma (NSCLC) (20).

Technical Advances

Volumetric measurements of lung cancer can modify the diagnostic and therapeu-tic evaluation of cancer patients under treatment. CAD volumetric measurements allow an easy and objective evaluation in the assessment of chemotherapy response, thus reducing interobserver variability (21). The utility of 3D Advanced Lung Analysis software (3D-ALA, GE Healthcare) in the estimation of pulmonary nodule volume is also useful in the volumetric evaluation of nodules (22).

Use of PET in the characterization of pulmonary nodules has superseded CT and MRI because of a greater diagnostic accuracy in both intra- and extrapul-monary lesions (Fig. 5). But, it is only used as a supplementary tool rather than as a primary tool for the assessment of lung cancers. Integration of MDCT and Tc-99m Sestamibi SPECT-CT can prove very useful in the management of soli-tary pulmonary nodules (SPNs), adding the diagnostic information of CT as well as PET (23).

MAGNETIC RESONANCE IMAGING

Although CT continues to be used more commonly in staging lung cancer, with recent advances in MRI techniques and Gadolinium-enhanced MRI, image quality and diagnostic capabilities of MRI are much more improved. MRI has proven useful in certain aspects of lung-cancer evaluation, particularly as a supplement to CT findings (24). These areas include the following: (*i*) evaluation of the local

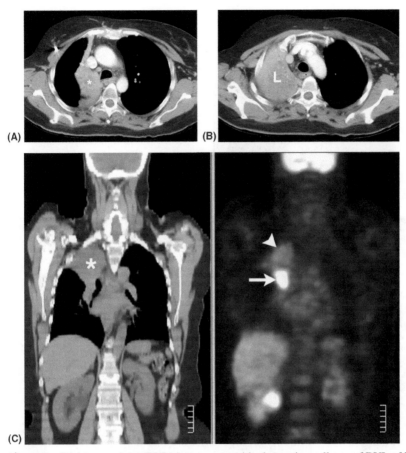

Figure 3 Right upper lobe (RUL) lung cancer with obstructive collapse of RUL of lung. of the lungs (**A**) demonstrates a large heterogeneous mass (*) located in the right hilar region. CECT of the chest (**B**) through the upper lobes of lungs shows complete collapse of the RUL (L). Corresponding computed tomography (CT) and positron emission tomography (PET) image in the coronal plane (**C**) clearly distinguishes the hypermetabolic tumor (*arrow*) from the collapsed RUL of lung (*arrowhead*) on the PET image as compared to the coronal CT image where it appears as a single mass (*). *Abbreviation*: CECT, contrast enhanced computed tomography.

extent of superior sulcus tumors, and (*ii*) distinction between stage IIIA (resectable) and stage IIIB (unresectable) tumors.

TUMOR DETECTION (SPN)

The SPN is the most common finding on chest radiographs and needs further characterization by the least invasive way possible to differentiate between benign and malignant (25–29) tumors. Although certain features such as stability or no

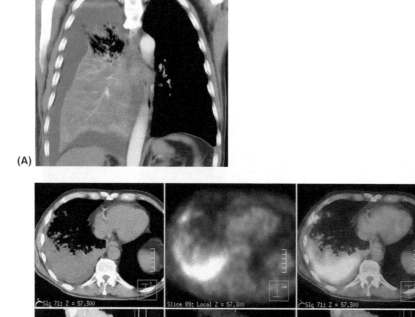

Figure 4 Consolidation of right lung masking malignancy. Contrast enhanced computed tomography of the chest (**A**) in coronal plane shows a large area of consolidation of the right lung with pleural effusion. Corresponding computed tomography (CT), positron emission tomography (PET), and fused CT–PET images (**B**) of the lungs in the axial and sagittal planes demonstrate an area of marked increased 18F-2-deoxy-D-glucose uptake in the posterior part of the consolidated lung, suggestive of underlying lung cancer not distinguishable on CT images.

growth for at least two years, presence of calcium in characteristic patterns, and age less than 35 years without any associated risk factors are reliable indicators of a benign process, indeterminate cases need to be differentiated by a confirmatory method.

Contrast-enhanced MRI plays a significant role in the evaluation of SPNs. Lung cancers lesser than 3 cm show a strong and homogeneous enhancement without necrosis. Gadolinium-enhanced MRI using T1-weighted spin echo and

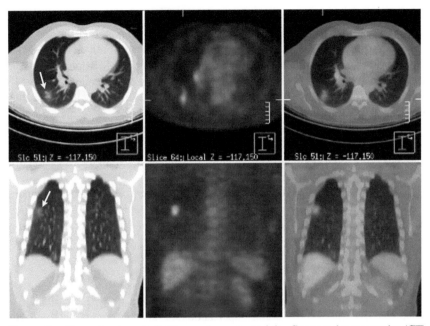

Figure 5 (*See color insert.*) Solitary pulmonary nodule. Computed tomography (CT), positron emission tomography (PET) and fused PET–CT images of the chest in axial and coronal planes demonstrate a faintly visible nodule (*arrow*) in the right lung, which shows increased uptake on PET and fused images.

snap shot gradient echo imaging may be helpful in differentiating between malignant and benign pulmonary masses, differentiating between hilar lung cancer and peripheral postobstructive atelectasis or pneumonia and tuberculomas (30), determining therapeutic effect after radiation therapy, and differentiating between recurrent or residual tumor and radiation pneumonitis (31). Further advances such as dynamic MRI based on MR pulmonary perfusion imaging help to evaluate the hemodynamics of SPN by improving benign or malignant characterization (32).

Locoregional Spread

MRI is superior to CT in detection of tumor invasion due to its primary multiplanar imaging capability and better soft-tissue resolution. MRI may thus be useful when CT findings are indefinite, particularly with regard to invasion of major cardiovascular structures (e.g., superior vena cava, pulmonary artery, pericardium, and heart) with cardiac-gated MRI; invasion of the tracheal carina or main bronchi; and in the evaluation of superior sulcus tumors with neurovascular invasion (33,34).

Diagnostic capability of MRI in detecting mediastinal and hilar invasion by lung cancer is particularly advanced by contrast-enhanced MR angiography (35,36). But, minimal mediastinal invasion is a limitation of MRI as it is for CT scanning (37).

For the evaluation of mediastinal lymphadenopathy, MRI and CT are equally sensitive, and PET is considered a better choice for lymph nodes' evaluation (34).

Chest-wall invasion is a diagnostic dilemma for both CT and MRI. Better contrast resolution and multiplanar capability gives MRI an upper hand theoretically, using T1- and T2-weighted imaging and dynamic cine MR imaging during breathing for determining chest-wall involvement of the lung cancer (38).

MRI should, therefore, be considered a primary imaging modality to evaluate lung cancers in patients with contraindications to intravenous contrast agents, and as a problem-solving modality when CT is inconclusive in the detection of a possible hilar or mediastinal mass.

The scope of MRI in the evaluation of lung cancers can be further expanded in the future with improvements in motion suppression techniques, use of ultrafast MRI (using echoplanar imaging), and further development of MRI spectroscopy and MRI contrast agents.

Distant Metastasis

Whole-body MRI is capable of detecting distant metastases, in particular, in organs at risk, that is, the brain, upper abdomen, and musculoskeletal system. With the advent of new fast sequences such as half-Fourier acquisition single-shot turbo spin echo and volumetric interpolated breath-hold examination, the spatial resolution comes close to that of CT, with an added advantage of outstanding soft-tissue contrast and no radiation exposure (39). New advances in chemical shift imaging with MRI are an excellent noninvasive method that can allow distinction of adrenal adenomas from metastases and help in the staging of lung cancer. Because MRI is vulnerable to motion artifacts from breathing and susceptibility artifacts from the air-tissue interfaces in the lung, it is mainly used as a problem-solving tool in the mediastinum and the chest wall.

POSITRON EMISSION TOMOGRAPHY

PET has now become a clinically useful, noninvasive study that complements conventional imaging studies (chest radiographs, CT, and MRI) in the evaluation of patients with lung cancer. PET imaging of lung cancer is typically performed with the radiopharmaceutical 18F-2-deoxy-D-glucose (FDG), a d-glucose analog (40). The principle used in PET in tumor detection is based on increased uptake and accumulation of FDG because of increased glucose metabolism by malignant cells. The PET camera reads the FDG distribution, thus allowing differentiation between normal and malignant tissues (41). The metabolic and physiologic abnormalities used in FDG-PET imaging, rather than conventional anatomic or morphologic characteristics used in other modalities, demonstrates tremendous potential in the advanced imaging of lung cancer (42). PET can also be used to define the target volume in radiation treatment planning and to evaluate treatment response. Incorporating PET seems to improve tumor coverage and spare normal tissues (43). Results are better with combined CT–PET evaluation; so, it is currently preferred for staging wherever available.

Tumor Detection (SPN)

FDG-PET can accurately characterize indeterminate SPNs suspicious of malignancy, thus reducing the need for invasive tissue biopsy (44). Nodules with low FDG uptake have minimal malignant potential and are followed up radiographically; nodules with increased FDG uptake are further evaluated with biopsy to confirm malignancy or are resected if strongly suspected to be malignant clinically (45). Of particular interest is the fact that PET is highly sensitive in detecting T1-stage (≤3 cm) lung cancers (Fig. 6) (46). It has been found accurate in differentiating benign from malignant lesions as small as 1 cm (46). But, with smaller lesions (<1 cm), there is also an increase in false-negative results because of the need of a critical mass of metabolically active malignant cells to produce a positive PET diagnosis (Fig. 7). Therefore, marked FDG uptake is required to lead to a relevant PET diagnosis in lesions smaller than 1 cm (41,44,47). False-negative results can also be seen in tumors with low metabolic activity such as carcinoid tumors and bronchioloalveolar carcinomas (41). Low FDG avid lung adenocarcinomas have also been seen (Fig. 8) and may give the impression of a benign lesion.

False-positive FDG uptake may be observed in inflammatory conditions due to increased granulocyte and macrophage activity (Figs. 9 and 10). These conditions include bacterial pneumonia, abscesses, aspergillosis, and granulomatous conditions of the lung such as tuberculosis, sarcoidosis, histoplasmosis, Wegener's granulomatosis, and pneumoconiosis (41).

Staging of Lung Cancer

Staging of cancer is the second step after detection of any kind of cancer, and imaging plays a key role. PET supplements the routine imaging techniques to assess the patient's prognosis as well as to decide upon the modality of treatment

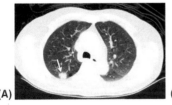 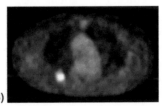

(A) (B)

Figure 6 Solitary pulmonary nodule. Axial computed tomography image (**A**) and corresponding positron emission tomography (PET) (**B**) image through the lungs demonstrate an solitary pulmonary nodule (2.6 cm) (*arrow* in **A**), which shows markedly increased 18F-2-deoxy-D-glucose uptake on PET, suggestive of lung cancer.

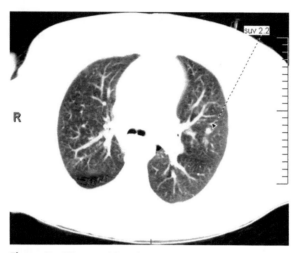

Figure 7 58-year-old male with known history of lung cancer. Axial computed tomography (CT) image of the lungs shows a small nodule in the left lung (*arrow*) with almost no increased uptake on positron emission tomography (not shown). The nodule was found to be positive for malignancy by CT criteria and showed progressive growth in size on follow-up CT.

that would give the best results for the patient's disease, in particular, to decide whether the patient is a good surgical candidate.

Evaluation of Metastatic Lung Cancer

Standard staging (48) of lung cancer is usually based on clinical factors and imaging tests such as CT, US, and scintigraphy. But despite the staging of cancer as a localized disease, about 20% of these patients subsequently have early distant relapse (Fig. 11) (49,50). This can be explained by the micrometastasis already present at the time of initial staging, which could not be detected by standard imaging. The metastases are usually present in the adrenal glands, bones, brain, and liver (51). Over the past few years, organ-specific studies have been performed to compare the efficacy of various imaging modalities, including PET, in the staging of lung cancer.

For bone metastases, PET has a much higher specificity than bone scintigraphy (98% vs. 61%) but an equivalent sensitivity (52). This is due to the ability of PET to better differentiate between benign and malignant lesions (Fig. 12) (53).

PET has a high sensitivity in the detection of adrenal metastasis (Fig. 13) (54–56), but false-positive results are common (54), therefore requiring further assessment before management of such patients is decided.

In the presence of liver metastasis, PET, with a better specificity as compared to US and CT, has a significant role when the findings from other modalities remain indeterminate (Fig. 14) (57).

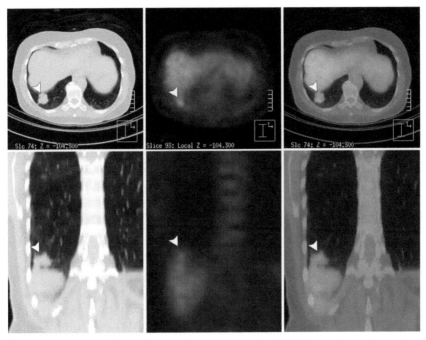

Figure 8 False-negative positron emission tomography (PET) in a confirmed case of lung adenocarcinoma. Computed tomography (CT)–PET images in axial and coronal planes demonstrate a spiculated 4 cm mass (*arrowheads*) in the right lower lobe, which shows minimal 18F-2-deoxy-D-glucose activity on PET images. Wedge resection was performed because of a high index of suspicion clinically and by CT criteria and was pathologically confirmed to be an adenocarcinoma.

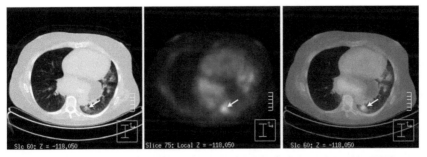

Figure 9 (*See color insert.*) False-positive positron emission tomography (PET). computed tomography (CT)–PET images of the lungs in the axial plane shows a nodule in the left lung (*arrows*), with marked 18F-2-deoxy-D-glucose uptake on PET and fusion images. Bronchoscopy confirmed the lesion to be nodular fibrosis that was nonmalignant.

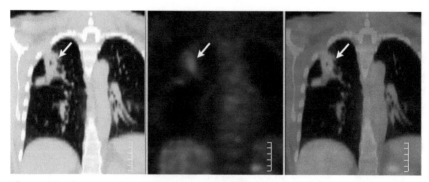

Figure 10 False-positive PET. Coronal CT–PET images of the chest shows a cavitary lesion (*arrows*) in the right lung, which shows mild activity on PET. This was thought of as a cavitary lung carcinoma. Bronchoscopy revealed absence of malignancy. Follow-up imaging showed progressive resolution of the lesion.

Besides, PET also can reveal the presence of metastasis in areas where standard staging failed to detect lesions, such as small nodules in the lungs, soft-tissue lesions (Fig. 15), and retroperitoneal (Fig. 16) or supraclavicular nodes (Fig. 17) (58). PET is not reliable in brain metastases and CT or MRI may be more helpful in detecting brain lesions.

Locoregional Disease Spread

Multislice CT, with its multiplanar reconstruction abilities, has improved the role of imaging tremendously by providing exquisite anatomic details in all desired planes. It is, therefore, considered a very useful tool in lung-cancer staging, particularly to assess locoregional spread of the cancer. But the limitation of CT lies in the assessment of lymph nodes and nodal staging of the lung cancer (59). PET, although limited in anatomic localization of the disease, is much more accurate than CT in detecting nodal disease (60–64). But, the accuracy can be further improved if PET and CT are interpreted together as a combined modality (Fig. 18) (65–67). This way the radiologist has the advantages of good anatomical details as well as metabolic information, particularly in nodal involvement. Histologic confirmation of metastasis is still essential in PET-positive mediastinal nodes, due to false-positive results in infectious and granulomatous diseases such as tuberculosis and sarcoidosis (58). EBUS, described later in this chapter, can be very helpful as a less-invasive procedure in confirmation of nodal spread of the malignancy (67).

Thus, in the overall staging of lung cancer, PET can be extremely useful in both intra- and extrathoracic staging. Its better accuracy as compared to standard staging methods, and a good negative predictive value in lymph-node staging, can have an important impact on staging of lung cancer and the subsequent treatment and may even prevent unnecessary surgery in some patients (68).

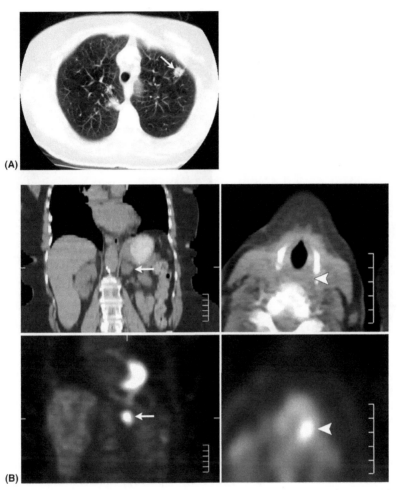

Figure 11 Early distant relapse of lung carcinoma. Axial computed tomography (CT) image of the chest (**A**) demonstrates a spiculated lung nodule (*arrow*) in the left lung, which was subsequently resected. CT–positron emission tomography (PET) images (**B**) of the adrenal (coronal) and the vocal cords (axial) in follow-up imaging after one year of resection shows presence of left adrenal metastasis (*arrows*) and left vocal-cord metastasis (*arrowheads*). Patient also had soft-tissue and brain metastases.

ENDOBRONCHIAL US

Optimal management of patients with lung cancer requires pathological confirmation of malignancy, tumor classification, and accurate staging in order to allow treatment planning. Appropriate tissue sampling identifies patients who will benefit from potentially curative radical therapy. CT, integrated with PET, has significantly improved the accuracy of staging mediastinal lymphadenopathy in lung

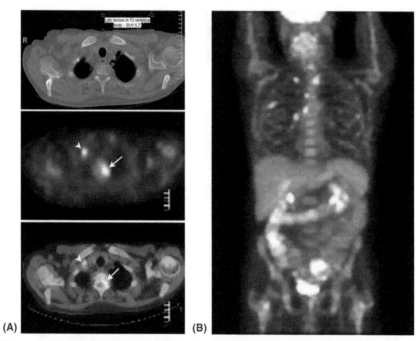

Figure 12 Metastases to bone. Axial computed tomography (CT)-positron emission tomography (PET) images (**A**) in this patient status post resection lung carcinoma show a lytic lesion in the T2 vertebral body (*arrows*), which shows increased activity on PET images. Also seen is a right supraclavicular metastatic node (*arrowheads*). Corresponding coronal PET image (**B**) shows presence of multiple bone metastases in the vertebral bodies and ribs.

cancer (69). However, it is critical to confirm by histological or cytological means the presence of metastatic malignancy in order to plan appropriate therapy (70).

Mediastinoscopy remains a gold standard for sampling mediastinal lymph nodes in staging of lung cancer prior to surgical resection (71) but it has the disadvantage of being invasive, requires general anesthesia, and only superior-anterior mediastinal lymph nodes can be accessed during this procedure (stations 2, 4, and the anterior-superior part of station 7). Moreover, mediastinoscopy is usually performed only once and therefore it is not used in monitoring the treatment after chemo- or chemoradiotherapy. Transbronchial needle aspiration has been used to provide tissue samples from hilar and mediastinal lymph nodes but it is a blind procedure, heavily operator dependent with low sensitivity (25–89%) (72,73).

Advances in endoluminal US technology have led to the development of endoscopic US gastroscope (EUS) and EBUS bronchoscope, whereby lymph nodes can be aspirated through either the esophageal wall or the airway. Both techniques allow for a real-time fine needle aspiration (FNA) and have the advantage of the real-time Doppler facility to exclude intervening blood vessels

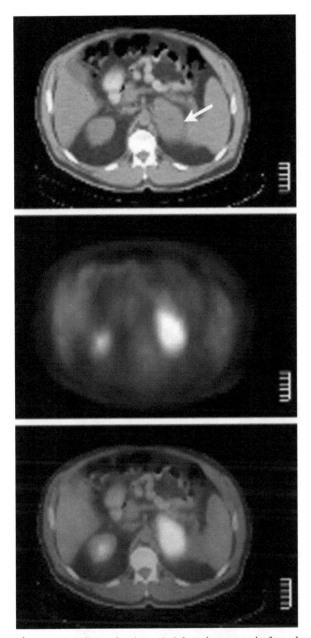

Figure 13 (*See color insert.*) Adrenal metastasis from lung cancer. Axial computed tomography (CT)-positron emission tomography (PET) images of the abdomen shows a large left adrenal mass (*arrow*) on CT, which shows marked uptake on PET images.

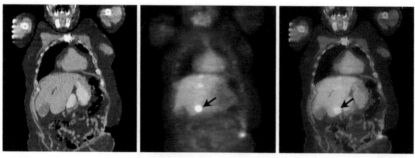

Figure 14 Liver metastases from lung carcinoma. Coronal computed tomography (CT)-positron emission tomography (PET) images of the liver demonstrate multiple bright foci in the liver on PET images, suggestive of increased activity; maximum uptake seen in the lesion in the left lobe of the liver (*arrows*).

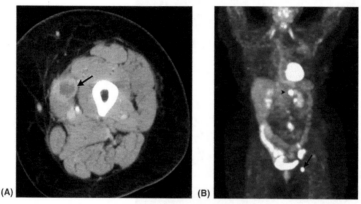

(A)   (B)

Figure 15 Soft-tissue metastasis from lung cancer. Axial CECT image (**A**) of the left thigh in this patient with resected lung cancer shows a hypodense lesion with peripheral enhancing wall (*arrow*) in the medial aspect of the left thigh. Corresponding coronal positron emission tomography image (**B**) demonstrates an increased uptake in the left thigh (*arrow*), which corresponds to the lesion seen on computed tomography (CT) and is suggestive of metastasis. This patient also had left adrenal (*arrowhead*) and brain metastasis.

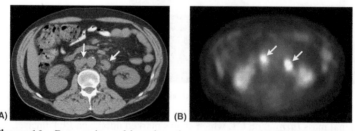

(A)   (B)

Figure 16 Retroperitoneal lymph-node metastases. Axial CECT (**A**) and corresponding positron emission tomography image (**B**) of the abdomen in this patient with resected lung carcinoma shows hypermetabolic left para-aortic and interaorto-caval lymph nodes (*arrows*), suggestive of retroperitoneal lymph-node metastases.

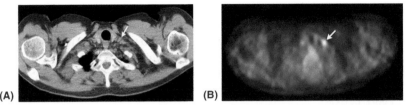

Figure 17 Supraclavicular lymph-node metastasis. Axial contrast enhanced computed tomography (**A**) and corresponding positron emission tomography image (**B**) of the supra-clavicular region in this patient with confirmed lung carcinoma shows hypermetabolic left supraclavicular lymph node (7 mm) (*arrow*) suggestive of metastasis.

immediately prior to lymph-node aspiration. Both techniques are performed on an outpatient basis under conscious sedation with Medazolam and Fentanyl. EUS allows an easy access to inferoposterior mediastinum (stations L4, 5, 7, 8, and 9), whereas EBUS gives an access to hilar stations 10 and 11 and to the mediastinal lymph-node stations 2, 3, 4, and 7 (74). EUS, in the staging of mediastinal lymph-adenopathy, carries a sensitivity approaching 90% (75).

EBUS bronchoscope (Olympus Ltd.) is similar to a standard fiber optic bronchoscope, with a maximum outer diameter of 6.9 mm, 30° oblique forward-viewing optics, and a 2.0 mm biopsy channel. An electronic convex array US

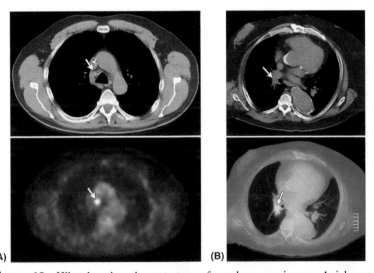

Figure 18 Hilar lymph-node metastases from lung carcinoma. Axial non-contrast enhanced computed tomography and corresponding positron emission tormography (PET) image (**A**) of the chest shows a 7 mm right hilar lymph node (*arrow*), which shows increased activity on positron emission tomography (PET), suggestive of presence of metastases. Axial NECT and fused PET–Computel tomography (CT) image (**B**) shows a right hilar mass lesion a part of which shows increased activity (*arrows*). Fused CT–PET image allows an exact localization of the malignant focus within an abnormal mass lesion.

transducer is mounted at the distal tip and is covered with a water-inflatable balloon sheath for better penetration of the US signal. Scanning is performed at a frequency of 7.5 MHz and allows a penetration of 20 to 50 mm. The aspiration is performed using a 21-gauge special needle (Olympus Ltd.) (Fig. 19). We and others (76–79) have previously reported the use of EBUS-FNA in the assessment of patients with lung cancer. The sensitivity reported by various authors varies from 89% to 95%.

We have analyzed data on our first 125 EBUS procedures performed in the Royal Infirmary of Edinburgh, U.K. A positive histology for lung malignancy was obtained in 64 cases. Sixty-one aspirates were negative for cancer. There were five false-negative samples (confirmed by mediastinoscopy or during surgical resection) and 38 true negative aspirates confirmed either by mediastinoscopy, by surgical resection, or at least by a six-month follow-up period without radiological or clinical progression of the disease. The most frequently sampled lymph nodes were from stations 7, 4, 10, 11, 2, and 3 (in order of frequency) (Figs. 20 and 21). The number of passes from aspirated lymph node varied between two and four. The specimens were processed using liquid-base, thin-layer technology as described in our previous paper (80). Calculated sensitivity was 92%, accuracy 95%, and specificity 100%. Fifty-one primary tissue diagnoses were obtained and 70 mediastinoscopies were avoided. We have not observed any complications from this procedure.

It is believed that EBUS-FNA and EUS-FNA are complimentary. When combined, these procedures provide easy and safe access to the majority of hilar and mediastinal lymph-node stations (except station 6), and when used together with CT–PET they should be regarded as an alternative for mediastinoscopy in the

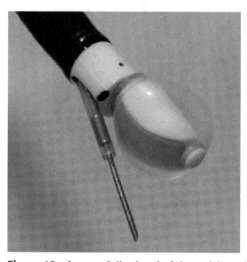

Figure 19 Image of distal end of the endobronchial ultrasound bronchoscope showing the curved array ultrasound transducer with balloon inflated around it and the aspiration needle protruding from the biopsy channel.

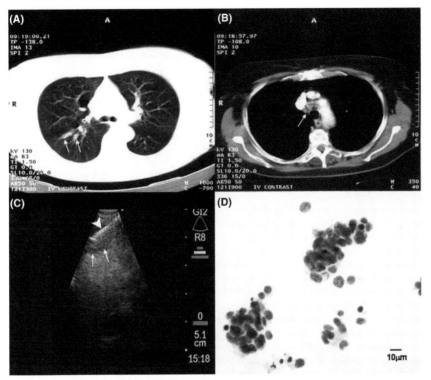

Figure 20 Non-contrast enhanced computed tomography image (**A**) of chest shows two small primary nodules (*arrows*), inaccessible by standard percutaneous biopsy or broncho-scopic techniques. Contrast enhanced computed tomography image (**B**) shows a solitary lymph node (*arrow*) positioned anterior to the trachea in the lymph-node station 4R. Endobronchial ultrasound image (**C**) of the same lymph node (*arrows*) as in (**B**), showing the aspiration needle (*arrowhead*) lying within the node. Fine needle aspiration cytology specimen (**D**) from the same lymph node confirms small-cell lung cancer.

staging algorithm of lung cancer. It is predicted that when the new staging algorithm of lung cancer featuring EUS/EBUS procedures is fully operational, a significant proportion of routine mediastinoscopies will be avoided.

MOLECULAR IMAGING

Despite improvements in preexisting imaging modalities and the introduction of newer imaging methods such as PET, the ability to detect microscopic tumor deposits remains limited. Additionally, distinguishing between inflammation and cancer is also limited because CT, MRI, or PET is unable to make a tissue diagnosis.

Molecular imaging has a great potential in accurate staging of the tumor because it increases the accuracy of detection of both primary tumors and metastasis

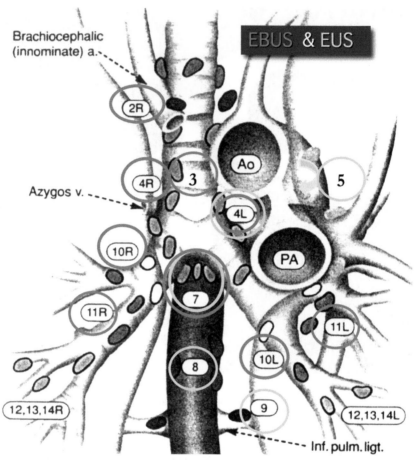

Figure 21 (*See color insert.*) Schematic representation of the hilar and mediastinal lymph-node stations (after Mountain et al.) showing nodal stations accessible for fine needle aspiration by endobronchial ultrasound (stations: 2, 3, 4, 7, 10 and 11—*red circles*) and by EUS (L4, 5, 7, 8 and 9—*yellow circles*).

secondary to its ability to detect micrometastasis that would otherwise be missed by other modalities of imaging.

Molecular imaging in oncology utilizes the principle of noninvasive imaging of the key molecules and molecularly based events responsible for the characteristic phenotype of human malignancy. It enables us to image molecules and biochemical pathways, explaining the facts such as why the cancer cell metastasizes, whether it is hypoxic, how fast it is proliferating, and whether it contains molecules that are amenable to cancer therapy or would resist cancer therapy and, also, to follow up after treatment to view how such molecules may be modulated during treatment (81). In fact, molecular imaging is not a completely new technique because some of its principles have been applied in nuclear medicine (radiotracers) for many years. But, the current enthusiasm in the field of imaging is due to the emerging applications of molecular imaging and the development of high-resolution imaging techniques, helping to understand the physiology of cancer at the molecular level.

Gene Expression Imaging

The concept of gene expression imaging was first introduced by Blasberg and Gelovani-Tjuvajev (82,83); their work is primarily based on the presence of a reporter gene and a reporter substrate. Subsequent modifications and refinements to the above methods led to the application of this technique in oncology. The expression of regulatory and system-control genes that are targets for drug treatment can be readily imaged with gene-expression imaging. These gene imaging methods have big potential in the development of novel cancer therapeutics (82,83).

Cancer Phenotype Imaging

Cancer phenotypic characteristics include angiogenesis, hypoxia, altered apoptosis, unchecked growth, and insensitivity to growth signals, invasion, and metastases. The biochemistry of cancer can be used as a basis for "functional" tumor imaging to image the molecular alterations associated with phenotypic features of cancer. Some of the characteristic biochemical alterations of malignancy, such as accelerated glycolysis and amino acid transport, are associated with an increased proliferation of the malignant state (81). Functional tumor imaging is performed by PET, SPECT, and MRI/MR spectroscopy.

Anticancer Agents

Molecular imaging also has potential in the development of new anticancer therapies. In antibody-based drugs, the use of radiotracers can demonstrate the degree of targeting to the tumors, thus providing direct information about the therapeutic index in vivo. Tracing the biodistribution of the radiopharmaceutical in the body and in cancer cells can lead to the development of active new therapies for cancers (81). Imaging can detect the presence of the target and determine the quantity of expression in vivo in the tumor tissue. Such studies can be useful as a baseline before therapy and during therapy to determine efficacy of the drug in vivo (81).

CONCLUSION

Imaging is an invaluable component of lung-cancer management. With recent advances in imaging, as described in this chapter, staging of lung cancer, assessment of response to treatment and recurrence can be done with much more confidence than it was a few years ago. Early detection of malignancy can improve the survival in patients. Introduction of PET has revolutionized the imaging of lung cancer. With an improvement in the accuracy of imaging through the use of PET, possibilities of understaging and overstaging have reduced tremendously, leading to an appropriate treatment for that particular stage. Molecular imaging, although still in a developmental stage, holds tremendous potential in the detection of lung cancer and metastases at a very early stage as well as in the development of anti-cancer drugs.

ACKNOWLEDGMENT

The authors would like to thank Margaret Kowaluk for her assistance with graphics preparation for the chapter.

REFERENCES

1. Schaefer-Prokop C, Prokop M. New imaging techniques in the treatment guidelines for lung cancer. Eur Respir J Suppl 2002; 35:71s–83s.
2. Valencia R, Denecke T, Lehmkuhl L, Fischbach F, Felix R, Knollmann F. Value of axial and coronal maximum intensity projection images in the detection of pulmonary nodules by multislice spiral CT: comparison with axial 1-mm and 5-mm slices. Eur Radiol 2006; 16:325–332.
3. Eibel R, Turk TR, Kulinna C, Herrmann K, Reiser MF. Multidetector-row CT of the lungs: multiplanar reconstructions and maximum intensity projections for the detection of pulmonary nodules. Rofo 2001; 173:815–821.
4. Fischbach F, Knollmann F, Griesshaber V, Freund T, Akkol E, Felix R. Detection of pulmonary nodules by multislice computed tomography: improved detection rate with reduced slice thickness. Eur Radiol 2003; 13:2378–2383.
5. Gurung J, Maataoui A, Khan M, et al. Automated detection of lung nodules in multidetector CT: influence of different reconstruction protocols on performance of a software prototype. Rofo 2006; 178:71–77.
6. Wormanns D, Ludwig K, Beyer F, Heindel W, Diederich S. Detection of pulmonary nodules at multirow-detector CT: effectiveness of double reading to improve sensitivity at standard-dose and low-dose chest CT. Eur Radiol 2005; 15:14–22.
7. Wormanns D, Beyer F, Diederich S, Ludwig K, Heindel W. Diagnostic performance of a commercially available computer-aided diagnosis system for automatic detection of pulmonary nodules: comparison with single and double reading. Rofo 2004; 176:953–958.
8. Rubin GD, Lyo JK, Paik DS, et al. Pulmonary nodules on multi-detector row CT scans: performance comparison of radiologists and computer-aided detection. Radiology 2005; 234:274–283.
9. Armato SG 3rd, Roy AS, Macmahon H, et al. Evaluation of automated lung nodule detection on low-dose computed tomography scans from a lung cancer screening program(1). Acad Radiol 2005; 12:337–346.
10. Armato SG 3rd, Li F, Giger ML, MacMahon H, Sone S, Doi K. Lung cancer: performance of automated lung nodule detection applied to cancers missed in a CT screening program. Radiology 2002; 225:685–692.
11. Li F, Sone S, Abe H, MacMahon H, Armato SG 3rd, Doi K. Lung cancers missed at low-dose helical CT screening in a general population: comparison of clinical, histopathologic, and imaging findings. Radiology 2002; 225:673–683.

12. Greene F, Page DL, Fleming ID. AJCC Cancer Staging Manual. 6th ed. New York: Springer, 2002.
13. Laurent F, Montaudon M, Corneloup O. CT and MRI of lung cancer. Respiration 2006; 73:133–142.
14. Higashino T, Ohno Y, Takenaka D, et al. Thin-section multiplanar reformats from multidetector-row CT data: utility for assessment of regional tumor extent in non-small cell lung cancer. Eur J Radiol 2005; 56:48–55.
15. Chooi WK, Matthews S, Bull MJ, Morcos SK. Multislice computed tomography in staging lung cancer: the role of multiplanar image reconstruction. J Comput Assist Tomogr 2005; 29:357–360.
16. Shim SS, Lee KS, Chung MJ, Kim H, Kwon OJ, Kim S. Do hemodynamic studies of stage T1 lung cancer enable the prediction of hilar or mediastinal nodal metastasis? AJR Am J Roentgenol 2006; 186:981–988.
17. von Schulthess GK, Steinert HC, Hany TF. Integrated PET/CT: current applications and future directions. Radiology 2006; 238:405–422.
18. De Wever W, Ceyssens S, Mortelmans L, et al. Additional value of PET-CT in the staging of lung cancer: comparison with CT alone, PET alone and visual correlation of PET and CT. Eur Radiol 2006.
19. Fischer BM, Mortensen J. The future in diagnosis and staging of lung cancer: positron emission tomography. Respiration 2006; 73:267–276.
20. Shiraishi S, Tomiguchi S, Utsunomiya D, et al. Quantitative analysis and effect of attenuation correction on lymph node staging of non-small cell lung cancer on SPECT and CT. AJR Am J Roentgenol 2006; 186:1450–1457.
21. Fraioli F, Bertoletti L, Napoli A, et al. Volumetric evaluation of therapy response in patients with lung metastases. Preliminary results with a computer system (CAD) and comparison with unidimensional measurements. Radiol Med (Torino) 2006; 111:365–375.
22. Volterrani L, Mazzei MA, Scialpi M, et al. Three-dimensional analysis of pulmonary nodules by MSCT with Advanced Lung Analysis (ALA1) software. Radiol Med (Torino) 2006; 111:343–354.
23. Sergiacomi G, Schillaci O, Leporace M, et al. Integrated multislice CT and Tc-99m Sestamibi SPECT-CT evaluation of solitary pulmonary nodules. Radiol Med (Torino) 2006; 111:213–224.
24. Gefter WB. Magnetic resonance imaging in the evaluation of lung cancer. Semin Roentgenol 1990; 25:73–84.
25. Swensen SJ, Morin RL, Schueler BA, et al. Solitary pulmonary nodule: CT evaluation of enhancement with iodinated contrast material—a preliminary report. Radiology 1992; 182:343–347.
26. Yamashita K, Matsunobe S, Tsuda T, et al. Solitary pulmonary nodule: preliminary study of evaluation with incremental dynamic CT. Radiology 1995; 194:399–405.
27. Zhang M, Kono M. Solitary pulmonary nodules: evaluation of blood flow patterns with dynamic CT. Radiology 1997; 205:471–478.
28. Patz EF Jr, Lowe VJ, Hoffman JM, et al. Focal pulmonary abnormalities: evaluation with F-18 fluorodeoxyglucose PET scanning. Radiology 1993; 188:487–490.
29. Guckel C, Schnabel K, Deimling M, Steinbrich W. Solitary pulmonary nodules: MR evaluation of enhancement patterns with contrast-enhanced dynamic snapshot gradient-echo imaging. Radiology 1996; 200:681–686.

30. Kusumoto M, Kono M, Adachi S, et al. Gadopentetate-dimeglumine-enhanced magnetic resonance imaging for lung nodules. Differentiation of lung cancer and tuberculoma. Invest Radiol 1994; 29(suppl 2):S255–S256.

31. Kono M, Adachi S, Kusumoto M, Sakai E. Clinical utility of Gd-DTPA-enhanced magnetic resonance imaging in lung cancer. J Thorac Imaging 1993; 8:18–26.

32. Ohno Y, Hatabu H, Takenaka D, Adachi S, Kono M, Sugimura K. Solitary pulmonary nodules: potential role of dynamic MR imaging in management initial experience. Radiology 2002; 224:503–511.

33. Heelan RT, Demas BE, Caravelli JF, et al. Superior sulcus tumors: CT and MR imaging. Radiology 1989; 170:637–641.

34. Thompson BH, Stanford W. MR imaging of pulmonary and mediastinal malignancies. Magn Reson Imaging Clin N Am 2000; 8:729–739.

35. Takahashi K, Furuse M, Hanaoka H, et al. Pulmonary vein and left atrial invasion by lung cancer: assessment by breath-hold gadolinium-enhanced three-dimensional MR angiography. J Comput Assist Tomogr 2000; 24:557–561.

36. Ohno Y, Adachi S, Motoyama A, et al. Multiphase ECG-triggered 3D contrast-enhanced MR angiography: utility for evaluation of hilar and mediastinal invasion of broncho-genic carcinoma. J Magn Reson Imaging 2001; 13:215–224.

37. Wong J, Haramati LB, Rozenshtein A, Yanez M, Austin JH. Non-small-cell lung cancer: practice patterns of extrathoracic imaging. Acad Radiol 1999; 6:211–215.

38. Sakai S, Murayama S, Murakami J, Hashiguchi N, Masuda K. Bronchogenic carci-noma invasion of the chest wall: evaluation with dynamic cine MRI during breathing. J Comput Assist Tomogr 1997; 21:595–600.

39. Hintze C, Biederer J, Wenz HW, Eberhardt R, Kauczor HU. MRI in staging of lung cancer. Radiologe 2006; 46:251–259.

40. Patz EF Jr, Erasmus JJ. Positron emission tomography imaging in lung cancer. Clin Lung Cancer 1999; 1:42–48; discussion 49.

41. Schrevens L, Lorent N, Dooms C, Vansteenkiste J. The role of PET scan in diagnosis, staging, and management of non-small cell lung cancer. Oncologist 2004; 9:633–643.

42. Erasmus JJ, Patz EF Jr. Positron emission tomography imaging in the thorax. Clin Chest Med 1999; 20:715–724.

43. van Baardwijk A, Baumert BG, Bosmans G, et al. The current status of FDG-PET in tumour volume definition in radiotherapy treatment planning. Cancer Treat Rev 2006; 32:245–260.

44. Lowe VJ, Fletcher JW, Gobar L, et al. Prospective investigation of positron emission tomography in lung nodules. J Clin Oncol 1998; 16:1075–1084.

45. Erasmus JJ, McAdams HP, Patz EF Jr, Goodman PC, Coleman RE. Thoracic FDG PET: state of the art. Radiographics 1998; 18:5–20.

46. Marom EM, Sarvis S, Herndon JE 2nd, Patz EF Jr. T1 lung cancers: sensitivity of diagnosis with fluorodeoxyglucose PET. Radiology 2002; 223:453–459.

47. Nomori H, Watanabe K, Ohtsuka T, Naruke T, Suemasu K, Uno K. Evaluation of F-18 fluorodeoxyglucose (FDG) PET scanning for pulmonary nodules less than 3 cm in diameter, with special reference to the CT images. Lung Cancer 2004; 45:19–27.

48. Silvestri GA, Tanoue LT, Margolis ML, Barker J, Detterbeck F. The noninvasive staging of non-small cell lung cancer: the guidelines. Chest 2003; 123:147S–156S.

49. Martini N, Bains MS, Burt ME, et al. Incidence of local recurrence and second primary tumors in resected stage I lung cancer. J Thorac Cardiovasc Surg 1995; 109:120–129.

50. Pairolero PC, Williams DE, Bergstralh EJ, Piehler JM, Bernatz PE, Payne WS. Postsurgical stage I bronchogenic carcinoma: morbid implications of recurrent disease. Ann Thorac Surg 1984; 38:331–338.

51. Quint LE, Tummala S, Brisson LJ, et al. Distribution of distant metastases from newly diagnosed non-small cell lung cancer. Ann Thorac Surg 1996; 62:246–250.

52. Bury T, Barreto A, Daenen F, Barthelemy N, Ghaye B, Rigo P. Fluorine-18 deoxyglucose positron emission tomography for the detection of bone metastases in patients with non-small cell lung cancer. Eur J Nucl Med 1998; 25:1244–1247.

53. Schirrmeister H, Guhlmann A, Elsner K, et al. Sensitivity in detecting osseous lesions depends on anatomic localization: planar bone scintigraphy versus 18F PET. J Nucl Med 1999; 40:1623–1629.

54. Erasmus JJ, Patz EF Jr, McAdams HP, et al. Evaluation of adrenal masses in patients with bronchogenic carcinoma using 18F-fluorodeoxyglucose positron emission tomography. AJR Am J Roentgenol 1997; 168:1357–1360.

55. Boland GW, Goldberg MA, Lee MJ, et al. Indeterminate adrenal mass in patients with cancer: evaluation at PET with 2-(F-18)-fluoro-2-deoxy-D-glucose. Radiology 1995; 194:131–134.

56. Maurea S, Mainolfi C, Bazzicalupo L, et al. Imaging of adrenal tumors using FDG PET: comparison of benign and malignant lesions. AJR Am J Roentgenol 1999; 173:25–29.

57. Weder W, Schmid RA, Bruchhaus H, Hillinger S, von Schulthess GK, Steinert HC. Detection of extrathoracic metastases by positron emission tomography in lung cancer. Ann Thorac Surg 1998; 66:886–892; discussion 892–883.

58. Vansteenkiste JF, Stroobants SG. Positron emission tomography in the management of non-small cell lung cancer. Hematol Oncol Clin North Am 2004; 18:269–288.

59. Dillemans B, Deneffe G, Verschakelen J, Decramer M. Value of computed tomography and mediastinoscopy in preoperative evaluation of mediastinal nodes in non-small cell lung cancer. A study of 569 patients. Eur J Cardiothorac Surg 1994; 8:37–42.

60. Wahl RL, Quint LE, Greenough RL, Meyer CR, White RI, Orringer MB. Staging of mediastinal non-small cell lung cancer with FDG PET, CT, and fusion images: preliminary prospective evaluation. Radiology 1994; 191:371–377.

61. Bury T, Paulus P, Dowlati A, et al. Staging of the mediastinum: value of positron emission tomography imaging in non-small cell lung cancer. Eur Respir J 1996; 9:2560–2564.

62. Scott WJ, Gobar LS, Terry JD, Dewan NA, Sunderland JJ. Mediastinal lymph node staging of non-small-cell lung cancer: a prospective comparison of computed tomography and positron emission tomography. J Thorac Cardiovasc Surg 1996; 111:642–648.

63. Dwamena BA, Sonnad SS, Angobaldo JO, Wahl RL. Metastases from non-small cell lung cancer: mediastinal staging in the 1990s—meta-analytic comparison of PET and CT. Radiology 1999; 213:530–536.

64. Fischer BM, Mortensen J, Hojgaard L. Positron emission tomography in the diagnosis and staging of lung cancer: a systematic, quantitative review. Lancet Oncol 2001; 2:659–666.

65. Vansteenkiste JF, Stroobants SG, De Leyn PR, et al. Mediastinal lymph node staging with FDG-PET scan in patients with potentially operable non-small cell lung cancer: a prospective analysis of 50 cases. Leuven Lung Cancer Group. Chest 1997; 112:1480–1486.

66. Weng E, Tran L, Rege S, et al. Accuracy and clinical impact of mediastinal lymph node staging with FDG-PET imaging in potentially resectable lung cancer. Am J Clin Oncol 2000; 23:47–52.

67. Fritscher-Ravens A, Bohuslavizki KH, Brandt L, et al. Mediastinal lymph node involvement in potentially resectable lung cancer: comparison of CT, positron emission tomography, and endoscopic ultrasonography with and without fine-needle aspiration. Chest 2003; 123:442–451.

68. van Tinteren H, Hoekstra OS, Smit EF, et al. Effectiveness of positron emission tomography in the preoperative assessment of patients with suspected non-small-cell lung cancer: the PLUS multicentre randomised trial. Lancet 2002; 359:1388–1393.

69. Shim SS, Lee KS, Kim BT, et al. Non-small cell lung cancer: prospective comparison of integrated FDG PET/CT and CT alone for preoperative staging. Radiology 2005; 236:1011–1019.

70. de Langen AJ, Raijmakers P, Riphagen I, Paul MA, Hoekstra OS. The size of mediastinal lymph nodes and its relation with metastatic involvement: a meta-analysis. Eur J Cardiothorac Surg 2006; 29:26–29.

71. Passlick B. Initial surgical staging of lung cancer. Lung Cancer 2003; 42(suppl 1): S21–S25.

72. Rajamani S, Mehta AC. Transbronchial needle aspiration of central and peripheral nodules. Monaldi Arch Chest Dis 2001; 56:436–445.

73. Hsu LH, Liu CC, Ko JS. Education and experience improve the performance of transbronchial needle aspiration: a learning curve at a cancer center. Chest 2004; 125:532–540.

74. Herth FJ. Mediastinal staging—the role of endobronchial and endo-oesophageal sonographic guided needle aspiration. Lung Cancer 2004; 45(suppl 2):S63–S67.

75. Wallace WA, Monaghan H, Salter DM, Gibbons MA, Skwarski KM. Endobronchial ultrasound guided fine needle aspiration and liquid based thin layer cytology. J Clin Pathol 2006.

76. Rintoul RC, Skwarski KM, Murchison JT, Wallace WA, Walker WS, Penman ID. Endobronchial and endoscopic ultrasound-guided real-time fine-needle aspiration for mediastinal staging. Eur Respir J 2005; 25:416–421.

77. Herth F, Becker HD, Ernst A. Conventional vs endobronchial ultrasound-guided transbronchial needle aspiration: a randomized trial. Chest 2004; 125:322–325.

78. Yasufuku K, Chiyo M, Koh E, et al. Endobronchial ultrasound guided transbronchial needle aspiration for staging of lung cancer. Lung Cancer 2005; 50:347–354.

79. Shannon JJ, Bude RO, Orens JB, et al. Endobronchial ultrasound-guided needle aspiration of mediastinal adenopathy. Am J Respir Crit Care Med 1996; 153:1424–1430.

80. Wallace MB, Silvestri GA, Sahai AV, et al. Endoscopic ultrasound-guided fine needle aspiration for staging patients with carcinoma of the lung. Ann Thorac Surg 2001; 72:1861–1867.

81. Hricak H AO, Bradbury MS, Liberman L, Schwartz LH, Larson SM. Functional and metabolic imaging. In: DeVita VT, Rosenberg SA, eds. Cancer-Principles and Practice of Oncology. Vol 1. Philadelphia: Lippincott Williams & Wilkins, 2005:589–616.

82. Blasberg RG, Gelovani-Tjuvajev J. In vivo molecular-genetic imaging. J Cell Biochem Suppl 2002; 39:172–183.

83. Gelovani Tjuvajev J, Blasberg RG. In vivo imaging of molecular-genetic targets for cancer therapy. Cancer Cell 2003; 3:327–332.

Index

T - #0221 - 111024 - C0 - 229/152/13 - PB - 9780367453091 - Gloss Lamination